THE BACTERIA MENACE

THE
Bacteria
Menace

Today's Emerging Infections and How to Protect Yourself

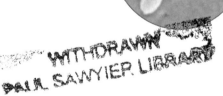

Skye Weintraub, N.D.

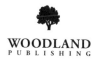

WOODLAND
PUBLISHING

The CIP record for this book is available from the Library of Congress.

For ordering information, contact:
Woodland Publishing, P.O. Box 160, Pleasant Grove, Utah 84062
(800) 777-2665

Note: The information in this book is for educational purposes only and is not
recommended as a means of diagnosing or treating an illness. All matters concerning physical and mental health should be supervised by a health practitioner knowledgeable in treating that particular condition. Neither the publish-
er nor author directly or indirectly dispenses medical advice, nor do they prescribe any remedies or assume any responsibility for those who choose to treat
themselves.

ISBN 1-58054-352-9

Printed in the United States of America

Please visit our website:
www.woodlandpublishing.com

Praise for *The Bacteria Menace*

"*The Bacteria Menace* has brought about much needed awareness regarding the problem of bacteria overgrowth in this country. Through my clinical experience as a colon therapist for the past twelve years, I have become acutely aware of this issue. This book details the issues of prevention and treatment, which is the most important step towards educating and helping people become more responsible for their health. I also recommend her previous book, *The Parasite Menace*, to all of our clients at my natural health clinics in Florida. I am so grateful for the valuable information Dr. Weintraub has written. I know digestive care is the crux of all disease in the body and my experience in working with clients is that cleansing and detoxification and restoring the good bacteria is a major help for all people."

Brenda Watson, C.T.
Owner of ReNew Life clinics, specializing in colon hydrotherapy, detoxification, acupuncture and homeopathy, and founder of ReNew Life Formulas

"Dr. Weintraub provides easily understood information detailing the risk factors and precautions to take in order to avoid contracting these worrisome organisms. From simple bacteria to complex parasites one appreciates how seemingly intelligent and survival-oriented these pathogens really are. She is fast becoming widely recognized by the public and among her fellow practitioners as an expert in the alternative medicine field due to her prolific writing of several best-selling books. Today's pathogens present a problem since they are more persistent due to their adaptability and resistance to antibiotic medications. As a naturopathic physician, Dr. Weintraub provides the reader with suggestions for healthy lifestyle choices and effective treatment alternatives. Books such as this provide a service by educating the public and health practitioner alike."

Stuart Wm. Russell, D.C.
National Manager for Professional Complementary Health Formulas and Natural Pharmaceutical Manufacturing

Dedication

I would like to give a big thanks to my father, Sig Weintraub, for being such a great inspiration to me. I have appreciated his guidance over the years. Without his support, I would not be practicing medicine or researching and writing books. Thank you, Dad.

"No disease can be comprehended without that what causes each person's individual susceptibility to disease—his constitution."

Paracelsus, Medical Alchemist, 1493-1541

"The idea of a microbe as a primary cause of disease is the greatest scientific silliness of the age."

Pierre Antoine Bechamp, Microbiologist, 1816-1908

"The unfortunate thing about this world is that the good habits are much easier to give up than the bad ones."

W. Somerset Maugham, Author, 1874-1965

"If you look at people they seem to be in good health and free from sickness, but in reality they have in their bodies the roots of illness which have not yet developed."

Lu K'uan Yu, Taoist Alchemy, 1898-1978

"One of the biggest tragedies of human civilization is the precedents of chemical therapy over nutrition. It is a substitution of artificial therapy over natural, of poisons over food, in which we are feeding people poisons trying to correct the reactions of starvation."

Dr. Royal Lee, 1951

"The situation results, in part at least, from the rather contemptuous attitude which certain chemists and pharmacologists in the West have developed toward both folk remedies and drugs of plant origin . . . They further fell into the error of supposing that because they had learned the trick of synthesizing certain substances, they were better chemists than Mother Nature who, besides creating compounds too numerous to mention, also synthesized the aforesaid chemist and pharmacologist."

Dr. Robert Ropp, Drugs and the Mind, 1960

Contents

Contents

Introduction

IF YOU ASKED most Americans what they considered to be the most serious threat to the survival of the human race, what would they say? Perhaps their concern would be pollution, global warming, or nuclear war; or maybe widespread famine or even a massive meteor. It is easy to think that our greatest threats come from things larger than we are. Conversely, just because something is smaller than us, it usually does not feel quite so threatening. Well, the ultimate threat to our health and way of life may be those tiny, invisible, and seemingly mindless organisms we call bacteria.

It is no secret that recent years have seen the emergence of numerous "super bugs" that have eluded the saving medicines of today's scientists and doctors. We see and hear reports every day of how a particular antibiotic is now ineffective against current strains of certain bacteria. There are incredible stories of individuals who have contracted a "mysterious" pathogen, causing symptoms and even death in ways never before seen.

According to the extensive advertising of antibacterial products for home use, it is necessary to destroy each and every bacterium in order to be safe. However, this is simply not the case. In some ways of thinking, all of these bacteria have a rightful place to exist. Additionally, we can't place germs into such easy categories as "good" and "bad." Maybe there is no such thing as a bad germ; rather, the principal reason we are seeing the emergence of so many bacteria-related diseases is that our collective state of health continues to decline year after year. This means that as our immune function worsens, as our dietary habits decline, as we suffer more stress and sleep less and less, that our bodies are not healthy enough to deal with these organisms.

Even though most of those who will read this book live in a "land of plenty," many of them (which means us, of course!) complain of constipation or diarrhea, bloating, abdominal pains, and other vague symptoms. Since World War II the modern world has witnessed the introduction of antibiotics, diets high in sugar and processed foods, environments that are teeming with chemicals, and the proliferation of pharmaceutical drugs. All of these factors, combined with declining health practices, have created in many of us the perfect environment for harmful organisms to grow, overrunning the body and suppressing the immune system. But how can we reverse this—is it even possible? The answer is "yes," though it may be difficult to do. When one considers the many years of poor nutrition, environmental toxins, devitalized foods sprayed with chemicals, little or no exercise, high-stress lifestyles, poor sleeping habits, and drinking water laden with metals and other chemicals, it is easy to see why taking a few supplements or changing your diet a bit isn't going to revitalize your health. It will take months, possibly years, of real and widespread lifestyle changes to see the desired benefits.

Because the human body is extremely intricate and complex in nature, it takes a relatively long time for it to adapt to even the smallest of environmental changes. On the other hand, the less complex bacteria can change rather quickly since they are masters at adapting to their environment. In a single day a bacterium can produce hundreds of generations with the strongest ones having the best chance of survival.

New organisms appear every year to make people sick. In spite of all the advances of modern medicine and the wonders of technology, this "enemy" just keeps getting stronger and more deadly. The miracle antibiotics are not working anymore. Every day articles appear discussing the emerging new strains of antibiotic-resistant microorganisms. We now know that more than 70 percent of the bacteria that cause hospital-acquired infections are resistant to at least one antibiotic. And this is not just happening in the United States—these "super bugs" are now a global problem. It may seem that we are fighting a losing battle if antibiotics are failing us.

The incidence of some type of infectious disease now accounts for 25 percent of all visits to the doctor. There is an accumulation of evidence that bacteria are playing a role in many unsuspected chronic diseases, from cancer to gallstones. Disease-causing microorganisms are able to transform and adapt to their changing environments very quickly when necessary, often avoiding detection as a result. Modern medicine has been reluctant to believe that hidden microbes are far more prevalent than commonly believed, and at the core of many chronic diseases.

In the past, lifestyle and stress alone were thought to cause ulcers. Now it is known that bacteria may be the more likely culprit. Scientists have also linked Alzheimer's disease with the presence of the bacterium *Chlamydia pneumoniae* in the brain. This same bacterium may be infecting many people suffering from heart disease. It has been suggested that as much as 80 percent of heart disease may be linked to infectious organisms. The *Clostridium* bacterium is linked to gallstones, and nanobacteria to kidney stones. *Mycoplasma pneumoniae* is being found in many people diagnosed with Crohn's disease, chronic fatigue, fibromyalgia, and Gulf War syndrome. Many experts also believe that rheumatoid arthritis (and related conditions) might be the result of the presence of a highly adaptive microorganism residing somewhere in the body. And don't bet on figuring out how you contracted a particular bacteria that is causing your chronic illness. Thinking back to something you recently ate or drank may work for some types of food poisoning, but it does not usually work for the chronic overgrowth of bacteria. You have probably hosted these organisms for years.

Autoimmune Dysfunction: A Symptom of Bacterial Overgrowth?

When a harmful pathogen, such as a virus or bacteria, sets up housekeeping in the body, the brain alerts the immune system to continuously send out attacks on areas on or around the part of the body where the pathogen has colonized. This may include muscles, joints, cartilage, and other tissue. If the pathogen has successfully hidden itself, and the body is unable to discern between it and healthy cells, the pattern of attacks usually becomes increasingly more intense, going ever deeper and wider, and may eventually destroy healthy tissue. Pain, inflammation, swelling and other symptoms are usually the result of this type of condition, generally known as autoimmune dysfunction. Autoimmune diseases include lupus, Crohn's disease, fibromyalgia, rheumatoid arthritis and multiple sclerosis. The problem with this definition is that it does not account for the causative factor—in other words, what was the body trying to attack before it began attacking itself? I believe, as do many other experts in the area of health and science, that chronic infections of bacteria and other microbes are at the root of these and other common health conditions.

More Than Food Poisoning

In the last twenty years over a dozen new disease-causing organisms have been linked to food poisoning. Bacteria account for a large percentage of these cases. *Campylobacter jejuni*, a recently recognized food pathogen, is now a very common cause of some intestinal diseases. *Listeria monocytogenes* is able to multiply in refrigerated foods, unlike most other foodborne pathogens. In Seattle, Washington, a virulent strain of *E. coli* killed three children and caused hundreds of people to seek hospital attention. And recently, there were several cases of *E. coli* contamination occurring in my state alone. One was at a Wendy's restaurant with about 70 getting sick; one campground had it in the drinking water; and vacationers at another campground contracted it from nearby swimming water. An *E. coli* outbreak also occurred at a retirement home, resulting in the deaths of five elderly people with many more becoming sick. One important thing to note is that after the acute symptoms of food poisoning disappear, some of these bacteria can remain in the intestinal tract, overgrowing, and later causing or contributing to chronic illness.

Bacterial Infection and Today's Emerging Diseases

The facts speak for themselves. Today's typical lifestyle—including diet, exercise habits, and stress levels—is far less healthy than it was twenty, fifty or one hundred years ago. Our environments are suffering from increasing levels of every kind of toxin. The rates of certain chronic and deadly diseases continue to skyrocket. Many mysterious diseases have emerged in recent years, most of which remain "unsolvable" by today's medical world. Various bacteria continue to change, remaining one step ahead of the latest antibiotic drug. And more and more evidence is linking the presence of bacteria and other pathogens with many chronic health conditions.

If you are ill today, the only way to really get better is to eliminate the cause of the illness. Despite what your doctor tells you, your real "opponent" may be bacteria, or possibly a yeast, virus, or parasite, that is overgrowing and causing "symptoms" which are ultimately the real disease. Illness does not just magically occur in people. You do not want to mask it with drugs or painkillers, or hope that a few vitamin or herbal supplements will do the trick. You need to know if you have harmful organisms living in your body. You cannot live a healthy life with pathogens overgrowing in your intestinal tract or elsewhere. If they are alive and thriving in your body today, they can bring about some type of illness tomorrow.

This Book's Message

The main message of this book is to tell you that the overgrowth of bacteria may be more involved in illness, especially chronic illness, than previously thought. This book will explain how the best route to defeating bacterial infection, and most diseases for that matter, is to build your immune system and turn your inner environment into a healthy and vibrant one. And ultimately, the book will provide you with valuable information regarding solutions to bacterial overgrowth: how to change your diet, proper hygiene practices, helpful tips on personal environment care, dietary supplements and other natural therapies.

Of course, often it is difficult to discern by yourself what your problem may be and what steps to take. I strongly suggest consulting with a physician—either a medical doctor that is familiar with and open to the ideas in this book, or a doctor trained in alternative/complementary medicine—that can guide you to an accurate diagnosis and proper treatment. It is my hope that the pages of this book will both expand your knowledge of bacterial infection and overgrowth and ultimately help you revitalize your health.

SECTION 1

Fighting Bacteria from the Inside Out

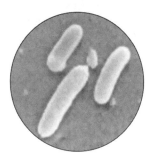

CHAPTER 1

It's All In the Terrain

EVERY DAY, EACH of us is exposed to various types of pathogens, such as bacteria, viruses and fungus. However, only a small percentage of us actually contract the flu, or a cold, or other infection on a regular basis. Every day, our bodies "create" thousands of cancerous cells, yet throughout our collective lifetimes, only a relatively low percentage will develop cancer. And every day, each of our bodies faces the onslaught of other toxins, chemicals, and deleterious agents too numerous to name. Yet again, most of us maintain an overall healthy state in spite of this daily and unending barrage.

Why? Is it because of antibiotics or other moderns drugs? Is it simply in our genes? Or is it just luck? The answer to each of these questions is a resounding "no." The reason that most of us are able to withstand the constant attack of pathogenic agents such as bacteria and cancer is our healthy internal "terrain"—the body's immune system and organs, tissues and cells. And it is this "terrain" that defends us from the dangers found both inside and outside our bodies.

One of the principal focal points of this book is the importance of this internal terrain and how it can make our bodies either a welcome host or a danger zone for unwanted invaders. To illustrate this point, let's look at the experience of the Russian scientist Elie Metchnikoff, who discovered the white blood cell. Through his research and work, Dr. Metchnikoff believed that if the body's defenses, namely its "immunity" cells, were functioning at an optimal level, they could protect the body from most pathogenic agents. To prove this, he consumed a flask of millions of cholera bacteria. One would certainly expect him to develop the disease; however, he did not.

The rest of this section will detail what the immune system is, and how it is affected by our diet, lifestyle, and other factors. You will also learn some fascinating history regarding the "germ theory" that has mistakenly persisted for decades. And finally, you will discover why a dysfunctional immune system and unhealthy terrain can be the principal factor in bacterial overgrowth, which can ultimately lead to a multitude of chronic health conditions.

Immune System Basics

A key focus of this book is our immune system and the role it plays in defending us from bacterial infection. So what exactly is the immune system? It is a multifaceted collection of multiple organs and trillions of cells that weigh just over two pounds. Among these immune organs are the tonsils, the thymus, spleen, appendix, lymph nodes and bone marrow. They are called "lymphoid organs" because they are in charge of the growth, development and use of white blood cells called lymphocytes, which are essential to immune function. Although these organs are located in different parts of the body, they function together through the lymphatic system, a network of vessels (similar to blood vessels) where immune and foreign cells are channeled in clear fluid called lymph. To facilitate this process, small structures called lymph nodes are located at various check points where immune cells can collect and confront antigens (foreign cells and particles).

The intestinal tract is another valuable "member" of the immune system. The intestines are one of your best lines of defense as an immune barrier to foreign substances or organisms that enter the body. Why? The intestines produce a substance called secretory IgA (S-IgA), which prevents the adhesion, or sticking, of pathogenic bacteria (and other agents) to the cells lining the digestive tract. So, in simple terms, when the bacteria can't stick to the body's healthy cells, then they can't cause disease. Consequently, they are soon destroyed and eliminated from the body. S-IgA also neutralizes viruses and keeps parasites from taking over the intestinal tract. In people with S-IgA deficiency, this decreased resistance can lead to an increased risk for infection and allergies.

How Do Immune Cells Recognize Invaders?

The basic duties of the immune system are to identify invaders, distinguish them from the body's own cells and rid the body of any threats. Every cell in the body carries molecules called self markers that identify it as belonging to the body, and under normal conditions the body's immune cells do not attack cells with these markers.

Foreign bodies also have distinctive markers. Amazingly, the immune system not only recognizes and distinguishes among millions of different foreign molecules, but it also responds to and counteracts them individually by producing immune cells called antibodies. Antibodies are triggered by the presence of any foreign substance (called an antigen). Of course, bacteria are antigens, as are cells from someone else (which is why a transplanted organ can be rejected by the body).

A Closer Look at Immune Cells

There are various types of immune cells, but they can be divided into a few main groups. For instance, large white blood cells that devour cells and particles are called phagocytes (and include cells such as macrophages and monocytes) and are collectively known as myeloid cells. Phagocytes are just one type of myeloid cell. B and T cells are classes of small white blood cells called lymphocytes.

B cells are very important because they secrete antibodies, immune agents that belong to a family of protein molecules known as immunoglobulins. In fact, each B cell makes one specific antibody designed to react to one type of antigen. When a B cell is triggered by an antigen, large plasma cells respond and manufacture the necessary antibody. Each antibody has unique contours on one side that allow it to bind to its matching antigen. The antibody fits the antigen perfectly—like a key fits into a lock. The other side of the antibody is able to link to other immune cells.

Some immunoglobulins—such as IgG—may sound more familiar than others. There are four types of IgG immunoglobulins, and they are found mainly in the blood. T cells, probably one of the most well known immune cells, provide a dual immune defense—helping to regulate immune function and destroy foreign cells. Regulatory T cells activate or suppress other immune cells, while cytotoxic T cells are responsible for disposing of infected and cancerous cells.

Cytotoxic T cells are one type of immune killer cell; the other type is natural killer (NK) cells. Whereas cytotoxic T cells need to identify a particular antigen in order to attack, NK cells do not. Both types are potent destroyers, however, and kill on contact.

Another group of cells you may have heard of is the cytokines, which are messengers that recruit other cells in the event of an invader attack. They do this by attaching to certain sites on the cells. Once attached, they can encourage cell growth, activation and movement, or they can destroy targeted cells. One example of a cell targeted by cytokines would be a cancerous cell, which is a normal cell that has mutated. Cytokines are also called interleukins because they can send messages between white blood cells.

As mentioned earlier, phagocytes are large white blood cells that devour cells and particles, including monocytes (in blood), macrophages (in tissue) and neutrophils (in blood and tissue). Macrophages are probably the best known of these scavengers and they also activate T cells.

Immune Defense: Running the Gauntlet

But how do microbes and other invaders get into the body in the first place? Microbes must survive a number of barriers, the first of which is the skin, mucous membranes of the mouth, nose and throat, and the digestive tract, all of which not only physically impede the progress of invaders but also contain scavenger cells and antibodies. If the invader cells make it past these barriers, they are greeted with patrolling scavenger cells, complement proteins and various other defenses that attack anything that they determine is not supposed to be there. These defenses are nonspecific, meaning that they are not targeted toward any specific invader, but to foreign cells in general.

Foreign agents tough enough to survive these defenses are then greeted by weapons (antibodies and other immune cells) specifically targeted for them. In fact, almost every antigen triggers specific and nonspecific defense responses by the body. Cells are able to recognize their targets because of customized molecules called antigen receptors that they carry, which can function in simple or very sophisticated ways to identify and destroy threats.

Memory: A Key to Immunity

With so many foreign threats, how does the body keep track of all possible antigens? Moreover, how can it possibly defend against so many? Well, the immune system has developed ways to remember the invaders it encounters. Whenever T cells and B cells respond to a threat, some of them become memory cells, so that the next time the same invader shows up again, the immune system will recall how it originally defended itself. If there are long-term memory cells for an antigen, it can be destroyed very quickly. The immune system also has a "short-term memory," meaning that it can receive antibodies from another individual and use the memory of these antibodies to fight off an invader. A great example of this is the antibody protection an infant receives from its mother.

Modern Immunity

In today's world, we assault our immune systems from every angle: bad dietary habits, recreational or prescription drug use (including antibiotics), auto exhaust, heavy metal exposure, smoking, recurring or chronic illness, and other factors that we expose our body to daily. The following sections discuss the various factors that have an effect—for both bad and good—on our immune functions and our body's overall inner terrain. For more information on causes and factors leading to a dysfunctional immune system and ultimately bacterial overgrowth, see Section 2.

Nutrition: The Backbone of Immunity

Consider the following questions, all of which have the same answer:

- What, more than any one thing, boosts our immune system and contributes to a healthy inner environment?
- What is vital for the body to overcome disease and heal itself?
- What key factor prevents disease?
- What is lacking from today's conventional medicine?

The only possible answer to these questions is "nutrition." More than our lifestyle, more than medicines, even more than exercise, nutrition is the one thing that can improve our immune function and create a healthy inner environment that defends the body from foreign pathogens.

In our supposed medically "advanced" society, nutrition has been downplayed in favor of pharmaceutical drugs. It is easier to just take a pill or an injection than it is to change the diet. Ultimately, healing does not, and cannot, come from outside of us by man-made chemicals. It comes from nourishing the inner terrain and the body's innate ability to heal from within. Nevertheless, there is a bit of a revolution underway. Today, more and more physicians are investigating the benefits of a healthy diet and complementary/alternative health practices such as herbal medicine, acupuncture and homeopathy. Their patients will be the better for it. As more nutritionally oriented physicians become available, people will have a choice and a place to turn when medical treatment is needed.

Why is nutrition often ignored in today's medical industry? Sadly, the answers to this question generally have to do with money and politics. The profits that pharmaceutical companies make from the sales of their drugs usually bears more weight than the health of an individual. When all factors are considered, typically it is money that speaks loudest of all.

Food: the Greatest Challenge

Many knowledgeable people have maintained that a strong immune system begins with good nutrition, but this concept is often ignored. It is nutrition that helps the body defend itself from foreign pathogens. Herbs, foods, nutrients, and vitamin supplements are the backbone of our immunity, but virtually ignored by medical science in favor of drugs and chemicals. The reason why people get infected in the first place is based on the health of their internal environment. You create this environment with the food you eat, the stress you are under, your sleep patterns, your exercise regime or lack of it, and other lifestyle patterns.

Just as food can be of great benefit for a healthy immune function and inner terrain, it can also be a detriment to the immune system. When an individual consumes generally healthful food, experiences complete digestion, possesses an intact intestine, and consumes a minimal amount of toxins, then the immune system is not overwhelmed and all goes well. Weaknesses in one or more of these areas can result in immune attacks upon foods as if they were foreign invaders. The response to a food allergen can take hours or days to develop. By then the relationship between foods and symptoms is often hard to pin down. It is important to recognize and manage food allergies because more than 50 percent of the immune system takes its signals from the gastrointestinal system.

A long list of health conditions has been associated with food allergies/reactions including: ADD/ADHD, aphthous ulcers, arthritis, asthma, eczema, bed-wetting, epilepsy, fatigue, gallbladder disease, migraines, irritable bowel syndrome, inflammatory bowel disease, otitis media (ear infections), psoriasis, and chronic sinusitis. For more information on food allergies and other food problems, read my book *Allergies and Holistic Healing*.

Poor Digestion Affects Immune Function

Undigested food remnants provide fuel for harmful bacteria, as well as other pathogens overgrowing in the intestinal tract, resulting in significant effects throughout the body due to the absorption of toxic by-products. The result is a worsening of symptoms such as bloating, skin rashes, mucus, fatigue, inflammation, and foul smelling flatulence. This process drains the immune system and complicates the picture.

The immune function relies on a proper combination of food, all of which are completely digested. If there are inadequate digestive enzymes, the body must draw on immune enzymes by moving them from their normal posts and transporting them to the digestive tract. This pattern leaves our immune systems unguarded. Having good digestion leaves the immune system free to do its job of defending us from foreign invaders.

For more information on how poor diet and digestion problems contribute to bacterial overgrowth, see Sections 2 and 4.

The Mind-Body Connection

Not only is your immune system influenced by the nutrition you put into your body and hormonal factors, It is also influenced by your mind. Your reaction to stressful events is entirely individual, reinforcing the fact that people differ greatly in their perceptions and responses to various life events. These variations account for the wide diversity of stress-induced illnesses. The suppression of the immune system is in proportion to the level of stress. Examples of stress-related conditions that could depress the immune system are mood disorders, chronic depression, or anxiety. Chronic stress does not have to be just emotional factors—they can be physical in nature as well. These include recurrent infections, weight gain, high blood pressure, high cholesterol, chronic yeast infections, allergies, chronic inflammatory syndromes, chronic fatigue, and even low blood pressure.

Autoimmune Diseases

As mentioned earlier, in order for the body to recognize an invader there must be some sort of recognition between the self and non-self. The non-self includes foreign material as well as damaged body tissue. If the two reach enough similarity, the body may not be able to distinguish between them. This may be the beginning of what is called an "autoimmune disease." These conditions result in the body attacking its own healthy cells rather than true invading pathogens or toxins. This can result in joint pain and inflammation, problems of the liver and other organs, and various other symptoms, some of which are serious. Autoimmune diseases are commonplace today, but were very rare just a few years ago. Some examples are rheumatoid arthritis, multiple sclerosis, and lupus. Amyotrophic lateral sclerosis (ALS) may be autoimmune in nature as well.

Autoimmune diseases may also be the result of a hyper-vigilant immune system. An immune error occurs when the system overreacts to something harmless, as in the case of hay fever. The immune system mistakes pollen for a dangerous invader and responds with a powerful and sometimes severe reaction. Some types of infection or overgrowth may precede the onset of autoimmune diseases. A pathogen will use some sort of tactic that fools the body into not attacking it. Fortunately, not all people are susceptible to this type of mimicry.

There has been some remarkable research on the link between vaccines and autoimmune diseases, especially Diabetes mellitus. It seems that the more often children are vaccinated, the more likely diabetes appears. The theory is that the structure of the measles or mumps virus is similar to the structure of the beta cells (which produce insulin) in the pancreas. So when someone is vaccinated against childhood diseases, the immune system makes antibodies to fight off the measles virus. Then those same antibodies attack and damage the pancreatic beta cells, resulting in diabetes. It is interesting to note that autoimmune conditions have increased right along with massive vaccination programs beginning in the 1940s.

What Part Does the Liver Play?

The liver is part of our body's immune system and plays a major role in protecting the body from toxic chemicals and heavy metals. Improving the health of the liver and promoting detoxification may be one of the most critical factors in the successful treatment of immune dysfunction. When the liver is even slightly damaged by a toxic chemical, the immune function is compromised. Should the liver be overloaded, or if the co-factors for necessary enzymes are missing, then toxins end up in the body's tissue instead of being escorted out of the body. Before doing a detoxification program, it may be important to see if the liver has the capacity to accomplish detoxification successfully. If it cannot, then a person just gets sicker. There are tests available to see if your liver has the ability to detoxify properly.

Probiotics Help

As discussed before, the intestinal tract is an important part of our body's defense system. Beneficial intestinal bacteria, or probiotics, contain substances in their cell walls that tend to have a major impact upon immunity. These "good" bacteria may prime immune cells and reduce the need for antibiotics.

Supplementing with probiotics may be helpful for anyone. In children, it could help to reduce health care costs associated with the rate of respiratory and gastrointestinal infections in day care. Reducing this rate even by 10 to 20 percent could have important benefits. A healthy balance of beneficial bacteria in the gut may help prevent recurrent infections and reduce their complication. Short-term probiotics appear to reduce symptoms of diarrhea from bacteria and viruses.

A new Finnish study in the *British Medical Journal* evaluated the long-term impact of using probiotics to prevent infections in healthy children. The children receiving *Lactobacillus GG* had 17 percent fewer respiratory infections. The length of the infections was also shorter, and there was about a 15 percent drop in days absent from daycare due to illness. This may seem like modest gains, but many of the children not receiving the probiotic had beneficial *Lactobacillus* bacteria in their guts anyway, altering the study. This probably occurred when they inadvertently consumed other substances containing beneficial bacteria, as probiotic products are widespread in Finland. Beneficial bacteria, such as *Lactobacillus GG*, may indirectly combat infection by selectively stimulating the activity of cytokine cells, which are important for proper immune function.

Antibiotics: Killing the Good with the Bad

Today's antibiotics, long-thought to be the best way to defend against bacterial infection, are actually harmful to all of the body's bacteria, the "good" and the "bad." Antibiotics destroy the beneficial bacteria and create the perfect environment for harmful bacteria to grow. Since the "good" bacteria keep the "bad" bacteria in check, the body becomes overrun with harmful germs. Now the immune system becomes dysfunctional and unable to help us when it is needed.

Almost all drugs suppress the body's natural immunities in one way or another. Even something as seemingly harmless as an antihistamine suppresses your body's natural defenses. Antibiotic overuse when you were growing up may have changed your intestinal environment to the point that you are almost defenseless against incoming germs.

Antibiotic treatment causes the first line of defense to collapse. This means that the friendly non-pathogenic bacteria are killed, resulting in a depressed immune system. The immune system is critically involved in intestinal pathology, and overall health is directly influenced by our immune system. This is the circle of health.

Sunshine Influences Your Risk of Infections

A point worthy of investigation concerns sunlight and lower rates of infections. Studies indicate that levels of bacterial and viral infections seem to peak on the shortest, darkest days of the year, not because of the cold weather of winter, but because of the reduction in sunlight. Sunlight drives melatonin secretion, which positively affects immune function. A lack of melatonin makes humans more susceptible to infections. Adequate amounts of unfiltered sunlight is critical to good health. Most people need about one hour each day to stay healthy (*Emerg Infect Dis 2001*).

Pathogens may be present all the time in the general population, but epidemics occur when susceptibility increases enough to sustain them. Dr. Scott F. Dowell of the Centers for Disease Control and Prevention in Atlanta, proposed as a possible mechanism "changes in receptors on the surface of epithelial cells, some of which may be expressed more commonly in winter, some more in summer." He also felt that seasonal fluctuations in the immune system levels could also be contributing factors.

Dr. Dowell also points out that many outbreaks, such as measles and influenza, are similar in timing and duration from year to year. Supporting his theory is the simultaneous occurrence of pneumococcus and influenza outbreaks in widely dispersed locations. Latitude appears to be a critical determinant in the timing and magnitude of peaks for polio, rotavirus and influenza. Dr. Dowell said "if you have a pathogen that is highly contagious and present year-round, it would exhaust the population of those who are susceptible. Pathogens that could sweep through for several months, then lie dormant until the group of susceptible individuals is renewed, would be at an evolutionary advantage."

An important thing to remember is that you will miss some of the many wavelengths present in sunshine if you wear glasses or just sit in front of a glass window. The sun's rays will never reach your retina and nourish your brain. If taken in moderate amounts, the ultraviolet wavelengths provide health benefits and do not promote skin cancers. One way to compensate for the lack of sunshine in the winter is by using full-spectrum lights. Be sure that they are fluorescent lights.

Incandescent bulbs frequently advertised as full-spectrum are color corrected and will not provide the same benefits.

A lack of sunshine also means that it is best to get to sleep earlier in winter months than in the summer months. You should be in bed soon after sunset. That can be as early as five in the afternoon in the dark of winter! Most people go to bed five to seven hours later than is ideal. This impairs the adrenal glands and ultimately the immune system.

Another thing to consider during the dark winter months is that most holidays dictate the consumption of sugar-laden foods and an increase in stress. People who do not have family during this time often feel lonely and depressed. Others feel stressed because of all the additional work they have to do. Changes in your lifestyle can make a big difference in how susceptible you are to bacteria and other germs.

Early Infections Are Needed

A recent Italian study found that exposure to bacteria early in life is essential for development of an infant's immune system. A baby must be exposed to germs during its first year in order to develop antibodies needed to fight infection later in life. It is dangerous for anyone, especially children, to live in a sterile environment. There is a natural and beneficial symbiotic relationship that exists between humans and microorganisms.

Better living standards are linked to more diseases, not less. Leukemia cases among young British children are increasing and doctors suspect improved living standards could be the cause. Children are exposed to fewer common childhood infections than they used to be so their immune systems are weaker and not as good at combating illnesses. Cases of acute lymphoblastic leukemia, the most common cancer in children, rose dramatically in northwest England from 1980 to 1998.

Clean living is linked to dramatic rises in childhood asthma. Early exposure to bacteria, fungi, dust, and animal dander, may help to explain lower rates of asthma and allergies among children raised on farms. We may be living in an environment that is too antiseptic. Of course, the increase in pollution in the cities could also be a factor.

In order for an infant's immune system to function properly, he or she must be breastfed. The mother transfers immunoglobulins to the newborn in her first milk, colostrum. The benefits of breastfeeding are numerous and extend well beyond the breastfeeding period. For non-breastfeeding parents, their fear of microbes affecting their children might be justified in some cases. I recently saw a five-month-old baby with an ear infection who had a bowel movement once only every three to four days. Even then, the bowel movements had to be triggered with suppositories. It turns out that instead of breastfeeding, the baby was taking cow's milk formula, which was the cause of the problems. By changing the formula to goat's milk (fortified with vitamin B12 and folate), the baby began to have regular bowel movements again. Soon, the ear infection cleared up as well, which indicates that there is a clear link between proper digestive function and immunity.

Vaccines and Immune Suppression

Another often-debated and intriguing point regarding our immunity concerns the affect vaccines have on our bodies. Studies indicate that many white blood cells needed for a healthy immune system are significantly reduced after vaccinations are given and do not return to normal for months. All vaccines have, to some extent, a depressant effect on our immune systems. From one perspective, we are often encouraging complete immune system depression for temporary immunity against a few diseases, usually innocuous childhood diseases. If we consider the benefits of vaccines, is this a fair trade? Are we trading mumps and measles for cancer and chronic illnesses?

Another example is the yearly flu shot ritual. There may be only two or three varieties of flu viruses in each shot, but there are many flu-causing viruses. Many people report getting the flu even after taking a flu shot. We do not know which variety of flu will affect us each year, and in each locale. Therefore, in my estimation, the best method to avoid the flu is to strengthen your immune system by eating properly, exercising and improving your overall lifestyle. In other words, pathogenic organisms will not grow where the conditions will not allow them. Remember that it is the terrain that dictates our health and not the germs themselves.

Vaccines are the only way conventional medicine can "prevent" disease since they seldom promote a healthy diet, herbal and other supplement therapies, or changes in lifestyle. Conventional medicine tries to force health by giving the body more toxins in a futile and erroneous attempt at preventing disease. Yet, vaccines set the stage for the depression of our immune system to fight off the very pathogens we had hoped to prevent.

Vaccinations reduce our immunity in various ways:

• Vaccines may contain many chemicals and heavy metals, such as mercury and aluminum, both of which are immune suppressing.

- Vaccines may contain foreign tissues and foreign DNA/RNA that can suppress the immune system or assist in gene-jumping.
- Vaccines alter our T-cell helper/suppressor ratio. This ratio is a key indicator of a proper functioning immune system.
- Vaccines alter the ability of our white blood cells to defend us against pathogenic bacteria and viruses.
- Vaccines suppress our immunity merely by over-taxing our immune system with foreign materials and pathogens.
- Vaccines clog the lymphatic system and lymph nodes with large protein molecules that have not been adequately broken down by our digestive processes. That is because vaccines bypass digestion when injected.
- Vaccines may deplete our body of vital immune-enhancing nutrients, like vitamins C and A, and zinc.
- Vaccines are neurotoxic and slow the level of nervous transmission and communications to the brain and other tissues.

The Effects Of Stress and Pain

New research shows that relatively brief stress and pain, such as that experienced during a root canal, can suppress the body's ability to fight off disease. We've known for some time that chronic pain can have an influence on immune function, but it's less clear whether short-term procedures, such as medical and dental procedures, could do the same.

One study suggests that those who contracted an infection reported higher levels of pain during a previously performed dental procedure, and these same individuals showed more suppressed immune function afterward. It appears that stress and pain make healthy people more vulnerable to infection, especially to mild illnesses such as colds. The greater concern is for people who already have compromised health, such as the elderly or those with heart disease, cancer, or AIDS. What happens to these people when they undergo painful and stressful procedures?

We Have an Elegant System

Even for people who are generally healthy, it is possible for the immune system to become temporarily depressed. When this happens, the body becomes more susceptible to infections and the overgrowth of pathogens. Many people have become dependent on pharmaceutical drugs and have forgotten that the human body has a complex, elegant, and efficient system of healing built right into it. Pharmaceutical drugs often interfere with this healing process. It would be better to use other methods and approaches to protect your health whenever possible. Amplify your immunity so disease does not have a chance. Instead of damaging your defenses, supercharge them. Your body has the capacity to heal itself, if given a chance. For more information on improving your immune function and promoting a healthy inner terrain, see Section 4.

CHAPTER 2

Bechamp vs. Pasteur: The Road Less Traveled

EARLIER, I DISCUSSED the idea that bacteria, viruses and other pathogens are usually defenseless against us if our immune systems and inner environment are inhospitable to such invaders. For the last 100 years or so, intelligent researchers, learned doctors and dedicated students have thought that bacteria, viruses, fungi and other pathogens were the sole cause of infectious diseases. However, if we examine the lessons history has preserved, we see that this premise is at least partially mistaken. Let's travel back to the late 1800s to analyze the work of one man, which showed that diseases "caused" by bacterial infections are largely a result of an imbalanced internal terrain and dysfunctional immune system.

Bechamp and the "True" Germ Theory

When considering the idea that germs are the sole cause of disease, we must first look at the nineteenth-century scientific genius, Antoine Bechamp (1816-1908). Bechamp was a respected researcher and teacher in France, but too busy to be bothered with conventions, awards, and politics. He dedicated himself to science and medicine until his death at 93. Bechamp made one of the greatest contributions to the science of microbiology. He, above all that came before him, stated that it is not the germ that causes disease, but rather the internal environment, or the terrain, in which the germs live that is the principal contributing factor to disease. He believed that disease, especially those marked by a pathogenic overgrowth, occurs when an imbalanced internal environment and weak immune system allow these pathological organisms to essentially "take over." This is really the foundation of the whole controversy of internal terrain versus germ theory.

Even before Bechamp's time, the theory of the cell being the basic unit of life was well-established. His investigations showed that the cell itself was made up of smaller living entities capable of intelligent behavior and self-reproduction. He gave them the name of microzymas, which he said were the real basic units of life. Bechamp described how in certain conditions microzymas could develop into bacteria within a cell. If the right conditions persisted, infection could develop in the body without the acquisition of germs from an outside source.

Bechamp had an incredible list of achievements. It was stated that on his death, it took eight pages in a scientific journal to record all of them. In spite of all that he had discovered and taught in his day, few people are aware of him today. His truths have been virtually ignored by traditional Western medicine. Did his information threaten the status quo or did it threaten the path that was more profitable by the medical establishment? How could someone with his magnitude and number of discoveries and achievements be so ignored in medical history?

Let's turn back the clock for a moment and go to the European continent during 1350 A.D. In less than two years' time, bubonic plague wiped out half the population of Europe. Fleas bit rats, which then bit humans. The rats had flourished because their natural predator, the cat, had been killed due to the belief of the time that cats were connected to witchcraft. An estimated 25 million people died in fourteen months. The mortality rate grew as high as 90 percent in some cities. Bodies were piled into carts and dragged away to be burned in common graves. It was a most grotesque way to die: bleeding and screaming and having one's organs literally liquefy. From infection to death took perhaps one week. Prior to that outbreak, bubonic plague had not been seen for nearly a thousand years. Scholars of the day attributed the cause to evil spirits, divine retribution, or other such nonsense. One question that came from this horror is why did some people die and some survive? Today we know the answer. It was the internal terrain and it was the strength of an individual's immune system.

Go forward now a few centuries to France in the 1870s. Some scientists were conducting experiments in the area of chemistry, particularly having to do with fermentation, yeast, and the new discovery of little organisms called bacteria. There was much competition and "borrowing" of discoveries, always with the undercurrent of politics and influence. Two of these men were Louis Pasteur and Antoine Bechamp. These men were not colleagues, but worked independently. A new area of human discovery was close at hand. Scientists in both France and

Germany were grappling with mankind's first look at fundamental questions about the nature of living matter itself.

Louis Pasteur and the Emergence of the "Germ Theory"

Louis Pasteur (1822-1895) had a gift for public relations. He rarely let his research keep him away from an opportunity to address royalty or medical society in the most prestigious university settings. He was often quoted, published, and offered practically every honorary title and chair in Europe. When the Emperor Napoleon decorated Pasteur early in his career, Pasteur's position as a scientist was thereby secured. But Pasteur was only trained as a chemist with no credentials at all in medicine or physiology.

It was perfect timing for an ambitious opportunist to take advantage of the general uncertainty and lack of understanding of the science being undertaken at that time. Pasteur claimed that he understood all the issues involved. Furthermore, he convinced others that he had thought of them first. Pasteur was noted for his habit of playing both sides of the fence on issues. He made claims that he had written these facts before anyone else. This is how Pasteur put himself into a position he did not deserve. He was not the trailblazer of science that we thought he was. Later, we find out how dishonest he really was, even by his own words.

The records show that Pasteur plagiarized much of Bechamp's work and his popularity survived largely because of the favor from Napoleon and the High Church. On the other hand, Bechamp was immersed entirely in his work, seeking neither favor nor fortune. Although devout in his religious faith, Bechamp was held in disfavor by the bishops of the Church. Pasteur may have won the race of politics and influence of his day, but many of his theories were not accurate or had been discovered by others. He even admitted his deception in papers released long after his death. What exactly was his primary germ theory? Very simply, it stated that a particular microorganism caused each disease. It was the job of science to find the right drug or vaccine that would selectively kill off the offending bug without killing the patient.

The record also establishes that Pasteur "borrowed" the research for some of his most famous discoveries, and then capitalized on the celebrity of being there first. According to Ethel Douglas Hume's 1923 book (reprinted in 1989) *Bechamp or Pasteur? A Lost Chapter in the History of Biology,* Louis Pasteur repeatedly plagiarized Bechamp's work, distorted it, and submitted it to the French Academy of Science as his own work. Pasteur worked the political system to his advantage whereas Antoine Bechamp, a man of science, did not. This book states that the ambitious Pasteur stole or misinterpreted many of his claims from this barely known, but eminent scientist. Ultimately, Pasteur would become world-famous, but the name of Bechamp would fall into obscurity.

Pasteur was more a merchant than a scientist, with his frequent reporting of false test findings and data. He seemed to have two motives—the self-promotion and profiteering from the sale of drugs and vaccines. The French government helped his success, because these substances were often made mandatory by legislators. It is quite interesting to note that Hume believed that had it not been for the mass selling of vaccines, Pasteur's germ theory of disease would probably have collapsed into obscurity.

From the beginning, the whole idea of piercing the skin with a needle for any reason was suspect, let alone introducing new proteins and agents into what was supposed to be an inviolable environment: the circulatory system. Injections are a total violation of nature. Normally, nothing is introduced into the bloodstream without going through the entire digestive system first. That is how nature protects the blood from external intrusions. Bechamp stated that "The most serious disorders may be provoked by the injection of living organisms into the body into a medium not intended for them and may provoke redoubtable manifestations of the gravest morbid phenomena."

In the early part of the twentieth century, a medical doctor reporting from the battlefields of South Africa during the Boer War notes that the war itself killed 86,000 men. With a 100 percent inoculation rate, there were an additional 96,000 casualties from disease alone. This was written by Walter Hadwen, M.D., in his book *Microbes and War.*

In 1915, another medical doctor wrote an article for the British medical journal *Lancet.* Dr. Montais studied twenty-one cases of tetanus, each of which had received Pasteurian inoculation. The conclusion of the article, which appeared in a 1915 issue, was that in every case, the tetanus was caused by the inoculation. Dr. Montais said, "Pasteur had created a new form of disease." We should be reminded that it was Pasteur who began the fashion of studying artificial disease conditions by inducing sickness by morbid injections in human and animal subjects, instead of studying naturally diseased subjects.

Pasteur's Monomorphism vs. Bechamp's Polymorphism

As far as Pasteur's "germ theory" goes, there was opposition to it among many researchers of his own time. Bechamp was only the first in a long line of researchers who have found evidence of pleomorphism and refuted Pasteur's germ theory. During a lecture given in London in

1911, M.L. Leverson, M.D., stated: "The entire fabric of the germ theory of disease rests upon assumptions that not only have not been proved, but which are incapable of proof, and many of them can be proved to be the reverse of truth. The basic one of these unproven assumptions is the hypothesis that all the so-called infectious and contagious disorders are caused by germs."

Pasteur's monomorphism is the theory that one germ creates one illness. Eliminate the germ and the illness disappears. He had not observed the changes in form capable by various microbes. Bechamp's theory of polymorphism (which today is called pleomorphism), stands in opposition to Pasteur. Bechamp identified extremely small corpuscles known as microzymes that are always present, but are only transformed into a pathogenic state when the system becomes imbalanced. The primary disagreement between them was that Bechamp said that disease came from within the body and Pasteur said that disease came from outside the body. As the nineteenth century came to a close, two schools of thought existed: the polymorphism of Bechamp and monomorphism according to Pasteur.

According to Pasteur, the following was true:

- Diseases arise from microorganisms originating outside of the body.
- The appearance and function of a specific microorganism are constant.
- Every disease is associated with a particular microorganism.
- Microorganisms are primary causal agents of disease.
- Disease is inevitable and can strike anybody.
- To prevent and cure diseases, it is necessary to destroy pathogenic microorganisms.

On the other hand, Bechamp's view was that the susceptibility to disease arises from conditions within the cells of the body. Bechamp believed the following:

- Microorganisms are generally beneficial and life sustaining if the body is kept clean from toxins.
- The appearance and function of microorganisms changes when the host organism is injured whether mechanically, biochemically, or emotionally.
- Every disease is associated with a particular underlying condition.
- Microorganisms only become associated with disease when the cells become toxified. Disease arises from conditions of increased toxicity.
- Preventing or curing consists of cleaning toxins from the body in a way that does no harm to the immune system and internal environment.

Bacteria, viruses, and other living organisms tend to be environmentally specific. This means that they can only survive certain kinds of surroundings. That is why some people get colds and others do not. That is why some survived the bubonic plague and others did not. That is why some doctors and nurses seem to be immune to disease even though they are surrounded by it every day. For example, when faced with a mosquito plague we try to destroy the mosquitoes with chemicals, but after 50 years of spraying pesticides the problem still exists. Mosquitoes just develop more resistance to the pesticides used. The only effective way to solve this problem is to eliminate the real cause—the swampy environment that promotes their ability to survive and reproduce. Changing the environment by drying out the swamp is the only way to really solve the problem. These principles can also be applied to our internal environment. Detoxify the system, create an inhospitable environment for pathogens, and disease is less likely to occur. Germs do not always cause disease but are an effect, or consequence, of it. This principle has enormous implications for the treatment of disease in the human body.

In the end Pasteur agreed that pathogens alone do not cause disease. In one of the most quoted deathbed statements, perhaps of all time, Pasteur recanted his germ theory. He admitted that his rivals had been right. It was not the germ that caused the disease, but rather the environment (the terrain) in which the germ was found. He finally admitted "the [human] terrain is everything, the germ [virus, bacteria, etc.] means nothing." Sadly, he did not give credit to Antoine Bechamp for the discoveries he had stolen from him. Before he died, Pasteur instructed his family not to release 10,000 pages of lab notes he had compiled over the years. However, after his grandson's death in 1975, Pasteur's secrets became public, showing him a man of serious scientific misconduct. He violated the medical, ethical, and scientific rules, and published fraudulent data. Money seemed to be the primary motivation.

Besides Bechamp, many famous names in history believed that the real issue surrounding the causes of disease was not the germ, but rather the human environment or internal terrain. These include Francois Voltaire, Rudolph Virchow, Christopher Bird, Gaston Naessens, Robert Ingersoll, Claude Bernard, Gunther Enderlein, Royal Rife, Anton van Leeuwenhoek, Henry Lindlahr, and even Florence Nightengale. How is it that so much of the medical community still acts as though "germ theory" is carved in stone, and why do most people still believe in it?

Bechamp had proven, after extensive observations and experimentation, that germs are not necessarily causing disease, but are the consequence of the underlying condition of immune dysfunction and an unhealthy inner environment. But Pasteur's theory was more simple to understand, had better economic perspectives, and was more in accordance with the old concepts of disease. About this time, Germany became predominant in world medical research. They focused more on medical problems than on the general study of biology. The germ theory became firmly entrenched in the minds of most doctors, and medicine followed the doctrines of Pasteur. This view dominated medical science and its philosophy.

The American Pharmaceutical Movement

About the same time that Pasteur and Bechamp were completing their work, the pharmaceutical industry was beginning to develop in the United States. With drug interests increasing, there was a push to move in a different direction than the competing homeopathic and nature cure medical profession of the day. Also, the doctrines of Pasteur were more profitable for America's medical and industrial complex that was developing around the beginning of the twentieth century. Two figures dominated this era, wielding more power over science, industry, finance, and politics, than possibly anyone else in history. They were Andrew Carnegie and J.D. Rockefeller. Their control over most aspects of American life was taking place quickly by the rise of organized medicine. Among many other things, Carnegie and Rockefeller controlled the oil and coal industries. By 1900, they became aware that these industries were producing mountains of waste each year. How would they turn these chemical waste materials into something that would make them a profit? Believe it or not, it turned out to be medicines. They began producing medicines like the world had never seen before. These medicines derived from waste chemicals are what today we call "pharmaceuticals."

How were the industrial empires of Carnegie and Rockefeller going to convince the public to accept these new forms of medicine? Until then, most people throughout the world simply used natural treatments, such as herbal products, and occasionally consulted the country or local doctor if they had something more serious. The way to gain general acceptance of the new pharmaceuticals soon became obvious to Carnegie and Rockefeller. They would standardize the education, training, and licensing of medical doctors. They would also raise the doctors' economic status to a level where they would follow policies dictated by the powers that be, namely Carnegie and Rockefeller.

About 1904, Andrew Carnegie noticed that the workers in his factories were making better wages than most medical doctors were making. Consulting with the president of MIT, Henry Pritchett, they set up the

Carnegie Foundation with $10 million. Its original purpose was to provide a pension fund for retiring professors. Now they would expand it to control education. In order to qualify for money from the foundation, a participating institution had to meet certain guidelines that ultimately would increase the profits of Carnegie's developing drug empire.

The Rockefeller Foundation also came into existence about this time. The foundation developed national standards for medical schools that were seeking "philanthropic" support. The medical school had to be connected to a large university. Universities had to be linked to clinical departments with laboratories and a university hospital. A small group of clinically oriented elite medical schools then became the recipients of the money. The raw materials for the new drugs were there. What had been lacking was an academic power-base to legitimize their development and general use.

This infrastructure for education, funding, research, and the organization of medicine, persists even today. Under the guidance and specifications of these two giant economic forces in history, Carnegie and Rockefeller's organized medicine became an immense industry, with its focus on market growth. An industry that is profit driven is not about to abolish itself by curing the diseases that have made them rich. This is why effective, inexpensive, non-pharmaceutical remedies, and holistic treatments have been systematically suppressed. It is just good business for the other side.

The germ theory fits too well with the market-oriented paradigm of medicine. If there are bad bugs out there causing diseases, people need drugs to kill them. New drugs mean new research funding, government money, the need for prescriptions, and an entire profession that can be financed and educated to write those prescriptions. The fact that the founder of germ theory, Pasteur himself, repudiated this concept, has not stopped anyone who expects to gain from next year's funding or who makes their living within the established medical industry. Economic factors are responsible for the continued use of this path in modern medicine today.

Penicillin: The Birth of the Antibiotic

In the 1920s, this burgeoning medical industry began to decline because infectious diseases decreased due to improved sanitation, for which medicine still took credit. However, in 1928, the germ theory got a big boost that has lasted to the present day. Dr. Alexander Fleming, a British scientist, had recently discovered penicillin and outlined its possible health benefits. Shortly after, there was a terrible fire in Boston that killed and injured hundreds of people. Penicillin was rushed to the area with the idea of preventing infections in the burned survivors. It was extremely successful, and the news exploded, ushering in the era of the "wonder drug." The discovery of the miracle antibiotic penicillin did more to bring credibility to the newly organized industry of Western medicine than anything else.

Even early in his research, Dr. Fleming knew very well that living things could change or adapt when stressful substances were added. He knew the dangers of resistance from the overuse of penicillin. He warned against that very overuse as expressed in an interview he gave to the *New York Times* in 1945. He was right. In 1952, almost 100 percent of *Staphylococcus* infections could be cured by penicillin. In 1982, fewer than 10 percent could be cured; today it is less than 5 percent. Bacteria and viruses have been around for billions of years. They have persisted through many different environments: hot, cold, wet, dry, without oxygen, with oxygen, etc. Yet they are still here and more visible than ever. It appears that bacteria and viruses are the ultimate masters of adaptation.

The strength of modern conventional medicine is the development of emergency treatments for external wounds, trauma, and deadly infectious diseases. In particular, modern medicine has made extensive strides in the conquest of many communicable diseases, which can easily and quickly kill many people. For the majority of health conditions, however, today's doctors do not possess any cure. They simply look to suppress symptoms. More importantly, today's conventional medical world does not promote the need to balance the internal terrain so that disease will not have a place to develop in the first place.

The day will come when there will be absolute proof that Professor Bechamp has interpreted nature's laws correctly. Nature desires that germs and humans should coexist harmoniously. This is available to us right now and always has been. Whether germs behave like dangerous bits of alien life or as non-pathogenic particles is entirely up to us. It depends on how we choose to look after our internal terrain. In case you think that antibiotics and vaccines offer a way to cheat the system, you are taking a dangerous path. Ultimately, nature cannot be fooled.

CHAPTER 3

Out of Balance:
The Overgrowth of Bacteria

NOW THAT WE have covered some of the basics regarding immune function and how modern medicine has mistakenly come to believe that simply eradicating a particular microbe will cure a disease, we can discuss this book's central notion that microbial overgrowth, particularly of bacteria, is linked to many more illnesses than previously thought.

It is a well-known fact that microbes are at the root of acute illnesses like sinusitis and food poisoning. However, more and more evidence is pointing to the fact that unsuspected infectious agents are principal contributors to chronic illnesses as well. The reason this fact has been so elusive is because these microbes usually are not diagnosed by ordinary laboratory tests and because the symptoms often mimic other disorders. Of course, stool analysis panels and specialized blood tests are now available to help identify the offending microbes, but diagnosis often remains difficult. For instance, there can be a mix of bacteria and fungus, which presents a very complex symptom picture for a physician. The mix could also contain organisms such as parasites and viruses. Mixed infections are the most difficult conditions to diagnose and treat because they are so complex and varied.

Furthermore, many doctors don't even consider the possibility that chronic illness may be the result of microbial overgrowth, especially in the digestive system. Because they do not believe in such overgrowths, they don't perform tests to check for this condition in the first place. The link between the ecology of the digestive tract and a person's level of health (and risk for disease) is often overlooked, despite the fact that proper digestion is essential to immune function. When normal function is interrupted, the whole body suffers. For more information on how bacterial overgrowth can lead to disease, see Section 3.

Bacterial Overgrowth in the Intestines

Normally, relatively few bacteria inhabit the small intestine (compared with the ample growth found in the colon). Digestive enzymes from the stomach and upper bowel, as well as intestinal motility, keep the small intestine relatively free of bacteria. However, a wide range of abnormalities and malfunctions can encourage bacteria to multiply here. The most common causes of bacterial overgrowth are from people who do not produce enough digestive enzymes, those who misuse antibiotics, and those with poor diets.

The presence of too many pathogens among the bowel microflora causes far more than intestinal symptoms like flatulence or diarrhea. Toxins from these pathogens can damage the intestinal tract by weakening the lining of the intestines. The injured lining then leaks toxins into the blood and lymph system, spreading them all over the body. If these toxins are absorbed by the body, they can produce varied symptoms almost anywhere in the body. As the physical and chemical structure of the stool continues to change as a result of the overgrowth, the environment of the colon also changes. When a critical level of tissue damage is reached, essential nutrients will not be properly absorbed, leading to deficiencies, immune weakness and even more symptoms.

These colonies of pathogenic bacteria act like small biochemical factories, feeding on carbohydrates and producing toxic products not usually found in the intestines. Many people suffering with bacterial overgrowths tell me that they feel as if they have been poisoned. I tell them that they have been. The poison is being manufactured within their own intestinal tract.

Dysbiosis: A System Out of Balance

Of course, not all microorganisms are bad. The digestive tract (especially the intestines) harbors trillions of microbes. The microflora of the gastrointestinal tract constitute a complex ecosystem of aerobic (oxygen living) and anaerobic (non-oxygen living) microorganisms. Surprisingly, this microflora system is stable over time, but is affected by diet, antibiotic use, and general health status. These microflora can be viewed as another organ of the body, since they profoundly influence the health of their human host.

Are They Pathogens?

It is not always clear if an organism is a pathogen or not. By definition, if an agent or microorganism causes disease than it is considered a pathogen. It might be better to use the categories "weak" and "strong" pathogens instead. Weak pathogens cause diseases in some people some of the time. If a susceptible individual is exposed for a long period to a weak pathogen, it is likely to cause health problems. This might suggest that many organisms become weak pathogens at the right time and in the right place. Strong pathogens cause diseases in most people most of the time.

Some strains of the same bacteria are harmless and some are potentially deadly, such as the case with *E. coli*. One strain is a normal inhabitant of human intestines, as well as other animals. It usually serves a useful function in the body by synthesizing appreciable amounts of vitamins. It also suppresses the growth of harmful bacterial species. Then there is a strain (called *E. coli* 0157:H7) that has the potential to kill. Other strains fall somewhere in between these two and only cause mild symptoms in most people who ingest them.

Among the hundreds of different types of intestinal microflora, many are beneficial to humans, acting in concert with the cells that line the intestines. They benefit their human host as well as derive benefits. This is what produces an optimally functional intestinal system. Provided with food and shelter by their human host, the beneficial intestinal microflora help produce nutrients, vitamins and hormones. Sometimes they also assist in the detoxification of toxins, produce anti-cancer substances, and stimulate the immune system.

These "friendly" microorganisms are not without competition, however. They must fight for food and space against potentially harmful microorganisms also trying to make their home in the intestines. As long as the "friendly" bacteria predominate, the intestines can maintain optimum health. If the "bad guys" take over, imbalances occur. The results are called "dysbiosis."

Dysbiosis is a state of imbalance that allows harmful bacteria the opportunity to multiply and overgrow at the expense of beneficial bacteria. Dysbiosis can exist in the mouth, gastrointestinal tract or vaginal cavity. Even "weak" pathogens can induce disease by altering the nutritional health or immune responses of their host. It is amazing just how much damage these pathogens are capable of producing. Their enzymes can destroy pancreatic enzymes necessary for digestion, damage the intestinal lining and alter the intestinal terrain in many ways. The toxins that they produce may cause dysfunction of the immune system, contributing to autoimmune and connective tissue diseases. The development of inflammatory diseases, cancer, degenerative diseases, allergies, and a host of chronic illnesses may all be attributed to intestinal dysbiosis. The solution is a relationship of balance; bacteria living in balance with each other and with us as the host.

How Do I Know If I Have Dysbiosis?

Individuals with intestinal dysbiosis will likely experience abdominal gas, bloating and diarrhea, usually within one hour after eating. You may also suffer from abdominal cramps, anemia, chronic intestinal infections, weight loss, greasy stools, foul-smelling flatulence, an inability to tolerate carbohydrates or starchy foods, a vitamin B12 deficiency, and sluggish bowels. Intestinal dysbiosis is known to contribute to other medical conditions: irritable bowel syndrome, food allergies, inflammatory bowel disease, colon and breast cancer, psoriasis, eczema, cystic acne and chronic fatigue, to name just a few. Bacteria overgrowth also contributes to poor digestion and malabsorption of nutrients. It may also be the major cause of significant malabsorption in the elderly.

The severity of dysbiosis can be easily measured in a properly collected stool sample and a laboratory that specializes in detecting these bacteria. Lab reports showing too many bacterial pathogens living in the intestinal tract should be regarded with much seriousness. Too often, doctors fail to appreciate the significance of this problem.

What Is Fermentation Dysbiosis?

Too much fermentation in the gut can be caused by a carbohydrate intolerance. This type of intolerance may be the only symptom of bacterial overgrowth, making it indistinguishable from other intestinal diseases, such as a yeast overgrowth. The symptoms that are commonly described are abdominal distention, fatigue, impaired cognitive function, flatulence, diarrhea, constipation and feelings of malaise.

People with fermentation excess are usually intolerant to starch, soluble fiber and fiber supplements. Simple sugars may also need to be avoided. A diet free of cereal grains and added sugar is generally the most helpful. Fruit, fat, and starchy vegetables may be tolerated to some degree, depending on the case. Some fibrous vegetables, carrots in particular, keep pathogens from attaching themselves to the intestinal lining.

What Is Putrefaction Dysbiosis?

The classic Western diet is high in fat and animal products, and low in insoluble fiber. This diet produces an increased concentration of pathogens in the intestines, resulting in a decreased concentration of the beneficial bacteria. Colon and breast cancer have been linked to this type of dysbiosis.

Bacterial imbalances caused by putrefaction are usually treated with a diet high in both soluble and insoluble fiber and low in saturated fat and animal protein. Insoluble fiber decreases bacterial concentration and microbial enzyme activity. Soluble fiber tends to raise the levels of beneficial short-chain fatty acids, which in turn helps to keep colon cells healthy. This may explain why fiber aids in the prevention of colon cancer.

How Do Low Hydrochloric Acid Levels Lead to Dysbiosis?

Low levels of hydrochloric acid in the stomach encourage the overgrowth and imbalance of bacteria both in the stomach and through the entire intestinal tract. Hydrochloric acid sterilizes the stomach. The low pH of the stomach is key to the entire body's nutritional state and to the ability of the intestinal tract to keep pathogens out. If there is decreased stomach acid with an unhealthy pH level, then all types of organisms, including bacteria, are allowed to pass on where they can cause damage or release their toxins.

The symptoms of deficient hydrochloric acid are bad breath, stomach distress, fullness, distension, gas, nausea, vomiting, diarrhea, constipation, severe heartburn, a loss of taste for meat, and epigastric pain.

Is Dysbiosis Difficult To Treat?

As mentioned earlier, "mixed" overgrowths consisting of more than one type of pathogen are probably the most difficult to diagnose and treat. People with mixed bacterial and yeast overgrowths are probably suffering a multitude of symptoms, yet their doctor may find nothing wrong with them. It is often difficult to detect yeast in some lab cultures

What If I Have a Sluggish Metabolism?

A sluggish digestive tract keeps food lingering in the intestinal system too long and feeds pathogens. Inadequate water intake, a low-fiber diet, or insufficient levels of digestive enzymes may cause reduced bowel movements. The addition of insoluble fiber helps create bulk and encourages a more normal transit time. Other conditions, such as low thyroid function, can reduce transit time as well. It is very important to have at least one to two normal bowel movements every day. It becomes even more important when taking products to eliminate dysbiosis.

because doctors usually don't know how to look for it. Some people might harbor mold overgrowth as well. Instead of being invasive the way yeast can be, molds live on the surfaces of things and produce many toxins. The treatment for mold overgrowth is difficult because it may require a different antifungal medication than the more popular ones used for yeast overgrowth. It is also possible to have parasites present in the mix. These people are probably the sickest of all, and treatment is even more difficult.

Moreover, bacteria overgrowths can be extremely difficult to diagnose. For instance, most of the major U.S. labs do not have the ability to identify anaerobic bacteria. One of the reasons for this is that the equipment for culturing anaerobes is too expensive. Even your doctor may not be aware of this fact and could send specimens to the wrong lab. Furthermore, many people do not receive the necessary treatment because their doctors do not believe that dysbiosis exists, even if stool cultures show the presence of yeast, fungus and bacterial overgrowth.

Can Drinking Water Contribute to Bacterial Overgrowth?

The safety of our drinking water is a concern shared by many, many people. Between 1994 and 1995, over 18,000 drinking water systems in the United States reported violations of health standards for microbial contaminants (besides toxic chemicals, lead and other violations). It is doubtful that this situation has improved. In fact, it is estimated that one out of every five Americans unknowingly drinks tap water contaminated with feces, lead, radiation, or other contaminants. Of course,

What Are Contributing Factors for Dysbiosis?

- Medication such as antibiotics or non-steroidal anti-inflammatory medications (NSAIDs)
- Chronic maldigestion, which includes pancreatic insufficiency, low levels of hydrochloric acid in the stomach and other digestive enzyme deficiencies
- Compromised intestinal immune function (low secretory IgA) or decreased immune status in general
- Inadequate water intake
- Inadequate fiber intake (soluble and insoluble fiber)
- A poor diet; a diet too high in meat, saturated fat, or refined carbohydrates especially sugar
- Nutrient deficiencies
- Inflammatory bowel diseases
- Chronic exposure to toxins or impaired intestinal detoxification
- Bowel pH is too alkaline
- Slow transit time or intestinal obstructions
- Excess stress

contaminated drinking water is only one possible contributing factor for dysbiosis.

How Does Dysbiosis Lead To Food Allergies?

Many speculate that food allergies are not an immune problem, but a disorder of bacterial fermentation in the colon. If you combine a reduction of digestive enzymes with an imbalanced bacterial microflora and increased intestinal permeability, you have a good candidate for food allergies. Food allergies are another symptom of imbalance, not the underlying cause.

Am I Lactose Intolerant?

When someone is lactose intolerant this means that they cannot produce enough of the enzyme needed to break down this carbohydrate into simpler sugars. The whole carbohydrate travels into the colon. Once there, bacteria fermenting the carbohydrate produce gas. Because the carbohydrate has not been digested, imbalances are created causing diarrhea, abdominal cramps or discomfort, gas and bloating. Over time, the intestinal lining becomes irritated, which can lead to malabsorption. Lactose intolerance is very different from a milk allergy, however. Individuals who do not produce sufficient quantities of the lactase enzyme are not necessarily allergic to milk proteins.

There are more than fifty million people in the U.S. that cannot digest lactose (milk sugar) because of inadequate lactase. It is estimated that 70 percent of people with lactase deficiency never associate their symptoms with their diet. Many people continue to eat foods they cannot digest properly. Unchecked, lactose intolerance will eventually compromise the digestive system and possibly affect other areas of the body as well.

Many unsuspected processed foods contain lactose, making it difficult to detect. Lactose can also be found in some supplements, prescription drugs, protein powders, and artificial sweeteners. If you are using these products, then you will experience ongoing symptoms. Lactose intolerance should be considered in anyone with undiagnosed abdominal complaints. Most ethnic groups are lactose intolerant to some extent. If other types of sugars are causing the problem then removing milk from the diet will not resolve the underlying problem.

Lactose intolerance is the most common type of malabsorption because milk sugar is so common in the modern diet. At the same time, it is possible to be intolerant to other types of sugars such as fructose, sucrose, and maltose. There are also degrees of carbohydrate intolerance. Some people produce a small amount of lactase, but others lack the enzyme completely. Any degree of decreased enzyme production will result in malabsorption.

Any condition that damages the intestinal lining can create lactose malabsorption. This could include intestinal parasites or inflammatory bowel disease. Other triggers of lactose malabsorption include alcoholism, gluten intolerance, malnutrition, pelvic radiation therapy, and antibiotics. Lactose intolerance may not only have the same appearance as dysbiosis, but it can lead to dysbiosis as well. For more information about foods that contain lactose and lactose intolerance in general, consult my book *Allergies and Holistic Healing*.

Can I Cure Dysbiosis by Fasting?

If you suffer from intestinal overgrowth of bacteria and try to treat yourself by diet or fasting alone, you may worsen the problem in the long run. Although some people do feel better when they first start fasting or begin a low-carbohydrate diet, these same individuals may have a more difficult recovery if they relapse later. It is not possible to starve out bacteria, yeast, or any other pathogen.

Some experts have suggested that an overly strict reduction in dietary carbohydrates, without effective antimicrobial therapy at the same time, simply causes the infection to retreat into the deeper tissue layers of the intestinal tract. Pathogens will just adjust their metabolism from carbohydrate to protein as an energy source. Whenever their favorite food supply is reduced, the bacteria will naturally switch to another source of fuel, sometimes becoming more invasive as they go foraging for new sources of food. As a result, the bacteria can be much harder to eradicate.

What Is the Dysbiosis Relapse Rate?

There is a high rate of relapse among people with dysbiosis. These individuals may experience a recovery that lasts for many months or even longer, only to relapse after they readopt old habits such as increased sugar intake, or after taking an antibiotic or suffering an accident. However, if a person is really in balance, such events should not be harmful enough to cause such major setbacks.

Why are relapses so common in seemingly healthy individuals? Pathogens can exist deep within the intestinal tissues without producing symptoms. Some organisms can hide inside other cells, waiting for the right moment to become active again. There may appear to be fewer bacteria because they cannot be detected on most conventional tests, but that does not mean they aren't there. Only when the latent pathogens are given the opportunity to begin overgrowing again do the previously seen symptoms reappear. In these cases, the individual had never truly recovered from the overgrowth.

Why Don't We Hear More about Bacterial Overgrowth?

Many doctors have adopted a position that the overgrowth of bacteria, yeast, or parasites does not exist. Many of the individuals that I consult with tell me that their doctors do not take them seriously when it comes to digestive complaints. Doctors do not usually look for bacteria overgrowth, or any other organism, as the cause of chronic illness. One of the reasons may be because many of these bacteria grow without oxygen (anaerobic), making it difficult to find them on lab tests. Not much research is being done on this subject, and doctors are rarely knowledgeable about dysbiosis anyway. They often believe that anyone who treats these conditions is a "quack." If you suffer from these conditions and have been successfully treated with the so-called "quack" medicine, however, you know how narrowed-minded conventional medicine can be.

Technology is just now understanding what these bacteria have been doing all along. The development of PCR (polymerase chain reaction) technology has pinpointed the genetic fingerprints of these bacteria in human tissue. However, since most doctors do not suspect an overgrowth of bacteria as the culprit of disease, they probably will not do the tests, even as they become available, until more research is done proving the links between bacterial overgrowth and chronic illness.

SECTION 2

Our Toxic Environment: Causes & Factors for Bacterial Overgrowth

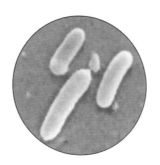

CHAPTER 4

Antibiotics & Bacterial Resistance

ALTHOUGH ONCE WORSHIPPED as the miracle cure of modern medicine, antibiotics are now credited for creating resistant and unstoppable "super bugs." In fact, the situation is so serious that the World Health Organization has made antibiotic resistance a top priority. As is discussed elsewhere in this book, the flawed logic of germ theory may be partially to blame for the current state of healthcare. Although many lives have been (and still are) saved with antibiotics and other drugs, antibiotic overuse and misuse is causing more bacterial strains to mutate and develop antibiotic resistance. I believe the solution to this problem is a careful shift in our focus from eradicating germs to building our immunity, our inner terrain.

Unfortunately, most people would rather pop a pill than eat correctly and do what is necessary to recover from their illnesses. This "health in a pill" mindset is supported and perpetuated by traditional medicine. For the last fifty years, we have been told that the only way to get rid of an infection is to use antibiotics. If the first course of antibiotics did not work, the doctor would prescribe a second or third batch, each being more powerful. In fact, it is estimated that the average person will consume at least one thousand doses of antibiotics by the time they are fifty, and the average child has already received many of those doses by the time they are three years old. It simply does not occur to many people that there are other ways to get well and stay well.

From Wonder Drugs to Wonder Bugs

The problem is that although we have developed a number of "wonder drugs" to fight bacteria since Pasteur's time, our battle for terrain with dangerous bacteria continues to occur—in our bodies, in animals, in agriculture fields and even on our antibacterial-soaked kitchen counters. After all of these years of overusing and misusing antibiotics, we are now confronting bacteria that have mutated, changed and built defenses against many antibacterial drugs and chemicals. These once treatable organisms become infectious bacteria or "wonder bugs" capable of causing extreme illness in vulnerable people. Miracle drugs are destroying the miracle.

When Did Bacterial Resistance Begin?

Bacterial resistance has been developing for many years, but it was first noticed during World War II. In 1940, an enzyme that destroyed penicillin was discovered in a strain of *Escherichia col*i (*E.coli*). At that time, this strain was a common and harmless bacterium found in the intestines of animals and humans. However, in 1946, just five years after penicillin came into wide use, another bacteria, *Staphylococcus aureus*, became resistant to the antibiotic. In the 1950s, there were already instances of resistant staph infections showing up in U.S. hospitals, but few people took notice. After all, new antibiotics were being discovered that could replace penicillin, and modern medicine could certainly stay one step ahead.

Reports of resistant *E. coli* and *Salmonella* surfaced during the 1970s. Then, two dangerous organisms became resistant to penicillin: *Haemophilus influenzae*, which produces respiratory infections, and *Neisseria gonorrhoeae*, the cause of gonorrhea. Moreover, scientists realized that both pathogens had the same resistance gene, implying that they most likely received it from bacteria living in the gastrointestinal tract.

Antibiotic-resistant strains of gonorrhea were first discovered in the Philippines among prostitutes who had been given penicillin regularly as a precautionary measure. That overexposure also caused drug resistance in U.S. servicemen suffering from gonorrhea. In fact, it is rumored that the infection of American GIs with drug-resistant gonorrhea was a deliberate act to weaken our armed forces. Even if the spread of gonorrhea was not deliberate, it reveals how quickly bacteria can become resistant and spread throughout the world. Today, every country in the world has drug-resistant gonorrhea.

Finally, in 1995, the American Medical Association declared the overuse of antibiotics by the U.S. medical community to be a serious health problem for everyone, not just people being given the antibiotics. Today, at least two dozen different kinds of bacteria have developed resistance to one or more antibiotics. Some strains of bacteria such as *Pseudomonas aeruginosa* and *Mycobacterium tuberculosis* now frustrate most known antibiotics. Ever-present pathogens that cause ear, nose and throat infections, as well as scarlet fever, meningitis and pneumonia, are becoming widely resistant as well. There is also a growing fear that some benign childhood diseases might eventually become unresponsive to treatment. We cannot deny that resistant and mutant strains of bacteria and viruses are here and can no longer be ignored.

The Antibiotic Incentive

Why then, with the growing problem of antibiotic resistance, has antibiotic treatment taken precedence over preventative healthcare practices? Regretfully, money has fueled some of the problem. To give you some idea how much money is involved, consider this: doctors prescribe over $500 million in antibiotics to treat childhood ear infections alone. Other childhood illnesses probably amount to another $500 million. Moreover, the increase of young children getting antibiotics has increased over 50 percent in recent years. In fact, nearly 1.5 million antibiotic prescriptions are given every week by internists and obstetricians, and gynecologists prescribe over 2.5 million antibiotic prescriptions weekly. To meet these demands, more than fifty million pounds of antibiotics are produced in this country each year for human, animal and agriculture uses.

Using Antibiotics Incorrectly

Antibiotic use is up, and so is misuse. Congressional hearings concluded that as much as 60 percent of all antibiotics are prescribed incorrectly in this country. And a 1997 study by the National Academy of Science estimated that almost half of the annual outpatient prescriptions for antibiotics are not medically justified, either because they are not indicated at all or the wrong antibiotic is prescribed. Dosage amounts and duration are often wrong as well.

Hospital patients are usually given some type of antibiotic prior to surgery in an effort to prevent post-surgical infections. In 1992, it was estimated that twenty-three million people received presurgical antibiotic therapy. Of those treated, almost one million still developed postsurgical infections. Because of this practice, hospitals have become a serious breeding ground for some of the most potent and resistant microorganisms.

Antibiotic overuse and misuse appears to play a large role in the resistance problem. When a strain of bacteria is first exposed to an antibiotic, most of the microbes are susceptible to the drug and die. But a few bacteria that already have some resistance to the antibiotic may survive, especially if the dosage of the drug is insufficient or if it is not used long enough. (This often occurs when people do not finish their prescriptions because they feel better.) In each subsequent generation, many more bacteria become resistant until the entire colony is resistant. This leads to a relapse of the disease in the individual and the spread of resistant bacteria to others.

A Flawed Medical System

If doctors and policy makers do not change the way antibiotics are dispensed, microbial resistance will continue to worsen. A report published in the *Archives of Internal Medicine* claims that healthcare economics has fueled this overuse and misuse. Hospital-acquired bacterial infections that do not respond to standard antibiotics now cost at least $1.3 billion each year.

Plus, drug resistance is not just happening in hospitals. Of the fifty-one million visits each year to the doctor's office for common illnesses, such as virus-caused colds and influenza (which cannot be treated with antibiotics), around 66 percent resulted in an antibiotic prescription. People's desire for "quick-fix" medications has pressured doctors to overprescribe antibiotics.

No parent likes to see their children sick, but some parents take it too far by pressuring pediatricians to prescribe oral antibiotics when such medications are not called for. In a survey of 610 pediatricians, 48 percent responded that parents were likely to pressure them to prescribe antibiotics when it was not clear that they were necessary. In addition, many physicians reported that parents requested an antibiotic over the phone, often asking for a specific antibiotic or a different prescription. About a third of the pediatricians said that they complied with the requests for antibiotics at least occasionally.

Physicians are also pressured by the health-care system. Doctors see their patients for such a short period of time and are encouraged to minimize return visits. So instead of solving the patient's underlying health problem, it is easier and faster to just treat the symptoms with drugs, and of course, this is also more economically profitable.

How Safe Are Antibiotics for Children?

Antibiotic use in children is a subject of particular debate since the number of prescriptions for children continues to rise. Some studies have shown the negative effects of antibiotics on children and especially infants. In one review of infants born in a California hospital between 1988 and 1996 who were infected early on with group B *Streptococcus* infections, researchers found that all of the infants exposed to antibiotics during birth again became ill within the first twenty-four hours of life. Some experts believe that this form of therapy predisposes infants to an increased risk of allergies, recurrent ear infections and all sorts of chronic illnesses, such as attention deficit/hyperactivity disorder (ADHD) and autism. Some critics of antibiotics advise the immediate and continued use of probiotics (beneficial bowel flora) if the decision is made to start an infant on antibiotic therapy. (It would probably be wise to continue giving the infant probiotics for at least four to eight weeks.)

Older children may suffer complications from antibiotic therapy as well. Children who are treated for *E. coli* infection with antibiotics are at a greater risk of developing a toxic condition leading to kidney failure, according to a study released by *The New England Journal of Medicine*. Researchers studied seventy-one children who had diarrhea from *E. coli* infection; nine received antibiotics. Five of the nine children treated with antibiotics developed a condition (more common in children than adults) that negatively affected their red blood cells and proper urine secretion. Study researchers recommended that children who may be infected with *E. coli* not receive antibiotics until they receive a stool culture indicating an infection treatable with an antibiotic.

Expecting mothers also need to consider the risks of antibiotics on their fetuses. Nearly one out of every three pregnant women will be treated with antibiotics, despite the fact that only around one in every 870 newborns has a group B *Streptococcus* infection.

Stay the Course

If you do decide to take an antibiotic or give one to your children, follow pharmacist and doctor instructions closely. Many individuals are tempted to stop taking their antibiotic as soon as they feel better. They think that they are doing something good for themselves by not taking the antibiotic for the entire duration. What they do not realize is that by preempting treatment, they only kill off the weak pathogens. Those organisms left behind are stronger and more dangerous. The untouched pathogens continue to reproduce, passing on their resistance to future generations, until the infection or overgrowth returns with a vengeance. Now the pathogen is resistant to the original antibiotic and may be harder to kill the second time around. To avoid a recurrence, keep the following in mind:

- Do not stop taking the antibiotic just because you are feeling better.
- Any time you have to take an antibiotic, you also need to take a probiotic. Start taking them as soon as you notice an infection and continue to take them for at least one month after stopping the antibiotic therapy. Also, be sure to let your doctor know that you are taking probiotics and any other medications or supplements you may be taking.

Understanding the Long-Term Effects of Antibiotics

Even if you do follow doctor's instructions when taking an antibiotic, taking them too often can also be a health hazard. Antibiotics typically wipe out weak bacteria but may let tougher bacteria survive and become stronger. In fact, it is almost impossible to destroy one hundred percent of the offending bacteria without extremely long courses of antibiotics. There will always be a number of drug-resistant survivors. Leaving just one percent of the harmful pathogens can have disastrous effects. Without competition from friendly bacteria, these resistant mutants double in population every few minutes and spread in record time, reinfecting with a superstrain of bacteria. Moreover, antibiotics weaken immune function, leaving vulnerable people less able to defend themselves against these tough pathogens.

To make matters worse, antibiotics do not kill just pathogenic bacteria. Antibiotics indiscriminately kill off bacteria in the intestines, including many beneficial bacteria that make up our normal bowel microflora. Many types of good bacteria in the colon are necessary for numerous life functions, such as complete digestion, nutrient absorption, and keeping potentially dangerous bacteria in check. Antibiotic therapy creates the ideal breeding ground for pathogens to reproduce without any healthy competition. In many of the recent outbreaks of food poisoning, the individuals who suffered the worst fates were those who just happened to be taking antibiotics for other problems, such as sore throats or other minor infections.

When friendly bacteria are killed and resistant pathogens take over, it may take weeks or months for the body to rebuild normal levels of beneficial bacteria. Despite this fact, most doctors never suggest that their patients replenish the beneficial microflora after prescribing antibiotics. This makes for incomplete digestion, putrefaction, rancidity or rotting of intestinal contents.

Remember also that broad-spectrum antibiotics that kill off anaerobic bacteria (those that live without oxygen) may be more harmful than other antibiotics. Also, antibiotics that are rapidly absorbed into the bloodstream are less harmful than those that are absorbed more slowly from the gastrointestinal tract.

Why We Need Bacterial Exposure

Perhaps the biggest argument against antibiotics and bacteria paranoia is that the vast majority of the bacteria and viruses we are exposed to are completely nonpathogenic and may be quite beneficial. In fact, our bodies are naturally covered in bacteria. This layer of friendly microbes helps keep out harmful ones. Nonpathogenic bacteria are essential to our body's natural defenses against invading infectious bacteria. Friendly bacteria limit the spread of more dangerous bacteria simply by being in the way. Without them, the playing field is wide open for the proliferation of resistant bugs.

Compounding the problem is the fact that harmless strains of bacteria can also cause disease after repeated exposure to antibiotics, particularly in people with weakened immune systems. These harmless bacteria can also become drug-resistant and pass their resistance genes to disease-causing species.

Even disease-causing organisms may provide benefits by allowing the immune system to develop properly, especially in children, thereby reducing the chance of developing conditions like allergies, asthma and eczema. Actually, the recurrence rate for some infections, including ear infections, are actually higher after taking an antibiotic than if no treatment is given. The effects of antibiotics on friendly bacteria allows yeast, disease-causing bacteria or parasites to take over, making the situation worse. That is why protecting our beneficial microflora is so important, whether it is inside or outside of us. For more information on replacing friendly bacteria using probiotics, see Section 4.

Antibiotics Don't Cure Disease

The real tragedy of antibiotics is the medical mindset they perpetuate. In reality, the degenerative diseases that plague our society are not going to be cured by pharmaceutical drugs because they do nothing to address the underlying cause of disease. They only mask or suppress symptoms. For instance, the cause of a strep infection is not simply the presence of the strep organism. The real question is what allowed the strep organism to proliferate in the first place. If the human body were in balance, there would be no fertile ground for the bacteria to invade and multiply.

Infectious agents are everywhere. There is no way to kill them all, and the drugs we use to treat them, like antibiotics, poison and weaken the body. A better approach to preventing bacterial infection is to strengthen the body so that it is no longer susceptible to pathogens. Eliminating a symptom without revitalizing the body as a whole is suppression, not a cure. There are many natural remedies that work more effectively, with no side effects, and at a fraction of the cost.

Sometimes You Need an Antibiotic

Of course, sometimes it is a good idea to take an antibiotic. I am not totally against antibiotics. When used appropriately, antibiotics can save lives. In severe bacterial and potentially life threatening infections, they may be the best choice. Still, it is hard to think about using an antibiotic when it was probably an antibiotic that got you in trouble in the first place, but there are times when the only way to reduce the numbers of internal pathogens is to initially use an antibiotic. It may need to be combined with an antifungal medication and a probiotic such as *Lactobacillus acidophilus*.

Prevention is still the best course of action, however, and will definitely reduce the number of times you will have to take antibiotics. Unfortunately, because of blatant overuse of antibiotics, you may have a difficult time finding an effective antibiotic when you finally do need one. Even individuals who intentionally avoid taking antibiotics may be surprised to find out how many times they are exposing themselves and their families without even knowing it.

Other Causes of Bacterial Resistance

I have already mentioned the ways in which the healthcare system and antibiotic misuse and overuse have contributed to resistant bacteria, but these are not the only factors contributing to the birth of super bugs. Antibiotics are used in a number of household products, including dish and hand soaps, which may also add to the problem. Antibiotics are also used in agriculture, and there is now evidence that these uses have created an environment in which bacteria rapidly develop anti-microbial resistance. As a result, a whole host of human diseases are essentially not treatable with the commercially available antibiotics. Let's take a few minutes to see how commercially advertised antibacterial products and the agricultural industry have contributed to the problem of super bugs.

Adaptation: The Key to Resistance

Bacteria become resistant by adapting to changes in their environment when exposed to antibiotics, chlorine, household chemicals or any substance that threatens their existence. Some bacteria become immune to these substances on their own, either through genetic mutations or by inheriting resistance traits from prior generations. Some bacterial genes produce a sort of pump that transports antibiotics out of the organism before they have a chance to do any harm. Others generate powerful enzymes that inactivate the drugs. Still others modify the antibiotic's targets within the microbes or provide decoys that divert and disable the drugs. In some extreme cases, antibiotic-resistant bacteria can actually thrive on the drugs developed to kill or suppress them.

Bacterial resistance is a serious problem worldwide. Of particular concern is the increasing frequency of multi-drug resistance within *Salmonella* strains isolated from foodborne infections. *Salmonella typhimurium* DT04 and many other organisms use integrons, which are gene expression elements that have the potential for rapid and efficient transmission of drug resistance. Seventy-four strains of *Salmonella* other than *Salmonella enteritidis* and *Salmonella typhimurium* are now resistant to three or more antibacterial drugs.

This ability to become resistant is found in many less prevalent strains of *Salmonella* with extensive reservoirs, including swine, poultry, domestic pets and environmental sites (rivers, sewage effluents). This resistance gene is spreading through the food chain because of pressure from the intensive use of antimicrobial agents in farming and

Antibiotic Allergies

Still not convinced of the risks? Consider this: It is estimated that 10 percent of Americans are allergic to penicillin but may be unknowingly consuming small but continuous amounts of it in many foods. Would you serve your family penicillin, tetracycline or some other drug-resistant bacteria for dinner? These and countless other substances are routinely found in our food supply. More than 40 percent of the fifty million pounds of antibiotics produced in the United States are used in or on animals, especially to promote growth. For years, in fact, it has been a practice to mix the antibiotic tetracycline into animal feed. This certainly may contribute to the increase problem of food allergies, fatigue syndromes, gastrointestinal upsets and the overgrowth of yeast.

animal husbandry (as growth promoters and for disease prevention and therapy) further underscoring the public health problems of antibiotic resistance.

The Trail of Sickness

Did you know that about 40 percent of all antibiotics produced in this country are given to animals, not to treat any particular illness, but to promote their growth so that they can be marketed sooner? After all, time is money. The use of antibiotics in livestock has caused the incidence of foodborne *Salmonella* to skyrocket. The germs become resistant to antibiotics used in animals. Then an antibiotic-resistant strain of *Salmonella* is transferred to the person who consumes the meat.

The number of antibiotics used to prevent and treat udder infections in dairy cows is staggering. The dairy farmer uses the genetically engineered growth hormone developed by Monsanto to increase milk production. This causes many of the cows to have udder infections, which are then treated with antibiotics. The residues of these antibiotics end up in the milk supply. In fact, a 1992 study by the Congressional General Accounting Office discovered traces of sixty-four antibiotics at health level concern. Maybe the saying "Got milk?" should be changed to, "Got milk fortified with antibiotics?"

High levels of antibiotics in food aren't the only risk. Rutgers

University found that antibiotics at levels considered safe by the FDA could still cause resistant bacteria to emerge in great numbers. Antibiotic use is rampant in farming as well. The drugs are sprayed onto fruit trees to control bacterial infections. I will discuss the relationship between pathogenic bacteria and the food industry in more detail in a later chapter.

Global Opinions about Antibiotics in Our Food

The first countries to initiate restrictions on agricultural use of antibiotics were Sweden and Finland who successfully persuaded other member countries to think likewise. Now this union has taken a bold step in dealing with the pervasive antibiotic problem by banning the use of antibiotics in agriculture that are also used in human medicine. Unfortunately, the U.S. has not followed suit.

The European Union now authorize four drugs for use in agriculture that are not used in human medicine. The CDC in Atlanta supports this move because it believes that agricultural use of antibiotics is a major cause of antibiotic resistance in food-related illnesses; however, the U.S. pharmaceutical and meat industries are threatening to challenge the ban as an illegal barrier to trade.

If you would like to express your concerns regarding the agricultural misuse of antibiotics, you can urge the FDA to follow the European Union's lead and ban animal use of growth-promoting antibiotics, which are used in human medicine. To do this, contact the FDA via their website: www.fda.org.

It's Still an Antibiotic

Whether an antibiotic is applied to the skin, swallowed or consumed in food, it is still an antibiotic. Yet, many people, especially parents, unknowingly use these products many times a day on themselves and their children. Antibacterials can be found in household cleaning products, soaps, toothpaste and even plastic toys and cutting boards. This massive exposure may ultimately be very harmful to all of us—even topical treatments. (Most people do not realize that the skin is the body's largest organ, capable of absorbing many substances.)

Even if you are spooked about reports of killer *E. coli* and other outbreaks of food poisoning, what you do with that fear could be dangerous to your health. When you try to kill every germ you come in contact with, you could be creating the very super bugs that you want to avoid.

Buying kitchen products or toys with built-in antimicrobials may appear to offer peace of mind, but the sense of security is a false one. Advertisers have us worried about the germs living in our houses, but are antimicrobial products a legitimate weapon in the battle against germs? Antibacterial soaps have become so popular that you literally cannot buy one marketed for children without an antibacterial agent in it.

Disinfectants were first used in hospitals to kill many microbes including bacteria, viruses and fungi. This makes sense in a hospital setting where germs can make the difference between life and death for an already ill patient. Disinfectants soon found their way into the consumer world when manufacturers developed antimicrobial cleaners in response to increased consumer awareness about bacteria. They put triclosan into products such as cutting boards and toys. It was also being used in some liquid dish and hand soaps, Colgate Total toothpaste and one variety of Reach toothbrushes.

As mentioned, the major concern with these products is that they will contribute to the development of hardier strains of microbes. Scientists have traditionally discounted this possibility, believing instead that these household products kill germs in so many different ways that no one organisms could ever develop full resistance. Well, they are wrong. Common household bacteria have begun to develop resistance prompting the World Health Organization to directly link antibacterial products with the rise in antibiotic resistance. The Centers for Disease Control and Prevention (CDC) currently recommends that people use ordinary soap and water instead of antibacterial products. Triclosan is also being phased out, but what will manufacturers think of next?

Aside from promoting resistant bacteria, experts are also concerned that people will assume that antibacterial products do not have to be washed as often because they contain an antibacterial agent. In reality, most household bacteria can be kept in check with little more than a vigorous scrub with any good soap and hot water. Strong antibacterial cleaners are needed only when someone in a household is seriously ill or has low immunity.

Stronger Bacteria: A Global Threat

What is the bottom line? New variations of bacteria and other pathogens are springing up all over the world and are becoming more difficult to treat. In addition, the world is getting smaller due to increased international travel and more food being shipped internationally. In many countries there are large populations in areas with unsanitary conditions and deteriorating health infrastructures, combined with an increase worldwide of diseases that compromise the immune system.

Dr. Michael Osterholm (formerly a state epidemiologist in Minnesota) has studied antimicrobial resistance for twenty-five years. He says that these bacteria get into our sewage, passing their genes for resistance to other bacteria (perhaps even a more lethal strain). All it takes is for one animal, like a bird, to pick up the raw sewage and pass it onto a produce crop. Just a little *Salmonella* on a tomato leaf is all it takes to incorporate the bacteria inside the tomato.

Even more unsettling, scientists have now found antibiotic-resistant bacteria in the bodies of African tribesmen who live in total isolation from civilization, with no access to drugs whatsoever. The resistant strains are now part of our "normal" bowel microflora. So the more we take broad-spectrum antibiotics, the more we destroy the old non-resistant strains. Eventually, this will only leave the resistant strains.

Another driving force is the continued inappropriate use of antibiotics for infections such as *Streptococcus pneumoniae,* the cause of upper respiratory tract infections. The proportion of these bacteria that are resistant to antibiotics continues to increase at an alarming rate, especially in the United States. Reliance by cost-conscious managed care organizations on the cheapest antibiotics to treat many illnesses is another factor. The results are increases in bacterial resistance to antibiotics. Simply put, this type of treatment is shortsighted and not the most effective way to treat these infections.

New Antibiotics in Development

In response to the growing danger of pathogenic bacteria, the medical community is developing new strategies for dealing with antibiotic resistance. A new antibiotic called Zyvox may now be approved. It would become the first entirely new antibiotic to hit the market since 1965. It is supposed to destroy bacteria that have become resistant to other standard medications, but Zyvox only works against gram-positive bacteria. Gram-negative organisms cause more than half of all serious infections treated in hospitals worldwide. These include bacteria that cause pneumonia and infections of the skin, bloodstream and urinary tract, among other things. Another new antibiotic called Linezolid will be used on serious infections in hospitalized children, especially pneumonia, if the infection is due to antibiotic-resistant gram-positive bacteria.

Often, individuals get these infections while they are in the hospital for other health problems. It will join another new antibiotic, Synercid, approved by the FDA last fall. However, at least two cases of Zyvox-resistant germs have already been seen in experimental use.

The costs of developing new drugs and the regulations being imposed by the U.S. Food and Drug Administration discouraged drug companies from developing new antibiotics. Halts in research coincided with the time bacteria resistance was getting out of control. By 1991, at least 50 percent of the pharmaceutical companies in this country and Japan were reducing or stopping their antibacterial research.

Altered Bacteria: Another Option?

Bacteriophages, or phages for short, do nothing but attack and destroy other bacteria. They thrive anywhere bacteria are abundant, such as in sewage, on food, in water, even in your body. Phages can keep pace with the bacteria they are attacking. Each kind of phage usually goes after only one species of bacterium. Phages can also evolve along with the bacteria, so that the bacteria cannot develop permanent resistance to them.

The former Soviet Union has been experimenting with phages for nearly seventy years, although phage therapy had been dismissed as a failure decades ago in the West because of its inherent dangers. When doctors first tried giving phages to patients, they sometimes accidentally included poisons from the bacteria in the medicine, making patients sicker. In other cases, the phages may have done their work too fast, bursting too many bacteria at once, and releasing an overwhelming dose of poison from the bacterial cells. As a result, many patients died. So, except for special instances, phage therapy has not been tried in the U.S. for sixty years.

Now, there is interest in phage therapy again. Some scientists in the United States and Europe hope to use these bacteria to fight outbreaks of antibiotic-resistant bacteria. Only animal studies are being conducted because there is concern that a person's immune system could interfere with the treatment. Investors see this type of therapy as a good investment, and several companies and one government lab hope to launch clinical trials soon so that they can begin manufacturing these bacteria.

Unlike the previous bacteriophage therapies, which attempted to kill targets directly, one new approach would make use of a delivery system to incorporate genes into host DNA that encode for proteins toxic to the bacteria. Another approach being developed is trying to engineer the phages to inject DNA into the bacteria that turns off a set of genes, allowing the bacteria to be engulfed by the phage system. One of the latest reports is about investigators looking into parasitic viruses that replicate inside bacteria and then break down the bacterial wall when the virus matures. They want to make a new class of antibiotics based on this ability by certain viruses to kill bacteria. When the bacteria cell tries to divide, it blows up instead (*Science* 2001).

I think it is important to include this information because you should know how popular it is to manipulate nature these days. One of the major reasons for this type of research is because of all the money it is going to make. There does not seem to be enough concern in case these experiments go wrong. Once we start manipulating DNA or using one pathogen to kill another one, we are certainly putting ourselves at risk for unknown and possibly irreversible consequences.

Pushing the Survival Envelope: What Can You Do?

It is unlikely that there will be major changes in the way Western medicine addresses the problem of pathogens. The current focus in medicine today is to develop new and more powerful drugs rather than improve a person's immune system and internal terrain. The odds are overwhelming that more dangerous drug-resistant strains of microbes will continue to emerge. Just how serious will this situation ultimately become?

Never before have bacteria encountered the explosion of drugs designed to kill them. We are pushing microbial evolution into overdrive, making bacteria resistant to new drugs that have not even been tried on them. Is there anything you can do to protect yourself? Cutting out antibiotics (or at least our dependence on them) is a good start. In the next few years we will probably see all kinds of novel drugs developed. Even if these new drugs prove to be effective, are we just stalling for time until the next problem develops? Maybe it would be better to take a different approach. You can start by enhancing your body's natural immunity. Your immune system is your first and best line of defense. Section 4 offers suggestions for boosting immune function.

CHAPTER 5

The Nasty Little Secrets
of the Food Industry

ALTHOUGH THE FOOD industry has been under increased scrutiny in recent years, especially with increased awareness about the dangers of pesticides, there is still a lot about the food industry that the general public does not know—but should. Ignorance about what is in our food may ultimately compromise our health and make us more susceptible to super bugs and bacterial overgrowth. It is estimated, for instance, that one-third of all chickens in the U.S. are now contaminated with *Salmonella* bacteria. Moreover, over 50 percent of livestock today are given antibiotics, leading to stronger strains of disease-causing bacteria. This chapter will explore the dangers of genetic engineering and list various toxic substances lurking in the food we eat.

What's Wrong with Fruits and Vegetables?

The number of outbreaks of foodborne disease related to fresh produce has nearly tripled since the 1970s. This is not surprising considering the growing emphasis on including fruits and vegetables in a proper diet. Foods as diverse as alfalfa sprouts, mangoes, orange juice, strawberries and raspberries have been linked to outbreaks of bacterial (and other) infections. Convenience foods such as preshredded lettuce have also been linked to outbreaks. Although it is important for the public to learn about the benefits of fruits and vegetables, gastrointestinal health may suffer severely as a result.

Bacteria cause the majority of these outbreaks, followed by parasites and viruses. Most of the problems occur because of fecal contamination.

One outbreak was traced to water contaminated with feces used to irrigate a berry patch in Guatemala. Another incident occurred in California where apple trees were contaminated with cow feces spread under them. The feces contained the potentially deadly bacteria, *E. coli* 0157:H7. When the apples fell to the ground they were contaminated with this bacterium. Also in California, a recent outbreak of *Salmonella* poisoning was linked to contaminated water that touched tomatoes. However it happens, pathogens grow on the surface of fruits or vegetables and may travel thousands of miles before arriving on your dinner table.

Briefly heating beverages and then rapidly cooling them can kill most fecal bacteria, making even contaminated drinks safe. Unfortunately, it can alter the taste and nutritional content. While this may be an issue, the safety benefits of pasteurization are not. The list of disease-causing organisms in fruits and vegetables is almost as varied as our supply of fresh produce. It may be safer to avoid unpasteurized foods that are suspected of contamination.

With several cases of food poisoning traced to raw sprouts, it is best to eat only cooked sprouts (including homegrown). Sprouts are one of the worst culprits, causing twenty outbreaks since 1973 (fourteen since 1995). The sprouting process is almost ideal for the growth of pathogenic microorganisms such as *Salmonella* since seeds are kept moist and warm for days. Any bacteria present on the seeds or in the water will be encouraged to grow. At the present time, there is not a good solution to the problem of contaminated sprouts. If you are eating out, ask restaurants not to add raw sprouts to your sandwich or salad.

Another common problem is fruit juice, including fruit juice "smoothies." There have been twelve reported outbreaks since 1974, and the majority of cases have been linked to unpasteurized orange juice and apple cider. Although scrubbing with soap or chlorine-based washes reduce bacterial counts, these approaches do not eliminate the problem. Some types of produce have complex, difficult-to-wash surfaces, which allow pathogens to adhere tightly to the surface. Contamination may also be internal.

In any event, consumers are at greater risk of foodborne infection than ever before, not only from eating more uncooked fruits and vegetables, but also because these foods, such as prepared salads and precut melons, undergo more processing. If you eat salads, juices or produce that is not peeled, cooked or washed properly, you risk a nasty upset stomach (or worse).

Genetic Engineering in the Food Industry

One of the biggest concerns currently with the produce industry is not just pesticides or food poisoning, but also the increase in genetically engineered plant foods. Genetic engineering involves the transfer of one or more genes from one organism to another, giving it specific characteristics. Since 1994, the amounts of new foods developed by using advanced biotechnology have risen dramatically. At least forty common vegetables, dairy products and hundreds of processed foods now contain genes from viruses, bacteria, insects, flowers and even animals. About 55 percent of the U.S. soybean crop planted in 1999 carries a gene that makes it resist the effects of a herbicide used to control weeds. Twenty-five percent of all U.S. corn planted in 1999 contains a gene that produces a protein toxic to certain caterpillars. More altered crops are being developed at this writing, including tomatoes, peas, peppers, apples, tropical fruit, broccoli, raspberries, melons, potatoes, corn, lettuce, coffee, squash, strawberries, lettuce, wheat, walnuts and cotton. Although undergoing varying degrees of genetic alteration, these unmarked and unlabeled foods account for about 60 to 70 percent of the foods currently on grocery shelves.

There are different reasons why foods are being altered. Some are designed to retain flavor and appearance while also having a longer shelf life. Agricultural researchers are looking at producing foods that are nutritionally enhanced or can deliver vaccines or medicine through gene splicing. Scientists at Cornell University, for instance, want to alter the common potato to create a vaccine against the pathogen bacteria *E. coli*. However, these scientists also say that tinkering with the immune system must be done carefully, because it could dampen important immune responses. Despite scientific enthusiasm, most informed consumers are concerned about potential health or safety issues associated with genetically engineered (GE) foods. There are many concerns that this new technology could be producing great harm to us and to our environment.

Labeling Genetically Engineered Foods

Even with strong scientific evidence of numerous potential health and environmental risks from GE foods, the Food and Drug Administration (FDA) does not require safety testing and mandatory labeling. The FDA recently announced new rules and guidance on GE foods, but they only require that food producers notify the agency before marketing a new GE food. Nevertheless, these foods could be toxic, cause allergic responses, lower nutritional value, and compromise the immune system in people who consume them.

Despite overwhelming consumer demand, the FDA has decided to make all labeling of GE foods voluntary. Not surprisingly, GE food producers have opted not to release this information. As a consumer, you have no way of knowing which foods have been genetically engineered, in violation of the consumer's right to know. Without labeling, neither consumers nor health professionals will know if an allergic or toxic reaction was the result of a GE food or from some other source. Why do food manufacturers resist labeling? The real reason they do not want to label their foods is because they are afraid consumers will avoid them.

The FDA also wants to make it more difficult for consumers to avoid GE foods by restricting label content for food producers of non-GE products. Clearly, the FDA is ignoring warnings about the adverse affects of genetically altered foods and instead is siding with the companies that make them. It is not surprising that companies who profit from GE foods have paid little attention to the potential hazards of these foods. What is astounding is that the FDA has not found it necessary to conduct comprehensive scientific reviews of foods derived from bioengineered plants, in violation of its 1992 policy. The policy states that genetically modified crops will receive the same consideration for potential health risks as any other new crop plant.

Critics of genetically engineered foods say consumers have a right to see labels stating that food has been altered. They also want the FDA to require more safety tests on both the food and environmental impacts. Consumers have a right to know what they are eating and being exposed to, don't they? In fact, in Europe, Japan, Russia, Australia and even South Korea and other countries, genetically engineered foods must be labeled. We may end up being the only country that does not require labeling of GE foods.

Consumer and environmental groups have demanded that the FDA follow the lead of the European Union, Japan and other nations by requiring labels on genetically modified foods so consumers know what they are buying. The U.S. government claims that such mandatory food labels are unnecessary because genetically modified food "poses no inherent safety risk." At a 2001 meeting of the FDA, consumer groups urged them to enact regulations that would require food manufacturers to list any ingredients known to trigger allergic reactions, such as peanuts, eggs and milk, on product labels, and to do so in simple language easily understandable by consumers. Often, labeling will use alternate names for these foods, such as "casein" for milk derivative or "semolina" for wheat.

In some cases, ingredients aren't on the labels at all. For example, companies that make products such as candy and cookies do not always properly disclose ingredients that cause allergic reactions, according to inspections at about eighty-five bakeries, ice cream makers and candy manufacturers. They found that about 25 percent failed to list possible ingredients that could result in allergic reactions.

For many people, eating a problem food can result in hives or rashes. For others, misunderstanding these words can be fatal. At least 150 deaths occur each year because people with food allergies ate foods they believed did not contain these ingredients. Representatives from the food industry, however, oppose strict labeling requirements, insisting that voluntary guidelines recently put in place are adequate to protect consumers.

Another issue is the increasing use of statements on labels like "may contain [particular allergen]." In one example, a box of raisins had raisins listed as the only ingredient, but the label contained a statement that the product "may contain peanuts." How can this be? It has been suggested that industry lawyers are advising companies not to test for allergens in their products and instead use "may contain" statements in order to avoid lawsuits. What are we to do if we cannot depend on the FDA and accurate labels to tell us if a product is safe to eat? If companies are deceiving us about allergens in foods, it is not hard to believe that many would also lie about genetically altered ingredients.

A recent survey by the International Food Information Council revealed that only 43 percent of the people in the U.S. even know that some of the foods they are consuming are genetically modified. One out of every four actually believes they are not eating this type of food, so be cautious of phrases such as "foods produced through biotechnology." It may sound nicer, but it is still genetically modified. Thankfully, Greenpeace has released the "True Foods Shopping List" to help frustrated shoppers. The list is a detailed report of thousands of foods made with GE ingredients. Find their list at www.OrganicConsumers.org.

What Are the USDA and the EPA Doing?

The FDA isn't the only government group under fire for its handling of the food industry and genetic engineering. The consumer watchdog group, U.S. Public Interest Research Group, recently accused the U.S. Department of Agriculture (USDA) of rubber-stamping approval of field tests of genetically engineered crops some believe could harm people and the environment: "Our environment is serving as the laboratory for widespread experimentation of genetically engineered organisms with profound risks that, once released, can never be recalled."

What about Food Allergies?

There is more and more evidence indicating that "biotech" plants may cause food allergies. Recently, a soybean modified with a gene from a Brazil nut proved allergic, but it was withdrawn before it reached the market. But are all potential allergens found before a product is found fit for human consumption? At this time, proper monitoring of these products is not enforced to identify potential allergens. Altered crops should to be held to standards at least as strict as those for food additives or pharmaceuticals, but better methods are needed to identify potential allergens.

Some more subtle allergens may be particularly difficult to determine. For instance, both the protein content and the viscosity of the starch molecules are changed whenever cereal grains are altered by genetic engineering. It has been suggested that altered grain may be less easily digested since it is more difficult for water or fluids to penetrate the inner core of the molecule, including digestive enzymes. Any food that cannot properly be digested can increase the risk of food allergies and sensitivities. These items also provide a wonderful food source for intestinal parasites and pathogenic bacteria and yeast.

Contrary to popular belief, the technology is not as precise as scientists would lead us to believe. They cannot control the location where the gene is inserted into the host's genetic code, nor can they guarantee stable expression of the gene in the new genetically engineered organism. Nevertheless, the USDA authorized nearly 29,000 field tests of genetically engineered organisms through 2000, mostly in Hawaii and Illinois. These experiments are being done in an open environment with little oversight or public notification. In fact, introducing non-native organisms into the environment is estimated to cost the United States $123 billion annually in ecosystem damage.

The report also claims that corporations and universities are becoming increasingly secretive about their genetic testing. From 1989 to 1999, the percentage of crops containing genes declared "confidential" increased nearly every year. Last year, 65 percent of the genetically engineered crops were declared confidential business information (*U.S. Public Interest Research Group "Raising Risk" Report;* June 14, 2001).

Concerns about genetically modified food became news in the United States when "StarLink" became a household word. Starlink is a genetically modified corn that was approved for animal feed, not for human consumption, yet it was discovered in a number of human food products. Aventis, the genetic engineering company that makes StarLink, was required to inform farmers that the corn produced from StarLink seeds was not approved for human consumption. However, for many months, farmers have insisted that Aventis never told them about these restrictions. As a result, corn designed for animal feed found its way onto our grocery store shelves in the form of Taco Bell taco shells and many other corn products.

Last fall, Greenpeace obtained an empty StarLink seed bag, which included a note to farmers stating that their crop could be used "for food, feed or processing." Charles Margulis, Genetic Engineering Campaigner for Greenpeace USA, was surprised to find that despite the many news articles, the EPA seemed unaware that farmers were facing this problem. Greenpeace supplied EPA officials with the StarLink bag and a stack of newspaper reports about farmers who were angry about being mislead by Aventis. For more information about StarLink, go to www.truefoodnow.org.

Exploring the Dangers of Biotech Foods

Of course, Starlink isn't the only genetically altered food that has made it into the food supply. Genetic engineering has been going on in agricultural research laboratories for over a decade, and the resulting foods reached grocery store shelves a few years ago. In fact, one of the arguments used to support biotech foods cites the fact that people have been unknowingly eating these foods for years and nothing has happened. Still, how do we know that the overwhelming increase in chronic diseases is not linked to food tampering? How do we know what the long-term effects will be?

Foreign proteins never before in the human food chain are being consumed in large amounts. For instance, the designers of the "new rice" used genes from a daffodil and a bacterium. They have also taken genes from fish and added them to strawberries to make them more tolerable to freezing. The same thing is being tried on tomatoes. It took sixty years to realize that the pesticide DDT had estrogenic activity that affected humans adversely. We are now being asked to believe that genetically modified foods are safe because people aren't dying immediately after eating them. Remember, however, that bioengineered foods were really not designed with your health in mind.

What Are Jumping Genes?

A big concern about some genetically modified crops, such as maize used as animal fodder, is that it includes a gene for antibiotic resistance. It is possible for genetically modified bacteria to transfer their antibiotic-resistance genes to other bacteria in the human gut, especially if they are from the same species. Now, once harmless bacteria have the ability to become antibiotic resistant. Since there are normally around a thousand billion gut bacteria, it seems possible and probable that many would be transformed. If some of the beneficial bacteria were killed off because of exposure to antibiotics, then the transfer rate from these antibiotic-resistant strains could increase even more.

The Toxic Side of Biotech Foods

Some researchers believe that GE foods could alter the flora of the intestines when ingested. In a 1999 issue of *The Lancet,* researchers from Aberdeen, Scotland, fed six rats potatoes that had been genetically altered to carry a gene that boosts the potatoes' resistance to attacks from worms and bugs. Ten days later, scientists found that the stomachs and intestines of these rats already had undergone widespread changes. Proponents of the research believe that this study shows the need for more research on the effects of ingested GE products. Critics say the study is flawed because too few animals were involved, making the findings insignificant.

I believe that we need to investigate the effects of GE foods on the human gastrointestinal tract, but we also need to know more about the effects of feeding biotech crops to the animals that humans eat. It is interesting that the government says that genetically altered foods sold in grocery stores are safe, but without any long-term studies how do they know this?

Moreover, how do we know that pest-resistant genes will not spread into the wild plant population and kill the harmless insect population and many other animals that depend on them to survive? There have been growing concerns, especially after researchers at Cornell University found that genetically modified corn killed the larvae of the beautiful monarch butterflies that fed on it. It also kills lacewings, which are natural predators of insect pests. Once genetically engineered bacteria and viruses are released into the environment it is impossible to contain or recall them.

Another risk of GE foods has nothing to do with genes. Monsanto, maker of the popular herbicide Roundup, also produces several genetically altered crops (including soy) designed to resist being killed by Roundup. As a result, farmers can now spray more Roundup on their crops, resulting in much higher levels of herbicide in the harvested product than before. On new leaf potatoes, farmers may use up to ten applications of chemical fertilizers and eight applications of potent fungicides, such as Bravo, in order to control fungal infection. This is what you are putting into your body when you eat red russet potatoes made into French fries in fast food franchises. In other cases, the pesticide may already be in the plant.

Are Plants Making Their Own Pesticides?

The public has been told that genetically altered plants will require fewer pesticides—now we know why. According to the journal *Nature*, one genetically engineered corn now makes its own pesticide. The toxin is supposed to kill only certain pests, but when ingested by a monarch butterfly in the caterpillar stage, it dies. The corn's toxin appears in the leaves, stock, pollen and roots, but lab tests show that the roots also discharge the poison into the soil. It was believed that soil bacteria would destroy the toxin, but investigators found that often this did not happen. In some cases, the toxin remained active for at least 234 days. Soil contamination is further perpetuated by fallen corn pollen. Plowing corn stocks into the soil contaminates it further.

How did researchers make a corn with pesticides? This new corn carries a gene that produces the active form of an insecticide made by using the bacterium, *Bacillus thuringiensis*, otherwise known as "Bt." This makes the corn toxic to pests and puts pressure on soil organisms to try to break it down. No one really knows what the consequences will be, but by using genetically engineered plants, farmers skip several pesticide sprayings at significant monetary savings.

Several groups fear future insect resistance to Bt. They are concerned that the widespread use of Bt crops will alter the environment, killing off food for certain animals and/or making insects resistant to Bt (or both). The biotech industry argues that Bt-resistant insects would most likely mate with nonresistant ones, thereby diluting any new Bt-resistant gene.

Moreover, because Bt is a pesticide, it is exempt from FDA regulation and excluded from food labels. New proteins engineered into foods are classified as "food additives," if they are not pesticides. The FDA has ruled that biotech foods labels are only needed if they contain an allergen or if they have been materially modified.

Monsanto's Canola Seed: Engineering Pesticide Resistance

If you spray Monsanto's weed killer, Roundup, onto a field, it kills everything growing there. To keep the pesticide from killing valuable crops, Monsanto has genetically engineered a canola seed so that Roundup will not harm it. That means that a farmer can spray this herbicide over an entire field, kill all the weeds growing there, and not hurt the GE canola crops. Farmers can buy the special seed, but Monsanto keeps the rights to the DNA itself.

Traditionally, farmers plant their fields using seeds saved from previous crops. They can do this year after year; however, farmers buying Monsanto's seed must sign a contract promising to buy fresh seed every year. Then, they must let Monsanto inspect their fields. Monsanto has put years of research into developing this technology and expects to recoup their investment by charging the farmer for the use of their special canola seeds.

Problems with this approach are already surfacing, however. Consider the case of Percy Schmeiser, who spent fifty years farming his land near Bruno, Saskatchewan, Canada. He has been growing this yellow-blossomed oil seed for forty years—doing his own experimenting, developing his own varieties and using his own seed. He says that he has never used Monsanto's canola seed but saves the seeds from his own crops and replants them, just like farmers have done for years. However, Monsanto investigators say that have found Monsanto DNA in Schmeiser's crops that he never paid for the right to use. They sued Schmeiser for the money they think they are owed. Now, there is a new threat to his farm, forcing him to fight for control of the seeds planted in his field.

How did the DNA get into Schmeiser's farm? It appears that the wind moved the DNA around, just like Mother Nature has been doing for thousands of years. Scientists from Agriculture Canada say that wind can blow seeds or pollen between fields, meaning the DNA of crops in one field often mix with another. Seeds or pollen can also be blown off uncovered trucks and off farm equipment. What are farmers to do? There is no way to tell regular crops from crops carrying the Monsanto DNA without testing each one. This means that even the seeds that farmers keep from their own crops may contain Monsanto's genetically altered gene. Nevertheless, Monsanto claims that Schmeiser deliberately stole their DNA.

Schmeiser defended himself against Monsanto in court saying that he is fighting back "because I believe what is happening to farmers is wrong. And I'm fighting this not just for myself, but for my children and my grandchildren, and for my farmer friends."

A Federal Court Judge in Canada ruled against Schmeiser. The judge said that no matter how Monsanto's patented DNA got into a farmer's field, whether it blows in or cross-pollinates, or comes in on farm machinery, it still belongs to Monsanto. The award figure Monsanto was seeking was $105,000, but who suffered the most damage? Not only have Schemiser's fields been contaminated and forty plus years of his own varieties of canola been destroyed, he now has to buy Monsanto's seed to prevent from being sued again. Farmer Schmeiser is still fighting back, however. He served Monsanto with his own lawsuit for more than $10 million.

Schmeiser isn't the only one accused. In fact, dozens of farmers have been accused of using Monsanto DNA illegally. Monsanto even asks farmers to call their toll-free phone line to turn in neighbors suspected of growing canola seed without paying. They also use private investigators to check crop samples for Monsanto's DNA. Court documents showed that Monsanto ordered its investigators to trespass into Schmeiser's fields and collect samples, even though Monsanto denies this.

In another Canadian case, Edward Zilinski traded seeds with a farmer from Prince Albert, an old farming tradition. Without his knowledge, the seeds he received from the farmer contained Monsanto's DNA. Now Monsanto says Zilinski and his wife owe them over $28,000 in penalties. Still another case concerned the Kram family in Raymore. They claim that planes have buzzed their fields dropping weed killer on their canola field to see if the crops had Monsanto's gene. Monsanto denies they had anything to do with this.

Herbicide-Resistant Wheat

As a result of the canola seed success, Monsanto is now about to release the first genetically engineered variety of wheat. It has been spliced with a gene that protects it from Monsanto's Roundup, allowing farmers to kill weeds without harming the wheat. The development of genetically modified wheat has taken longer because the plant is more complex, but the new wheat should soon be ready. Many foreign buyers are saying that they will not accept genetically modified wheat because of general fears about possible harm to the environment and human health, however.

Even without foreign buyers, some have speculated that the wheat's very presence on American farms could threaten the future of all U.S.

wheat sold abroad since the same thing could happen to wheat that happened to the canola in Canada—genetic drift. Half of all American wheat is now exported, accounting for $3.7 billion in sales and almost 20 percent of all agricultural commodities shipped abroad in 1999. What will happen to the farmers when contamination of this genetic material reaches other wheat farms, and they cannot sell their crops outside the United States either?

The Integrity of Monsanto

You may have noticed that Monsanto is a big name in genetic engineering, but what you may not know is that a corporation called Pharmacia owns Monsanto. (Pharmacia Corporation was created in April 2000 through the merger of Pharmacia & Upjohn with Monsanto Company and its G.D. Searly unit.) If the name Pharmacia sounds familiar, it is because they were involved in a recent scandal over the arthritis drug Celebrex. A study about the drug, which appeared in the *Journal of the American Medical Association,* apparently misrepresented the results of research on its effectiveness. It seems that all the sixteen authors of the article were either employees of the drug company, Pharmacia, Celebrex's manufacturer or paid consultants of the company. Should you trust a company with your food that publishes lies in a trusted medical journal just to make more money?

Who Is Promoting Biotech Foods?

With all the research surfacing about the dangers of genetically altered foods, it may seem surprising that anyone could support their use in our food supply. In fact, many prominent individuals are using their political muscle to promote genetically engineered food, including thirteen state governors who announced their loyalty to the industry in May 2000. What were their reasons for supporting GE crops? They were concerned that if they opposed this technology, it would hurt farmers and biotech companies. The governors in favor of biotech foods include those in North Dakota, Iowa, Missouri, Delaware, Idaho, Michigan, Nebraska, Nevada, Wisconsin, Illinois, Indiana, North Carolina and Washington. Interestingly, the states of Missouri and Delaware are home to two of the leading companies in the biotech industry, Monsanto and DuPont.

Worldwide Concern for Genetically Modified Foods

Although many influential people support the genetic engineering of crops, the use of genetically modified food is currently a subject of enormous global controversy. Arpad Pusztai, a scientist from the Rowett Research Institute in Aberdeen, UK, unwisely announced on television that experiments had shown intestinal changes in rats caused by eating genetically engineered potatoes. He said he would not eat such modified foods himself and that it was very unfair to use fellow citizens as guinea pigs. After this announcement, Pusztai was removed from his job, but it was too late. Shoppers across Europe took his announcement seriously. Within two months, seven European supermarket chains announced they would not sell genetically modified foods. Three large food multinationals followed suit. The Europeans and many other people in different parts of the world are fighting to keep genetically altered crops from entering their food chain, because many people there do not believe these foods are safe.

The plains of China may seem worlds away from technological revolution, but cotton farmers favor cutting-edge science to ensure a good harvest. Most of the cotton fields are sown with seeds genetically implanted with a bacterium that is toxic to the bollworm. With memories of famine and dwindling useable land to feed its 1.26 billion people, China has pursued genetically modified foods. Current controls on grain imports from China will change with China entering the World Trade Organization, possibly allowing these genetically altered crops to be consumed elsewhere.

In other Asia-Pacific nations, the controversy over biotech foods has increased. In India, Japan, New Zealand, Thailand and the Philippines, consumer movements are demanding controls on the use of genetically modified crops. Proponents contend that genetically altering crops to resist pests, drought or other adverse conditions, may be the only way to ensure food security in the developing world, particularly in densely populated Asia, home to more than half of humanity.

However, in Southeast Asia, only Singapore has come out strongly in favor of biotechnology, viewing it as a promising new industry. "If it is safe for the Americans, it is safe for us," says Lee Sing Kong, a member of the Singapore government. Some countries may not even have the final say about whether they produce GE crops. In the Philippines, for instance, seven out of ten farmers are landless, renting fields from landlords or working for large corporations such as Dole Foods. In these situations, big corporations can, and ultimately will, call the shots. People in some of these countries may not even be aware that animal genes—

maybe from cows or pigs—are being used in plants, creating a religious conflict for Hindus and Muslims.

The Global Arena: Presenting Evidence

As one of the many scientists presenting evidence to the Royal Commission on Genetic Engineering, Dr. Mae-Wan Ho hopes that New Zealand would assume moral and intellectual leadership in rejecting this technology that is so obviously serving the corporate agenda instead of the public good. Dr. Mae-Wan Ho is Director of the Institute of Science in Society in London. She says that it has become increasingly evident that genetically modified technology is inherently hazardous and unreliable both in agriculture and in medicine. GE crops are unstable, as noted in numerous new scientific publications. Even "Roundup Ready" soy is showing signs of breakdown: reduced yield, non-germination, and diseases and infestation by new pests. According to Dr. Ho, these dangerous genes may spread and wipe out other crops as well as wild plant species. It has become clear that GE agriculture cannot co-exist with other forms of agriculture.

Dr. Ho also believes that there is no way to prevent the spread of GE constructs to unrelated species, which can occur in all environments, including the digestive and respiratory tracts of animals. In fact, genetic modifications are designed to cross species barriers and invade genomes. Since they possess a wide combination of viral and bacterial DNA, they are much more likely to recombine with and transfer genes to all those agents. Actually, there is evidence that GE crops with viral genes are prone to give rise to recombinant viruses, including virulent strains. Dr. Ho believes that we have all the means to deliver genuine health and food security to the world without using GE technology and going against the wishes of the vast majority of people.

Genetically Modified Foods and Bacterial Overgrowth

If you are wondering what genetically modified crops have to do with the overgrowth of gut bacteria, one concern is that some of these crops, such as maize used in animal feed, include a gene for antibiotic resistance. These resistance genes are not expressed in the crops but could be incorporated into bacteria in the intestinal tract of animals and humans and create antibiotic-resistant pathogens. Some researchers say there is no such risk because the modified DNA breaks down quickly; however, a new study suggests that DNA lingers in the large intestine for several minutes.

Plants as Vaccines?

Researchers have investigated the idea of using plants as "factories" to produce and deliver vaccines, including a preventive and treatment vaccine currently in development for HIV. In fact, there have already been human trials involving plant-based delivery of a rabies vaccine, even though there are virtually no studies documenting the safety of these approaches. Isn't it bad enough that hormones, antibiotics, pesticides and other toxins are already in our food supply? Now they want to modify common healthy foods to deliver experimental, unproven vaccines. In the near future, it is entirely possible that you could ingest vaccines or even contraceptive agents without your knowledge or consent.

The foods that are being considered to deliver these vaccines are potatoes and tomatoes. One way they can do this is by developing a vaccine that can latch onto the lining of the gut without being destroyed by digestive juices. When they developed the cholera vaccine in potatoes, they took bits of the cholera toxin and joined them with proteins from two other infectious pathogens that invade the gastrointestinal tract. The thinking is that edible vaccines may be more practical, especially in developing countries. Food-based vaccines would not require syringes, medical equipment and personnel, nor would they need to be stored and transported the way ordinary vaccines must be.

Can we trust this industry to develop safe vaccines and would they tell us if there were something wrong with them? They certainly have not been up front so far about genetically altered food crops or the problems with other vaccines. If things go wrong, how will we ever be able to return to a harmless state? There should be extreme caution with this type of experimental biology. If the biotech industry's past record is any indication, we are heading for problems.

How is resistance transferred? Microbes can become genetic couriers with capabilities to store genetic information in the form of gene packets. Different capabilities can be stored and these capabilities can be shared with the community at large. When a particular capability is needed, it can be obtained from free-floating genetic material. Organisms can "borrow" resistance genes from each other via mobile snips of DNA that pass genetic information between them, even to non-related organisms. This is called "trans-kingdom genetic exchange." Genetic recombination is accelerated whenever a biological system is threatened, such as with pesticides or antibiotics. This set of events is called the "SOS Response." Medical procedures such as chemotherapy, radiation therapy and the use of pharmaceuticals, also accelerate this response.

Insecticides and the Birth of Chemical Farming

Of course, genetic engineering isn't the only danger in our food supply. Insecticides can also be hazardous to our health. The chemical farming era began in the early 1950s. Before then, farmers were still taught age-old methods that worked with nature, not against it. Pests and diseases were controlled naturally by what was known as "good husbandry." The premise was, if your soils are healthy, then your crops will be healthy. If your crops are healthy then your animals will be healthy. When you have healthy crops and animals, you have natural resistance to disease. Nature does not rely on drugs to control diseases. It relies on natural immunity. What we need to do is learn and practice "health creation" not "disease eradication" both in agriculture and in human health.

There are plans to ban certain uses of one of the most commonly used insecticides sold under the tradenames Dursban and Lorsban. The EPA say that this insecticide poses a great risk to children when used in the home. Its use in farming may also be restricted, but it will still be allowed. Farmers probably will not be permitted to spray crops such as apples once they have bloomed, but it can still be used prior to that point. In addition to being used on 75 percent of the nation's apple crop, it is also used heavily on grapes, wheat and corn crops. This is, of course, another great reason for eating only organic foods. Around the home it is used to kill termites, roaches, ants and fleas. The manufacturer of this chemical, Dow Agra-Sciences, disputes the EPA's claims of danger and maintains that the product is safe.

Synthetic Chemical Fertilizers

When you use synthetic chemical fertilizers you encourage once harmless bugs to mutate into antibiotic-resistant virulent strains. A chemically treated lawn or the playground that your children use may be a reservoir for deadly germs. More information on synthetic chemical fertilizers can be found in my book *Allergies and Holistic Healing*.

Sewer Sludge Used as Fertilizers

In 1986–87, there was an investigation into the disease-causing potential of sewage products in the island country of Bahrain in the Arabian Gulf. The dried sludge was being collected and stockpiled in the open for later use as fertilizer. Not only did researchers find pathogenic bacteria and viruses in the dried sludge samples, but also parasitic worms and protozoa.

If you think that cannot happen here, then you may be surprised to learn that New York sewer sludge ended up on Arizona farmland. It was comprised mainly of human fecal waste, domestic and industrial products, and storm water runoff. The sewage contained fecal coliform bacteria at 33.5 times the federal limit, yet some sludge stored for as little as three months is hauled away to private farms for use as fertilizer and soil conditioner.

Is It Safe for Human Consumption?

Plant crops aren't the only food supplies currently threatened. What the USDA considers safe for human consumption may surprise you. In 1998, they reclassified an array of animal diseases as being "defects" that they believe rarely or never present a direct public health risk. These defects, which include cancers, glandular swellings or lymphomas, sores, infectious arthritis, diseases caused by intestinal worms, and pneumonia, are not considered health hazards to humans and could easily be passed on to consumers. They consider these conditions aesthetic problems only, and animals with these conditions receive the government's seal of approval as food fit for humans to eat. These new, lowered food standards allow chickens with pneumonia or pus-filled meat to be considered edible.

The Agriculture Department is also proposing rules that would require federal food inspectors to monitor what the plant employees are doing, rather than inspecting each carcass individually. This means that federal inspectors would rely on scientific testing from samples of butchered meats to determine the wholesomeness of meat, rather than the traditional item-by-item scrutiny.

Delmer Jones, a federal food inspector for forty-one years who lives in Alabama, said he is so revolted by the lowering of food standards that he does not buy meat at the supermarket anymore. He does not trust that it is safe to eat: "I eat very little to no meat, but sardines and fish. When I started inspecting, inspectors were looking at thirteen birds a minute, then forty. Now it's ninety-one birds a minute with three inspectors present. You can't do your job with ninety-one birds a minute."

"They just cut off areas,'" said Carol Blake, spokeswoman for the Agriculture Department's inspection and safety system. "The production lines are moving so fast that they can't catch all the diseased carcasses, and some are ending up on supermarket shelves." If you need further convincing, consider the condemnation by former supervisor of U.S. Poultry inspection, Rodney Leonard: "I don't eat chicken anymore. I won't eat it. I won't allow it in my house." Who would want to have a diseased piece of meat on their dinner table, even if they couldn't catch the disease? It is very sad that our food is getting so unhealthy when so many of us are trying to improve our health.

Because consumers will not buy visibly defective products, such products will probably be sold to manufacturers, grinders or others who process or disguise the food. It will get harder to detect which foods contain these unwholesome products. Some government veterinarians have voiced their objection to the current food safety rules. They feel that there may be a threat to public health because untrained, uncertified and inexperienced company employees are expected to distinguish between localized conditions, which can be trimmed off, and systemic diseases, which could pose public health concerns. Previously, trained inspectors did the examinations, but under the new system, trained inspectors with scientific expertise are no longer required. If you are a meat eater, then this is just one more reason to eat certified organic meat. They must meet very high standards, and I for one, am very glad of this.

A recent preliminary survey of beef and poultry sold in U.S. supermarkets conducted by the FDA has found relatively high levels of antibiotic-resistant bacteria. Surveyers found *Enterococcus* strains in meat bought at several Washington, DC-area supermarkets, and the bacteria contained "fairly substantial amounts of resistance to a number of drugs," FDA microbiologist Dr. David Wagner said. *Enterococcus* strains were found in 67 percent of the chicken samples, 34 percent of the turkey samples and 66 percent of beef samples. The researchers also tested for resistance to twenty-nine different types of antibiotics, including six commonly used in animal feed. Strains of *Enterococci* taken from either chicken or turkey tended to be much more resistant to the antibiotics compared with strains taken from beef, the researchers concluded. The study sample was relatively small, but the findings suggest that our food supply is now generally contaminated with bacteria that are going to be harder to kill.

What's in the Chicken?

Even as far back as 1991, the *Atlanta Constitution* reported that the poultry industry was selling feces-contaminated and disease-containing meat. Out of eighty-four federal poultry inspectors interviewed in the report, eighty-one admitted to allowing thousands of contaminated birds to be rinsed off and sold. Any visible signs of disease are just cut off. In fact, one inspector said that they salvage practically every bird and that he avoids buying precut chicken parts. Diseased meat is often salvaged as breast fillets or buffalo wings.

In the past, inspectors would condemn any bird that had yellow fluids and mucus in the lungs. Yet in an 1989 article in *Southern Exposure*, a USDA inspector in Arkansas said that he was forced to approve approximately 40 percent of birds that would have been condemned ten years earlier. Another Arkansas plant inspector compared grocery store chicken to chicken dropped into a fresh manure pile. This is what we can expect from some chicken processing plants today.

The machines used to remove intestines from the carcasses move at such a fast speed that they rip the intestines open, spilling feces all over the body cavity. Feces and dirt are then pounded into the skin of the chicken by machines that are supposed to pluck feathers (but actually pound them off). Then they bathe thousands of dirty chickens together in a chill tank, creating a "fecal soup" that spreads contamination from bird to bird. Consumers end up paying for this in more ways that one when they buy chicken, since up to 15 percent of poultry weight consists of this fecal soup.

As a result of these lapses in safety, *Salmonella* contamination in chicken has steadily increased and may now be at 60 percent. The USDA released a study in 1988 saying that washing does not adequately remove *Salmonella* germs left behind by fecal contamination, even after forty consecutive rinses. The crowding and the stress on chickens also increase the risk. Beside *Salmonella*, chickens today also have a lot of health problems because they are forced to grow so fast.

Chicken safety has also been compromised in other ways. An issue of *The Touchstone* published an article describing the disregard for plant worker's health and hygiene. This is not a surprise. A system that disregards the health of its product would likely disregard the health of its workers. Some even described the work as modern slavery. Employees are not always allowed to leave the production line to go to the bathroom, so sometimes they urinate on the floor. According to inspectors at one Southern poultry plant, the management would not stop the production line even after a person vomited on it. Some poultry plants use chlorine to wash chickens in order to kill the germs—up to 70 percent chlorine. The heavy fumes from the solutions caused workers' eyes to water and their skin to peel from their hands, as well as lung problems, chronic headaches and sore throats.

School children in thirty-one states are being fed chicken nuggets made from diseased poultry, according to a 2000 report in the *American-Statesman*. Inspectors defended their actions by saying that the chicken nuggets would not hurt anyone since humans do not get poultry diseases. They did, however, admit that the food is not wholesome. Inspectors said the acceptable birds can even have pockets of jelly-like pus in various parts of the body (or covering virtually the entire cavity). "The skin's got sores and bruises and things on it," said Ellen Dingler, a federal food inspector. "They mix the skin with the meat and call it binder. It's been really terrible. This is the worst that I've ever seen."

What does the government think about these industry practices? John McCutcheon, who oversees the U.S. Agriculture Department's food-safety inspectors, said the government does not want diseased poultry going to consumers. He acknowledged that his agency approves a plant's product even though half the carcasses may have sores, scabs or some kind of infection, but he said that even with "100 percent inspection" diseased birds would still slip through.

At the same time, McCutcheon faulted any inspector who sees diseased poultry and does not condemn it. "When you know a carcass has a condition on it that shouldn't go into commerce, we expect our inspectors to act immediately," he said. Some inspectors are cynical and complain that the agency is speaking out of both sides of its mouth. On one hand, it is saying that regulations are still in place and diseased poultry ought to be thrown away. One the other hand, the agency believes that if diseased meat does go to the consumer, it will not hurt them if they just cook it properly.

In Texas alone, 172 public school districts, plus scores of other private and charter schools, get chicken from two Gold Kist plants in Alabama. The food comes from the U.S. Department of Agriculture's commodities program. The commodities program is a big part of the food service in school districts. The USDA buys the chicken, then the states and schools decide how to serve it, either as whole pieces or processed into chicken patties or nuggets. They try to choose forms they think will be kid friendly, such as nuggets. After learning that chicken skins were being processed into some of these chicken products as binders, several school districts contacted by the *American-Statesman* expressed concern. However, they said they would await more information from USDA or other officials before taking any action. Preston Ingram, a business manager involved in this situation said, "It may not be the most nutritious form, but it's in a form they'll eat. I don't know how we'd function if we stopped taking commodities. If we had to pay for everything, the meal prices would be substantially higher. The use of scabby chicken skins is certainly a cause of concern for school officials so why did the federal government ship us that chicken?"

Inspectors blame the conditions at the two Alabama plants on an experimental federal food-surveillance program that turns over poultry inspection to the company. "Inspectors are frustrated over what they are seeing," said Stan Painter, president of Local 2357 of the National Joint Council of Food Inspectors, whose Local represents government inspectors at the plants. "They are frustrated over what is going on, and they are frustrated that they cannot do anything. Every minute of the day, diseased products are going down the line [at plants where companies do their own inspections]." It is estimated that the amount of diseased products leaving the plant has increased by 50 percent because of the experimental program. To give you some idea of the products that make it through, consider the experimental inspection regulations which say that that an inspector can find sores on 52 percent of the birds, and the company still will pass inspection. Plus, if the company fails the inspection, nothing happens.

Tainted Eggs

Eggs are another safety concern. Over three million eggs each year are infected with *Salmonella* bacteria, causing thousands of cases of illness. The first contamination happens at the farm; the second happens at the packing plant. It is believed to be the cause of more than 800,000 cases of food poisoning every year. For years, food safety experts have warned us about the threat of foodborne illness caused by this organism. *Salmonella* is a worldwide problem, but it is most extensively reported in North America and Europe, with cases on the rise each year. Food poisoning from this organism may occur in small, localized outbreaks in the general population. It also occurs in large outbreaks in hospitals, restaurants, or institutions for children or the elderly. *Salmonella* is caused most often by drinking unpasteurized milk, eating undercooked poultry, and contaminated poultry products. Any food prepared on surfaces contaminated by raw chicken or turkey can become tainted. Less often, the illness may stem from food contaminated by a food worker.

What's in the Beef?

Poultry products aren't the only risky foods. A high percentage of the ground meat sold in supermarkets may contain toxin-producing bacteria that industry-screening methods do not adequately detect. In the *Journal of Food Protection*, it was reported that a quarter of the beef purchased at grocery stores in Boston and Cincinnati contained *E. coli* bacteria. (Although not all toxin-producing bacteria are hazardous to humans, some strains of *E. coli* can make people ill if they eat food that has not been handled or cooked properly.) Back in 1994, these bacteria occurred only in one out of every 2,000 carcasses at the slaughter plant, but some experts now think that half of all U.S. cattle may contain this bacterium.

According to one Agricultural Research Service study, during the summer peak season, 28 percent of live cattle entering the processing plants were actively shedding the potentially dangerous *E. coli* 0157:H7 in their feces. They also found that 43 percent of 341 carcasses were initially contaminated with the bacterium. Eleven percent of hide surfaces were also contaminated. This was higher than expected. Research also showed that processing plants could take measures to reduce the incidence of *E. coli* 0157:H7 on beef carcasses to less than 2 percent if good hygiene practices are incorporated. It doesn't help that feedlot cattle are typically fattened in a confined area just before going to slaughter. One of the ways that animals spread *E. coli* 0157:H7 is by defecating and drooling in shared water troughs.

Among cattle, *E. coli* 0157:H7 lives harmlessly in their digestive tract. The bacteria migrate when animals are slaughtered and skinned, moving from internal organs and hides in the flesh. It only takes a small dose of *E. coli* 0157:H7 bacteria and the right conditions to cause illness in humans. Symptoms include low-grade fever, bloody diarrhea, dehydration and even kidney failure. Most people recover on their own in about a week, but young children and the elderly are at a higher risk for more severe problems.

In 1993, the largest known beef-related *E. coli* outbreak occurred at Jack-in-the-Box restaurants in four Western states. More than 700 people became ill and four children died after eating hamburgers there. In fact, it is estimated that *E. coli* is responsible for thousands of illnesses and 250 deaths a year in the United States alone. At present, most outbreaks have involved *E. coli* 0157:H7; however, another strain has also developed the ability to produce dangerous toxins. Routine lab tests do not detect these new varieties, so consumers need to protect themselves by adopting food safety habits to use with any potentially bacteria-contaminated food.

Feeding Cows Grain and Bacterial Resistance

Most farmers feed their cattle grain, rather than less fattening hay. Cattle that are fed grain are estimated to have 300 times as much *E. coli* in their feces as cows fed hay. In a typical commercial beef production, steers are fed a 90–100 percent grain diet for several weeks in feedlots prior to slaughter so that tender, tasty fat marbling is added to the muscle. However, these ruminant animals are designed to consume and digest huge amounts of grass, not grains. That is why they have four stomachs. When you feed cows mostly grain, it creates an acid stomach, making the cattle prone to ulcers. Bacteria migrate through the ulcers and infect the liver, where they cause abscesses. Antibiotics then become necessary to treat these abscesses. These bacteria are also much more likely to withstand stomach acid. This is significant because stomach acid is a natural barrier that usually kills foodborne pathogens that might try to enter our digestive tract. Many people also take antacids, further decreasing the protection stomach acid provides.

Why would grain-fed cattle be more likely to have acid-resistant bacteria? Cattle produce only small quantities of enzyme that breaks down starch. Large quantities of starchy grain pass into the cow's intestines undigested, and then ferment. Bacteria raised in this acidic environment can become acid-resistant and then survive and multiply. If later they find their way into a human's stomach, they can survive there as well. Switching cattle from a grain diet to a hay diet quickly changes the intestinal environment and eliminates acid-resistant *E. coli* in their digestive tract within five days.

Recent research suggests that feeding cattle less grain and more grass would solve much of the need for antibiotics. Diets of starchy, high calorie grains trigger a condition favorable to the growth of the pathogen *E. coli*, which must be treated with antibiotics and other drugs. The overabundance of antibiotics given to these animals leads to antibiotic-resistant pathogens that causes disease in humans and resist traditional antibiotic therapies.

Antibiotic resistance microbes can spread easily to humans through the food chain. For example, a multi-drug-resistant strain of *Salmonella* found in hamburger meat was recently traced to a farm that used antibiotics in its cattle feed. The more people that buy and eat these antibiotic-fortified foods the more opportunity there is to develop bacteria resistance.

Another solution used to counteract the cattle's acidic stomachs is to give them bicarbonate of soda or lime. I think we call these substances antacids. Even this is not enough to compensate for the increase in infections that the cattle now have. It is estimated that half of all the antibiotics produced in this country go to cattle. Finding the healthier grass-fed beef at any commercial store is rare.

Yet much of the bacterial problem could be corrected by including beneficial forms of bacteria and yeast in animal feed instead of antibiotics. In one study, the probiotic yeast *Saccharymyces boulardii* was first added to the feed of half of a test group of chickens. Then all the chickens were inoculated with *Salmonella*. Usually *Salmonella* is in the intestines of most commercially grown chickens, but only 5 percent of chickens who ate feed containing probiotics tested positive for *Salmonella*.

New Agriculture Inspection System Actually Worse

In the 1950s we condemned carcasses with fecal contamination, in the 1970s disease and contamination was cut off of carcasses, in the 1980s it was washed off and now it is eaten. Yet instead of improving the old system, a new meat and poultry inspection system is being launched at some slaughterhouses that may pose further dangers to the public. The Department of Agriculture has started a company self-inspection program that will allow employees to be the inspectors instead of using trained and licensed federal inspectors. This system has never been tested before, but two pork plants and one chicken broiler plant will begin selling products inspected under the new system to the public with no warning labels. The pork plants are Hatfield Quality Meats, Inc. in Hatfield, Pennsylvania, and Quality Pork Producers, in Austin, Minnesota. The broiler plant is Goldkist, Inc. in Guntersville, Alabama.

It is unclear whether this new system will even ensure the same level of quality and safety as delivered by the previous, heavily flawed system. Delmer Jones, Chairman of the meat inspectors #146 union said of the new plan, "We will be vulnerable to more deaths and illnesses and no one seems to care." Under the new system, company employees will perform public health tasks formerly performed by federal inspectors. There will be no training requirements for company employees who will take over these tasks. Plus, unlike federal inspectors, company employees can be fired at will for stopping or slowing the line to prevent the release of dangerous product, or blowing the whistle on unsafe practices.

Moreover, public health standards have been reduced for some conditions, including pre-fecal contamination, feathers and organ remnants including lungs. Out of over 40,000 birds per line per shift, only sixty will be rechecked by government inspectors for food safety or aesthetic problems, such as sores, scabs, blisters, bruises and organ remnants. The rest will be shipped directly to consumers after receiving only a company examination. Tom Devine, Legal Director of the Government Accountability Project, said that the new standards are a fraud on American consumers. Unfortunately, the Department is not willing to equip inspectors to protect the health of the American people.

What can consumers do? According to Felicia Nestor, consumers should protest by avoiding poultry and pork unless consumer safeguards are substantially improved. There is no basis for American consumers to trust an industry honor system for meat and poultry inspection.

Congress plans to spend more for national defense abroad, but what about defending the American people at home? Without federal inspectors present, plants may further reduce the health of our food. The following list are just a few examples of conditions reported by whistle blowing inspectors since 1995 found in USDA records. If you have a weak stomach, it may be best to skip this part:

- Filth accumulates on equipment and plant floors, including human and animal excrement, blood, oil, grease, machine parts, glass, plastic, wood chips, rust, paint, cement, dust, insecticides, insects and their eggs, maggots and rodent droppings.
- Water and plumbing sources malfunction, and condensation accumulates, often spilling water onto the plant floor from backed up sink or floor drains; broken hoses or their nozzles; clogged toilets; or condensation dripping from coolers or dirty pipes overhead. This water mixes with the previously mentioned contaminants on the floor to create filthy soup.
- Plants fail to honor pre-operational building sanitation requirements, resulting in an accumulation of mold and bacteria-ridden residues on coolers, walls, floors and equipment that comes in direct contact with meat products. Company inspectors, who are required by law to check the plant for sanitation before production begins, repeatedly fail to have surfaces cleaned which are encrusted with potentially deadly residues like fat, blood, charcoal and fecal matter.
- Facilities violate pre-operational sanitation rules for their production equipment, such as knives, scabbards or clipboards, which the law requires to be kept sanitary at all times. Plant management fails to check that employee equipment is maintained, including items such as rubber belts, rubber aprons, mesh gloves and leather belly guards. These items can foster bacterial growth that can potentially leak into food products.
- Facilities carelessly hose down equipment, ceilings, walls or floors, and splash filthy water onto food products or the surfaces they come in contact with. Meat plants also fail to maintain sanitizing water tem-

peratures (180 degrees), and poultry plants often fail to maintain required chlorine levels (20 parts per million). As a result, rather than killing bacteria, the water spreads it over a larger area.

- Sometimes food product falls into this pathogenic soup on the floor and are returned to the line without being rinsed, affecting literally hundreds of pounds of meat that pile up on the floor.

- Flies and other insects gain easy access to meat products through large open doors. Maggots and other larvae breed in storage and transport tubs and boxes, on the floor, and in processing equipment and packaging.

- Needed repairs of employee bathrooms are often delayed until most toilets are unusable. Toilets back up and leak onto the floor. Employees must wade through sewage to use the toilet, and then they track the filth out onto the plant floor. Bathroom soap and towel supplies often run out. However, supervisors have instructed inspectors not to report conditions in employee bathrooms, because to do so would harass management.

- Abscesses and digestive organs are punctured during slaughter, releasing pus and fecal material over carcasses, onto conveyers, workers and the floor. Because these substances may contain dangerous bacteria, the law requires that affected meat and poultry be trimmed rather than rinsed. Plants repeatedly skip trimming and merely rinse the meat, which can force bacteria into the porous flesh. Up to 25 percent of slaughtered chickens on the inspection line are covered with feces and bile.

- Employees also fail to sanitize their equipment or hands, as required by law, after incidents of pus or fecal material contamination. As a result, employees become sources of cross-contamination.

- Facilities fail to trim abscesses from meat and allow them to be processed. Plant employees also miss hide, hair, ear canals and teeth in products approved by the facility. By failing to discover these defects, company inspectors who are required to check samples approve up to four times more product for consumer use.

- Red meat animals and poultry that are dead on arrival or die in the yard while awaiting slaughter are hidden from inspectors doing antemortem inspections and hung up to be butchered. Severed heads from cattle with eye cancer are switched to smaller carcasses so less meat will be condemned.

- Rancid, outdated and contaminated meat is often accepted for further processing or packaged for shipment. For example, in one enforcement action at a single facility, inspectors retained six tons of ground pork with rust, which was bound for a school lunch program in Indiana. There was also 14,000 pounds of chicken speckled with metal flakes and 5,000 pounds of rancid chicken necks. Seven hundred and twenty-one pounds of green chicken so spoiled that employees gagged from the smell was also confiscated. In fact, rancid meat is typically smoked to cover foul odor, or marinated and breaded to disguise slime and smell.

- Meat not stored at legally required temperatures (to prevent rapid bacteria growth) or obviously sour products are added to acceptable meat and then processed together.
- Chickens and hams are soaked in chlorine baths to remove slime and odor, and red dye is added to beef to make it appear fresh.
- Facilities repeatedly fail to respect personal hygiene rules such as adequate bathroom breaks. Consequences include reports of employee failure to wash hands, urination in carcass coolers or on the floor while working the line, and incidents of toilet paper covered with human feces on the bathroom floor.
- Plants repeatedly fail to adequately enforce the rule requiring employees to change uniforms and wash their hands when they switch from working with raw product to working with ready-to-eat product. Consequences include ready-to-eat food coming into contact with filth such as blood, meat scraps and germs that encrust the coats employees use while working with raw product. Employees also fail to wash their hands after working with unsanitary product or equipment.
- Sadly, employees may be fired for alerting inspectors about violations in the plants. Company inspectors are pressured to ignore defects.

For more information on reporting of unsafe practices in the food industry, go to this website: http://www.whistleblower.org/index.htm

What Can Be Done about Contaminated or Infested Foods?

At a government-sponsored conference on food safety, federal officials said that improving farming practices was the most promising way to prevent foodborne illnesses. This area gets the least amount of attention but is the most important way to improve food safety. But will cost-conscious farmers change farming practices unless the government forces them to do so? What options does the government have since the USDA doesn't have the authority to regulate how farmers raise their animals? Regardless of the ways in which farmers are encouraged to improve agricultural safety, most of these suggestions can be implemented at low cost, on a small scale (which probably makes more economic sense than the medium to large scale facilities required for irradiation to be cost effective):

- Do not contaminate food in the first place. Prevention is always the best method, and this can be achieved by keeping facilities clean and culling out infested fruits and vegetables.
- High pressure technology harnesses the natural and low-heat power of hydrostatic pressure to destroy pathogens such as *Salmonella, Listeria* and *E. coli* while maintaining the food's nutritional value, taste and color. Manufacturers of juices, sauces, meats and seafood are currently using this technology in the United States and abroad, which could replace traditional food safety systems such as pasteurization, irradiation or chemicals.
- Sulphur dioxide gas fumigation has been successful in reducing bacteria during preliminary trails. Within a few days the residue from the gas was negligible. This may be an option for some spices.
- Food extracts including vanilla, cinnamon, pepper and almond contain compounds that inhibit the growth of bacteria. For instance, cinnamon is a lethal weapon against *E. coli* in unpasteurized juice. Using these extracts in food safety is currently under investigation at the U.S. Department of Agriculture.
- The use of low concentrations of ozone for fresh juices is also under development.
- Cold treatments may also be used to kill pathogens by decreasing the temperature of the fruit or vegetable for short periods of time. Fruits may also be treated with bursts of hot forced air.
- By creating an atmosphere in shipping containers where CO_2 or nitrogen is kept high and oxygen is kept low, pathogens may also be killed.

What Is Food Irradiation?

Irradiated food is briefly exposed to ionizing radiation to kill microorganisms. The USDA has approved the use of three different irradiation technologies. The first uses gamma rays generated by a radioactive substance (such as cobalt 60 or cesium 137) and is routinely used to sterilize medical, dental and household goods. The second type shoots electron beams from an electron gun. The third and newest approach uses powerful X-rays. The FDA's approved meat radiation dosage of 450,000 rads is approximately 150 million times greater than that of a chest X-ray.

Despite the potential dangers, supporters of irradiation argue that it has been used for twenty years to sterilize commercial products such as

Food Sanitation Solutions: Current Testing

- About 98 percent of juices in the United States are now heat pasteurized, but carbon dioxide can kill bacteria without altering flavor. In tests, pressurized liquid carbon dioxide was added to room-temperature fruit tainted with *E. coli* or another pathogenic bacteria. After ten minutes, the mixture was decompressed (the carbon dioxide reverted to a gas and escaped), leaving behind a fizz-free juice without any bacteria.
- To make meat stay red longer, antioxidants have been added to the plastic wrapping, adding at least a couple of days to the normal shelf life. (Steaks typically turn brown before their germ count is high enough to be considered spoiled, however.)
- Pigs and cows are being fed sodium chlorate to reduce *Salmonella typhimurium* and *E. coli* O157:H7. Sodium chlorate, fed in low doses before slaughter, selectively kills these pathogens. Besides adding the chlorate to feed, the researchers suggest adding chlorate to drinking water for the animals upon arrival at the processing facility.
- A new antimicrobial spray is being tested on meat carcasses during processing to reduce microbial contamination. The product called Inspexx 200 is applied to each carcass at various processing points to reduce microbial, particularly pathogenic bacteria, contamination such as *E. coli*, *Salmonella and Listeria*. Inspexx 200 is unique in that it can be applied at concentration levels one hundred times lower than other treatments currently available.
- The FDA amended food additive regulations to provide for the safe use of a mixture of peroxyacetic acid, octanoic acid, acetic acid, hydrogen peroxide, peroxyoctanoic acid and ethylidene-1,1-diphosphonic acid as an antimicrobial agent on red meat carcasses.
- A proprietary *E. coli* inhibitor in the cow's gut is being tested by Nymox Pharmaceutical.
- Researchers are also working on portable prototype biosensors to detect and quantify bacteria.
- Research is under way on vaccines that would prevent cattle from carrying dangerous bacteria, as well as feed additives that would help eliminate it from infected animals and new methods of composting manure so it can be used as fertilizer without contaminating crops or ground water.

- U.S. poultry companies are testing various food safety measures, including treating drinking water with chlorine, hydrogen peroxide or ozone; litter (bedding) treatment; and hatchery disinfection.
- Essential oils such as carvacrol and thymol, available from common herbal plants, are being looked into to block the formation of foul-smelling volatile fatty acids in manure as well as reduce levels of E. coli and other potentially harmful bacteria.
- Ozonation uses water infused with ozone molecules to reduce/eliminate bacterial contamination. Ozone is an unstable three-atom form of oxygen. This atom is highly reactive, and it can burst the cell wall of a bacterium rapidly. For this reason, it is considered a better disinfectant than chlorine, a tried-and-true microbe killer that's used throughout the food industry. The Food and Drug Administration has put ozone in their "generally recognized as safe" category. Treatment with ozone-bearing water kills upwards of 90 percent of pathogens on surfaces.
- Steam pasteurization uses a burst of superheated steam for less than one second and effectively pasteurizes the exterior of the carcass just before it enters the cooler. Steam and hot water vacuums remove visible dirt or debris aseptically, replacing the previous practice of trimming off contaminated flesh.
- Research is under way on a variety of promising approaches, including pulsed energy, bright light, high pressure and other nonthermal technologies, but few are ready for immediate application.
- An Arkansas researcher has proposed that cetylpyridinium chloride, the active ingredient in some mouthwashes, may be used to clean pathogens from chicken carcasses and will soon be tested. The antimicrobial also kills Campylobacter and Listeria, and extends product shelf life by two to three days. It is anticipated that this substance will be used on fully cooked, ready-to-eat products because it kills Listeria.
- Lactoferrin, a milk protein, starves E. coli and other microbes. During a recent study, lactoferrin reduced E. coli O157:H7 and kept it from affixing itself to the surface of a meat sample when applied to raw meat surfaces. Laboratory results indicate the activated form of lactoferrin is effective against more than thirty different kinds of harmful bacteria, including E. coli O157:H7,

Salmonella and *Campylobacter*. The technique is reportedly inexpensive and could be used during slaughter, processing and packaging stages.

• Cold plasma technology may be able to prevent bacterial formation on the surfaces of food-industry materials, such as processing machines, preparation surfaces and packaging. Food pathogens can thrive in the nooks and crannies of food preparation implements, escaping even the most thorough cleaning. This technique changes the surface of materials to incorporate antimicrobial agents in extremely thin layers. It also provides a protective film over the surface so that bacteria are incapable of forming colonies on the surface.

Q-tips, baby pacifiers, bottles and feminine hygiene supplies. The technology is also used by commercial irradiators in the U.S. for sterilizing sutures, syringes, intravenous lines and other medical supplies. It is also used on billions of dollars worth of consumer goods, ranging from plastic wrap and milk cartons to contact lenses.

Is Irradiation a Cause for Concern?

Some critics, including consumer activist groups, charge that irradiation creates new and potentially hazardous dangers in foods. There is no requirement for the FDA to do human research for radiation-treated food, and we do not know what the long-term effects of irradiation are. Despite this, irradiation has been endorsed by numerous international and national health organizations, including the World Health Organization, the Food and Agricultural Organization of the United Nations, the American Dietetic Association and the American Medical Association. Such endorsements may bring a false sense of security that irradiated meat is safe to eat. However, in one animal study, mice and rats had a greater incidence of kidney disease after eating irradiated food. Another study found testicular damage in rats fed irradiated food. Moreover, malnourished children in India who ate irradiated wheat more often developed an increase in abnormal white blood cells.

Anti-irradiation activist Michael Colby of *Food & Water* says, "Irradiation is going to allow all the root causes of a contaminated food supply to flourish. This is inevitably going to lead to sloppier handling in the meat-processing facilities. Consumers also may feel a false sense of security from irradiation. There are people out there who say they can't wait until we get irradiation because they love rare burgers and steak tartar." In addition to fears that irradiation will simply cover up sloppy slaughterhouse procedures, there is concern that meat plants will irradiate, rather than dispose of heavily contaminated meat. This means that we will be served food that still contains the organisms that caused the food to spoil in the first place. Even with pathogens dead, the dangerous toxins they produced remain in the meat.

Furthermore, some scientists worry that irradiation will destroy the beneficial and harmless bacteria that compete for survival with the bad pathogens. If an illness-causing organism does make its way onto an irradiated food in a consumer's kitchen, it might multiply at a faster rate than it would if its competitors were still around. What should consumers do to improve the safety of the food production process? First, they should become knowledgeable about how to handle and prepare foods themselves. Second, they should encourage the food industry to do the same.

How Does Irradiation Change Food?

Irradiation changes the chemical makeup of food, prompting the formation of radiolytic compounds. Supporters of irradiation tell us that these compounds are inconsequential, but is this true? Even so, the irradiation process also changes the structure of protein, making it a far less healthy food. Irradiation also negatively affects nutrients in food. It leads to some loss of certain vitamins, particularly A, C, E and B vitamins (especially niacin and thiamin). Despite this, the FDA says that the nutritional content of irradiated foods is not altered and no harmful toxins are added. Of course, they said the same thing about pasteurized milk even though pasteurization is believed to contribute to making milk today's number one allergy-related food.

Even as far back as 1970, studies by India's National Institute of Nutrition reported that feeding freshly radiated wheat to monkeys, rats, mice and to a small group of malnourished children induced gross chromosomal abnormalities in blood or bone marrow cells and mutational damage in the rodents. Food irradiation results in major micronutrient losses. The USDA even admits that these losses are synergistically increased by cooking, resulting in empty-calorie food. This should be a major concern to us.

Irradiated meat also has higher levels of reactive free radicals and peroxides from unsaturated fats. As far back as 1977, the U.S. Army revealed major differences between volatile chemicals formed during irradiation. Levels of the carcinogen benzene in irradiated beef were ten times higher than in cooked beef. Other chemical products, which had been classified as carcinogens or carcinogenic under certain conditions, were also identified in irradiated meat.

Based on these findings, in 1980, the FDA advised that testing be done on concentrated extracts of irradiated foods, rather than on whole foods, to be sure that these chemicals could be adequately tested for safety. Until this is done, there is little scientific basis for accepting this industry's assurances of safety. Yet in an editorial comment, the FDA admitted that it is nearly impossible to detect and test these products with current techniques.

Instead of requiring standard toxicological and carcinogenic testing of by-products of irradiation, the FDA relies on studies published prior to the 1980s, which claim that irradiation is safe. Even the chair of FDA's Irradiated Food Task Committee insisted that none of the studies they use are adequate by today's standards. In fact, detailed analysis of these studies revealed that all were flawed, and a wide range of independent studies prior to 1986 identify mutagenic and carcinogenic products in irradiated food.

Who Is Promoting Irradiation Practices?

Most large companies have resisted irradiation because of opposition from activists and because they believe consumers will not buy irradiated food. However, the food and nuclear industries, with strong government support, have capitalized on recent outbreaks of pathogenic *E.coli* meat poisoning to mobilize public acceptance of large-scale food irradiation. It is easier and more profitable to sell the idea of irradiating our food products instead of using better hygiene practices so that our food is not contaminated with fecal matter in the first place. Already, the FDA is allowing the use of high-level radiation to treat vegetables, beef, pork, poultry, eggs, spices, fruit and flour. The USDA has also proposed that imported fruits and vegetables also undergo irradiation.

Additionally, the Department of Energy (DOE) continues its aggressive promotion of food irradiation as a way of reducing disposal costs of spent military and civilian nuclear fuel by providing a commercial market for cesium nuclear wastes. The DOE ignores the fact that irradiation facilities using pelletized isotopes pose risks of nuclear accidents to communities nationwide from the hundreds of facilities that would be built for the potentially enormous radiation market. Opponents of irradiation are concerned that these facilities would be minimally regulated and unsecured. They would also need regular replenishment of cobalt 60 or cesium 137 isotopes, thereby increasing nationwide transportation hazards.

The former DOE Senior Policy Advisor, Robert Alvarez, warned that the Nuclear Regulatory Commission files are bulging with unreported documents on radioactive spills, worker over-exposure and off-site radiation leakage. Furthermore, the EPA still does not require an Environmental Impact Statement prior to the use of food irradiation facilities.

Irradiated Foods in the Marketplace

Irradiated meat may already be showing up in supermarkets since new rules allowing the irradiation of raw beef, pork and lamb took effect in February 2000. Most meatpackers intend to start small, testing irradiated ground beef in select markets to see how it sells. Many are not sure how consumers will respond. Food companies and supermarkets that have tried to sell irradiated fruits and vegetables over the years have faced picket lines and threats of boycotts.

Some irradiated meats, such as sausages and bologna, must be labeled; however, the labeling requirements do not apply to meat bought through food service operations, such as restaurants, school cafeterias, or hospitals. Because of this, fast-food restaurants are expected to be major purchasers of irradiated meat.

Irradiation has long been allowed for poultry, as well as fruits, vegetables and spices. It is seldom used on poultry, however, partly because the primary poultry pathogens are not as dangerous as the *E. coli* that favors meat. Also, chicken processors do not think it is worth the expense. On the other hand, one big recall for *E. coli* could devastate a meatpacker financially.

Identifying Irradiated Foods

Originally, the "Radura" symbol, which looks like a flower surrounded by a broken circle, was proposed for labeling irradiated foods in the supermarket. Then it was proposed that the FDA sanitize it's already weakened labeling requirements for irradiated food by eliminating the word "irradiated" in favor of an "electronic pasteurization" label. This term was proposed by the San Diego based Titan corporation, a major defense contractor using the costly linear accelerator "E-beam" technology (originally designed for President Reagan's "Star Wars" program).

Due to powerful industry interests, Congress is considering putting yet another spin on the name used for the process of food irradiation by calling it "cold pasteurization."

SureBeam and other companies are attempting to make irradiation more acceptable to consumers by using the word "pasteurization" in the label because they want people to think that they are providing pasteurization services. This change in terms would be misleading because pasteurization and irradiation are very different processes. Pasteurization is a heat process that kills microorganisms while irradiation is an ionizing radiation process that utilizes a type of linear accelerator, which fires electrons nearly at the speed of light, killing microorganisms by disrupting their DNA.

Now, when you see the wording "electronically or cold pasteurized" you will know what it means and not be mislead. Consumers have a fundamental right to know what is in their food and how it has been treated. This label "softening" only serves to trick people, not to inform them. Rather than trying to fool the public in response to special interest groups, it would be better to focus on improving the sanitation of our nation's food supply.

What Are the Alternatives?

Researchers at California State Polytechnic University at Pomona and the giant packing company, Farmland National Beef Packing Company, say they have come up with a natural way to neutralize dangerous microbes in meat products. They have developed a spray using activated lactoferrin (a protein derived from cow's milk) that detaches the contaminants from meat, thereby preventing the bacteria from binding to iron. This method starves the bacteria so that they cannot reproduce. They claim that lactoferrin offers key advantages to ward off bacterial contamination for forty-five days or more. If this proves true, treated meat will remain safe long after it is bought or opened, meaning that it provides much better protection than irradiation. The protection irradiation provides ends when a package is opened. The spray works against *E. coli, Salmonella* and ten different radiation-resistant bacteria. Food-safety advocates and industry insiders are intrigued, but testing is still in the early stages. This technology may be used on the market in the coming years, however.

Another alternative is being tested at Kansas State University. Researchers there are testing a new steam-based pasteurization system that they say can wipe out deadly bacteria in ready-to-eat meats. The process uses condensed steam to sterilize already fully packaged and

Irradiated Foods: Just How Risky?

The debate over food irradiation would not be complete without an understanding of the risks associated with the technology itself. Supporters of food irradiation often say that irradiation facilities are safe and that the public is not in danger. The record says otherwise. Since the 1960s, dozens of accidents and numerous episodes of wrongdoings have been reported. Radioactive water has been flushed down toilets into the public sewer system; radioactive waste has been thrown into the garbage; facilities have caught fire; equipment has malfunctioned; and workers have been injured or killed. As if radiation leaks aren't bad enough, there have also been charges of fraud and cover-ups by company executives. How can we trust that this technology is safe when involved parties can't even police themselves adequately?

A proposed international food irradiation standard winding its way through legal channels in Europe could further jeopardize the quality and safety of food sold to United States consumers. Under an international plan endorsed in 2001, virtually every assurance that irradiated food will be of good quality, be handled by trained workers, and be processed under safe and clean conditions in government-inspected facilities would disappear. The proposal would also remove the international irradiation dosage limit. Yet the proposal has been endorsed in The Hague, Netherlands, and by the Codex Committee on Food Additives and Contaminants, which advise the Codex Alimentarius Commission. Operating under the auspices of the United Nations and World Health Organization (WHO), the Codex sets global food safety standards for more than 160 nations, representing about 97 percent of the world's population. The United States is one of these nations. For more information contact Public Citizen at www.citizen.org.

sealed meats like hot dogs, ham and bologna before they hit grocers' shelves. Why pasteurize at this stage? Though the meat itself is fully cooked before packaging, sometimes the packaging process contaminates the surface of the product, and harmful bacteria can then be spread when the consumer opens the package. The process does nothing to alter the meat product in appearance or taste, but it does decontaminate it. In fact, university data shows a 99.99 percent eradication of *Listeria* bacteria on tested products.

Listeria in ready-to-eat meat products is a significant health issue. Over 34,500 pounds of hot dogs were recalled in the year 2000 because of this bacteria in the United States alone. For some populations, it is extremely deadly. Still, I believe the focus is misdirected. Radiation and agribusiness industries direct their energies to the highly lucrative cleanup of contaminated food rather than preventing contamination at its source. Food poisoning from bacterial contamination could be prevented by basic sanitary measures.

For instance, feedlot sanitation, which includes reducing overcrowding, disinfecting drinking water, and fly control, would drastically reduce cattle infection rates. *E. coli* 0157:H7 infection rates could be virtually eliminated by feeding hay, rather than the standard unhealthy starchy grain diet, for seven days prior to slaughter. Improving sanitation would also prevent water contamination from feed lot runoff, incriminated in the recent outbreak of *E. coli* 0157:H7 poisoning in Walkerton, Ontario. Moreover, contaminated runoff will remain a continuing threat even if all meat is irradiated.

The Quick Fix

There is no question that there is a problem with contaminated meat today. The food industry uses irradiation as a short cut to avoid addressing the bigger problem: dirty slaughterhouses, rampant bacterial contamination, overuse of antibacterial agents and sloppy handling of our food products. Irradiation is just a substitute for poor hygiene and poor cooking practices in the food industry. Irradiation is not a magic bullet. Anything we do (from a food-safety standpoint) is only as good as what the end user does. Irradiated ground beef still needs to be refrigerated or frozen properly and cooked adequately.

CHAPTER 6

Risks for Bacterial Overgrowth in the Home

ALTHOUGH YOU MAY not be able to control safety measures on farms or slaughterhouses, there is a lot you can do to protect your own home from dangerous bacteria. Your home is not only your castle, it may be a haven for infectious bacteria. *Salmonella* isn't just found in uncooked meat or unwashed produce. It can thrive in human feces, and it only takes a tiny amount of contaminated stool on a person's hands to cause a problem. For instance, if those unwashed hands touch a phone, the next person that uses the phone could pick up thousands of bacteria. If this person places their fingers in their mouth, enough *Salmonella* bacteria may be ingested to trigger disease. Well, you get the picture.

Some common household items are particularly notorious for harboring germs, particularly telephones, faucets and sponges. The common household sponge may harbor hundreds of thousands of bacteria. Just picking up a sponge can result in the transfer of many of these bacteria to your hand. Obviously, the more often a sponge is handled, the greater the chances of spreading bacteria. You can reduce these risks by changing your sponge often. Telephones and sponges aren't the only items implicated in germ transfer.

Touching everyday objects, such as kitchen faucets or counters, is the easiest means of transferring high levels of potentially dangerous bacteria to people's hands. In one study, researchers looked for bacteria on the palms of volunteers' hands after making dinner, cleaning the house, doing laundry, using a public restroom, petting a dog or a cat, or returning home from elementary school. Surprisingly, people had the fewest microorganisms on their hands after leaving a public restroom and the most after making a meal.

The second easiest way to transfer bacteria is by cleaning the house. Not only will the individual who is cleaning touch object contaminated by other family members, they will often spread germs on cleaning sponges and rags. Germs can also be picked up by petting a dog or a cat (though dogs transmitted the most germs of the two). Other sites of bacterial transfer implicated in the study include schools, laundry (because of handling underwear), and public restrooms.

The investigators then added a viral and bacterial mixture to everyday objects, such as sponges and telephone receivers. They found that telephone receivers and kitchen faucets transferred high numbers of this mix of microbes, while squeezing out a sponge transferred even more organisms to the hands. When they added the mix of organisms to volunteers' fingertips, they found that 35 to 40 percent of the microbes were transferred to the mouth—a dose large enough to cause infection. Researchers concluded that an individual's bacterial exposure is greatly reduced if they wash their hands often and keep them away from the nose, eyes and mouth.

The Kitchen

The main source of disease-causing bacteria in the kitchen is raw meat. In some areas almost 100 percent of poultry contains organisms such as *Campylobacter* and *Salmonella* that can cause diarrhea or flu-like illness. Food poisoning makes headlines when cases are traced to restaurants or other public settings, but studies have shown that 50 to 80 percent of foodborne illness is caused by food prepared at home. Although people may be careful when storing and cooking meat, it is also important to disinfect cutting boards and countertops after they come in contact with raw meat.

Bacteria Love Sponges

You would not think of preparing food in the bathroom. Instead, you place food on a kitchen countertop, even though it harbors far more bacteria than a toilet seat. Why? Wiping a kitchen counter top with a sponge spreads germs all over your kitchen. Germs really like kitchen sponges, and squeezing out a sponge does not get rid of bacteria. It does, however, transfer germs to the sponge-holder's hands. You can also transfer germs to the sponge if you don't wash your hands before handling the sponge, especially after going to the bathroom or changing a diaper.

Kitchen sponges can host many different bacteria. After an investigation of fifty sponges used for only three weeks, they were tested for coliform or fecal coliform bacteria (found in soil, water and the intestinal tract). All of these bacteria can cause illness in humans. At least 70 percent of the sponges had high levels of coliform bacteria and 38 percent showed high levels of fecal coliform bacteria. What the researchers discovered was that most of the bacteria found on the sponges came from food left on dirty dishes, especially raw foods such as meat or poultry and even vegetables.

So, what are some ways to safely use sponges? Ensure your sponge is squeezed dry and free of food residue. Also, remember to clean the sponge after using it to wash dishes, and keep it away from the cutting board, especially if you have used it to cut raw meat. It is crucial to remember that you may even think you are cleaning your cutting board when you are not. Rather, you are simply moving the bacteria deeper into the board to grow and contaminate the next item put there.

Another way to maintain a clean sponge is to put it in the dishwasher with the dishes. Hopefully, the hot water will kill the bacteria. You can also rinse your sponge in a 10 percent solution of chlorine bleach or put it in the microwave at the high setting for five minutes. Finally, replace used sponges regularly—about every ten days is optimal.

"But It Looks and Smells Fine"

Have you ever smelled the leftovers in the refrigerator to see if it is still safe to eat? What you see and smell may provide some clues to the food's safety, but how that food was handled and stored may be more important. It is important to realize that taking just a little extra care with your food handling can significantly cut your risks of getting ill.

To illustrate this point, a new government survey found that 25 percent of men and 14 percent of women did not wash their hands with soap after handling raw meat. Half of those surveyed indicated that they ate undercooked eggs during the previous year—a risk factor for *Salmonella enteritidis*. Despite recent publicity about *E. coli* contamination linked to undercooked hamburger meat, 20 percent of the participants said they ate hamburgers without cooking them thoroughly. More men reported eating rare hamburgers compared to women, however. In fact, men generally had riskier food safety behavior than women, and younger people took more risks than older folks did. Additionally, people with higher incomes handled foods improperly more often than those with lower incomes. City residents were not as careful as rural residents were.

You may think that you are more savvy about food handling than those surveyed above, but are you really? Scientists put cameras in the kitchens of one hundred middle-class, well-educated, college town families. These families thought they were doing a pretty good job with food safety, so they were surprised by the research findings. For instance, cameras revealed that most people skipped using soap when washing their hands. They also used the same towel to dry their hands that they used to wipe up raw meat juice. Salad greens often went unwashed, and meatloaf was undercooked. One person even tasted the bacteria-ridden marinade where raw fish previously had soaked. One mom handled raw chicken and then fixed her infant a bottle without washing her hands. Another mom merely rinsed her baby's juice bottle after it fell into raw eggs, despite the fact that it could now be contaminated with *Salmonella*.

The purpose of this experiment was to improve the education of consumers by showing them how to better protect themselves from the food poisoning that strikes seventy-six million Americans each year. One of the greatest barriers in getting people to change is that they already think they are doing a good job. Most Americans blame restaurants for foodborne illnesses, not themselves. When asked if they follow basic bacteria-fighting tips, most insist they do in their own kitchens. This does not appear to be true, however, since most food poisonings occur at home.

Below are other disturbing habits that researchers caught on camera:

- Only 25 percent of those videotaped stored raw meat and seafood on the refrigerator's bottom shelf. Dripping juices could contaminate other foods.
- Before starting to cook, 45 percent washed their hands, but only 16 percent of these people used soap. On the average, each cook washed his or her hands seven times less than was thought necessary to observe good food safety. A third of them consistently used soap while the rest only rinsed and wiped their hands on a dish towel.
- The safest way to clean up raw meat juice is to use paper towels, but dozens wiped the countertop with a contaminated dishcloth, further spreading germs the next time they dried their hands.
- Thirty percent did not wash salad lettuce, while others placed salad ingredients on countertops where raw meat had been sitting.
- Finished meals were checked with a thermometer: 35 percent undercooked meat loaf, 42 percent undercooked chicken, and 17 percent undercooked fish. It is important to use a meat thermometer even if meat looks cooked enough, because it may not have reached a high enough temperature to kill the bacteria.

Researchers concluded that if people would simply wash their hands and clean food surfaces after handling raw meat, many would reduce the risks of pathogen contamination. Unfortunately, they did not stress the washing of fruits and vegetables.

Recycled Organic Household Waste

Household waste also has risks. You may be putting yourself and your family at risk when you dutifully segregate organic materials from the household waste for collection or recycling as compost. Organic leftovers release higher amounts of potentially harmful bacteria than those containing mixed garbage or garbage containing preservatives or antibiotics.

Some people with respiratory illnesses said that their symptoms became worse when they started collecting household waste for their compost pile. High levels of toxins released by bacteria can cause symptoms such as coughing, breathlessness and flu-like symptoms. The humid state of pure organic waste suits microorganisms much better than mixed waste, which dilutes organic material. In homes where organic bins are not emptied for a week or more, levels of bacterial toxins were three times as high as in homes where waste was not separated. The solution is to keep the organic waste bins outside, though this may not be possible in some situations (such as downtown areas with restricted space).

Sickness in the Home

THE HOME-CARE PATIENT

The home-care patient may be at substantial risk for catching an infectious agent. Several factors put them at risk including advanced age, chronic illness or immune suppression. Home-care is often provided by family members in a setting that is loosely structured. Sanitation and ventilation may be poor or absent, but the basic principles of hygiene need to be adapted and applied. Home-care workers should wash their hands often, especially upon entering the house or after they touch many things with unwashed hands. Stethoscopes and blood pressure cuffs should also be disinfected after each use. In most cases, the use of gowns, gloves and masks in the care of homebound patients is recommended to protect the health-care provider, not the patient. To reduce any risk of infection, medical supplies and foods should be properly refrigerated, and meticulous care of kitchen appliances and tools is also important.

Serving Bean Dip?

Last year the Food and Drug Administration advised Americans not to consume certain layered bean dips. The nationwide recall included dips containing layers of black or pinto beans, salsa, guacamole, nacho cheese and sour cream. These products were thought to be contaminated with *Shigella sonnei.* After being ingested, these bacteria can cause bloody diarrhea, cramps, fever, nausea and vomiting. Some people even need hospitalization. So far, there have been reports of forty-nine illnesses due to layered bean dip, including five hospitalizations from this outbreak of food poisoning.

If a home-care patient is infected with a multi-drug-resistant organism, they may be transmitted to other home-care patients through inanimate objects or by the hands of the healthcare worker. Home-care patients known to have a multi-drug-resistant organism should be cared for through disposable equipment when possible. Additionally, reusable equipment, such as stethoscopes and blood pressure cuffs, should remain in the home if they cannot be disinfected easily. If practical, these patients should be seen as the last appointment of the day. If this is not possible, visits should be scheduled to avoid seeing patients at risk, such as those requiring wound care, after seeing a patient with multi-drug-resistant organisms. If you are using oxygen equipment or an intravenous line at home, be sure to ask for instructions that clearly state how to clean the device and how it should be properly maintained.

BEING A CAREGIVER

One study shows that being the caregiver of someone with schizophrenia increases the stress levels high enough to be susceptibility to infectious illnesses. This points out the powerful influence of being around a continuous stressful situation as a predictor of illness. As a caregiver, it is important to find ways to decrease your stress levels with meditation and relaxation training. Developing a positive attitude and finding a support system may also be helpful. One consequence of this increased stress is on the immune system. Because there is a direct link between stress, the suppression of the immune system and the onset of infection, taking a holistic health approach is an important part of staying well.

Pets and Their Risks

TAKE PET BITES SERIOUSLY

In the United States, some two million people suffer animal bites each year with 90 percent coming from dogs. All bites from animals—domestic or wild—are potentially serious. Even bites that look superficial can sometimes involve damage to underlying nerves, tendons and blood vessels, or they can become infected. Any bite that breaks the skin deserves medical attention, regardless of how innocent it may appear. The longer the delay, the more time microorganisms have to multiply.

In one study, scientists analyzed animal bites and found bacteria not previously recognized as bite-wound organisms that cause disease in humans. The majority of the infections contained more than one type of bacteria, and treatment required carefully chosen antibiotics. The study identified more than 150 different kinds of bacteria, some dangerous, and some potentially fatal, without counting the potentially fatal rabies and tetanus bacteria. It may seem unnatural to make a big fuss about a couple of punctures from an otherwise friendly cat or dog, but animal bites are among the most infectious wounds a human can sustain.

Dog bites to the hands or arms are more likely to becoming infected as those to other parts of the body. Dog bites to the face and neck are dangerous because of their proximity to major blood vessels. They can cause serious lacerations requiring stitches and even reconstructive surgery. Dogs inflict fewer deep punctures. They are more likely to cause a rather wide, superficial wound that is generally easier to clean and less prone to infection, especially if it can be left open to the air. Still, dog bites become infected 15 to 20 percent of the time.

Cat's teeth generally do less damage to the tissues than dogs, but their bites are usually more infectious. Deep punctures made by a pair of stiletto-like teeth from a cat create a warm, dark, narrow, hard-to-clean environment perfect for rapid multiplication of microorganisms. And cat saliva carries some very virulent varieties. More than half of all cat bites become infected, regardless of location on the body. This includes any bite on the hands or feet; wounds involving joints, tendons, ligaments or bones; and bites occurring twelve or more hours before receiving medical attention.

After a bite, rinse the wound vigorously with warm water and wash it with soap, preferably an antibacterial one. Deep puncture wounds or lacerations accompanied by a lot of bleeding warrant an immediate visit to a doctor or emergency room; so do bites to the hands or feet, and those from wild animals. Less risky bites can be treated at home, but should be checked out by a physician within twelve hours to make sure the wound is thoroughly cleaned. Swelling surrounding a bite wound is a normal bodily reaction to injury, but persistent swelling accompanied by redness, throbbing pain, discharge from the wound, or fever, could indicate infection and requires immediate medical attention.

Dog Toys Also Pose a Threat

Animal bites aren't the only bacterial risks. That chew toy in your dog's mouth may be loaded with *Salmonella*. The FDA issued a warning saying some pet chew toys made from pig ears, beef jerky, smoked hooves and other animal products, may be contaminated with *Salmonella* and could pose a health threat to humans and their pets. The FDA urged pet owners to handle these products carefully and to be sure to wash your hands well with hot water and soap. The warning came after reports in Canada linking *Salmonella* outbreaks to pet toys. *Salmonella* poisoning can cause flu-like symptoms such as fever and muscle aches. It can be particularly dangerous for people with weak immune systems, small children and the elderly.

Domestic and wild animals can harbor the *Salmonella* bacterium, including poultry, pigs, cattle, and pets, such as turtles, iguanas, dogs and cats. Even without symptoms themselves, they can pass the infection on to humans.

Can You Get Ulcers from Your Cat?

In one case, a thirty-eight year-old man had a history of stomach problems and was diagnosed with ulcers. Testing revealed that he was infected with three different strains of *Helicobacter heilmannii*, a type of bacteria often found in animals, but rarely in humans. Later it was determined that one of the man's cats had an identical strain.

Other Factors

THE BUG ZAPPER

A bug zapper may do more than kill bugs. Investigators found that these devices, used to lure and electrocute insects, are spreading bacteria. Where do these bacteria come from? One example is houseflies. They pick up the bacteria from human or animal waste. Millions of bac-

A Warning Regarding Caged Animals

When animals in crowded cages are treated with antibiotics, resistant microbes can survive and multiply. This can cause the once harmless bacteria, *E. coli* and *Salmonella*, to mutate into virulent strains.

teria on the surface of these insects are scattered into the air when the zapper causes the insects to explode. The bacteria can be hurled as far as six feet in a still air environment. If the zapper is near a fan or an air conditioning vent, the bacteria can probably travel much further.

Moreover, one study conducted in the backyards of homeowners found that only a small percentage of the insects that were zapped were the intended victims, the female mosquitoes. It is only the female that bites. Many more beneficial insects were killed. If you decide to use a bug zapper, it would be best not to eat food that is placed anywhere near it. Be aware if a bug zapper is hanging over a condiment table, a take-out window, a barbecue grill or even where baby toys are stored.

FINGER PAINTS

Do not let children stick their hands into jars of finger paint that have been opened before and stored for any length of time. Prevent contamination by pouring the paint into a separate container to be used. Do not pour any remaining paint back into the original containers. Odors given off by bacteria growing in jars of outdated finger paints caused vomiting and have landed over sixty elementary school students and their teachers in the hospital. Even the preservatives used in the paints may not prevent bacterial overgrowth.

PRODUCTS THAT CONTAIN CHLORINE

A group of scientists are researching ways to pre-treat cotton clothing with chlorine to kill bacteria. This will be like wearing a designer pest strip. You could wear a sweater that defends you from *Salmonella* infections or a T-shirt that kills *E. coli*. What they are hoping will occur is that the chlorinated clothes will destroy bacteria and some viruses and reduce the risk of infection. The treated cotton could be worn by your health-care provider, used as hotel bedding or become sportswear that stays odor free. The technique may also be used to treat wooden cutting boards to kill bacteria in food.

A synthetic rubber product that kills microbes on contact has been developed at Auburn University. They used a process that holds chlorine molecules onto the surface of the rubber. When microbes come in contact with the chlorine, the molecule transfers to the organism and kills it. According to researchers, the antimicrobial rubber continues to kill microbes until the chlorine atoms are used up. You would place the product in bleach and the chlorine will again be taken up on the surface of the rubber. If companies develop this product, it could be incorporated into plastic, cloth and rubber-containing products to be used in hospitals and food service areas. Using it in condoms could prevent spread of sexually transmitted diseases. Around the home, the product could be used as a sponge to kill germs on countertops. It could also be used in pacifiers, baby bottles or bottle nipples.

What harm would it cause by putting us in constant exposure to chlorine? Would it be poisonous to babies chewing on the chlorine in their pacifier? Scientists still don't know what will happen to the bacteria that come into contact with these products. They may become just as resistant to chlorine as they were to antibiotics. Who knows what kind of microbe resistance we could ultimately cause. Chlorine is added to most water supplies because it kills *E. coli* and other microbes. Doesn't it do the same thing for the harmless and beneficial bacteria that are suppose to grow in our gastrointestinal tract?

POOR HYGIENE

Americans do not appear to be improving their hygiene even after all the reports telling us that the spread of pathogenic bacteria is increasing. Yet, hygiene (especially hand washing) is the best way for reducing contact and fecal-oral transmission of infectious organisms. According to a new survey conducted for the American Society of Microbiology, Americans continue to avoid washing their hands. Researchers found this to be true when they observed men and women who used public restrooms in Atlanta, New York, New Orleans, Chicago and San Francisco. A total of 7,836 people were observed. Researchers also did a telephone survey of another thousand or so people. Ninety-five percent of those surveyed over the phone said they regularly washed their hands after using a public bathroom, but only 67 percent of the people actually observed in public restrooms washed their hands.

From the telephone survey, researchers found women were also more likely than men to wash their hands after sneezing or coughing, after petting a dog or cat, and after handling a dirty diaper. We need to understand the significance of these findings and the importance of hand washing. The more people do their part to control the spread of infections, the less we have to rely on antibiotics, which continue to lose their potency as bacteria develop resistance to them.

Contaminated fingertips and fingernails transfer germs easily. This area accumulates dirt, makeup, oils, plus microscopic pieces of skin, hair, mucus, saliva, sexual fluids, feces and other body tissues. All this material combined with an enormous concentration of germs is self-inoculated constantly into the nose, eyes, mouth, ears and skin. Fingernails also damage the tissues and reduce the number of germs required to cause an infection. This can stress and overload the strongest immune system in the healthiest person. Since the fingertips and nails are used extensively in sexual contact, make sure you and your partner both have clean hands and clean fingernails.

CHAPTER 7

Risks for Bacterial Overgrowth in Public Places

Hospitals: Are They Healthy for You?

You check into the hospital thinking you will come out healthier than you went in, yet more and more people are picking up infections while they are hospitalized. Bacteria that cause serious illness have been found on medical equipment, lab coats, stethoscopes and even doctors' pens. They are also found on catheters, intravenous lines and breathing tubes, thereby allowing bacteria easy entry into the body.

These infections cost the healthcare system an estimated $4.5 billion a year. Part of the cost is picked up by hospitals themselves, because insurers, including the government, will not pay for a person's illness if they get sick from something contracted in the hospital. There should be an economic incentive to keep the place clean and sanitary. Still, the problem is getting worse.

About two million Americans contract an infection each year in a hospital (or other medical center). The U.S. Centers for Disease Control (CDC) estimates that about 88,000 people die each year directly from blood and other infections contracted in healthcare facilities. In fact, many hospital patients are now automatically given antibiotics prior to surgery in an effort to prevent post-surgical infections. However, it appears that this practice has not been very effective and has actually resulted in making the hospital a serious breeding ground for some very potent microorganisms. According to a CDC study, as many as 70 percent of the hospital infections examined involved organisms that were resistant to one or more antibiotics.

I believe a better solution to the problem would be for doctors, nurses and anyone else that handles patients to wash their hands after every patient contact. In fact, the rate of hospital infections fell about 40 percent in one study when medical personnel placed alcohol dispensers at each patient's bedside and used them to regularly disinfect their hands.

In 1993, researchers at a Paris hospital found out that about 21 percent of the patients admitted to their wound care center carried specific drug-resistant bacteria. Nine percent of these patients acquired the bacteria while at the hospital. Then a program was implemented in which nurses and other staff members were trained to vigorously wash their hands, use fresh gloves and gowns more frequently, and use disposable devices more often. The cases of hospital-acquired infections involving resistant bacteria dropped significantly. Sometimes we forget the importance of simple hand washing in preventing disease.

Fingernails: What Lies Beneath?

How a health-care worker maintains his or her hands can be a case of life or death for newborn babies and some vulnerable patients. Potentially lethal germs can lie under the fingernails of hospital workers. Hospitals should require their employees to maintain short, natural fingernails to reduce the risk of spreading bacteria, but there are no regulations in most hospitals that require employees to do this. It is shocking that even simple precautions are not being used to keep from spreading infectious agents from patient to patient, despite the risks.

For instance, a while back I heard a news report about three nurses in an Oklahoma City hospital who spread the bacteria *Proteus* to several newborn babies. The source of infection was lying under their long fingernails. Recent studies have noted the incredible efficiency of contaminated fingernails/fingertips to spread bacteria. Hidden cameras show that we all scratch our skin, our eyes, suck on our fingers, bite our nails and scratch our heads, even in our sleep. The area under and around the fingernails has an inexhaustible supply of germs and the hardest area to clean. Personal hygiene of the fingernails, hands and skin is the most important step in prevention of infection.

Computer keyboards and faucet handles in medical facilities are potential reservoirs for pathogens as well. Not only does hand washing need to be reinforced in medical facilities, but installing faucets that do not have to be touched would certainly reduce contact contamination. One study in the *American Journal of Infection Control* (2000) found that 26 percent of the computer keyboards and 15 percent of the faucets were contaminated. *Staphyloccus aureus* was the most frequently occurring pathogen, followed by *Enterococcus, Enterobacter* and other gram-negative bacteria. Plastic covers on keyboards that are cleaned daily would reduce this contamination.

One bacterium, *Pseudomonas aeruginosa,* breeds in moist places such as sinks, respiratory equipment, incubators and even hand lotion. Infants, burn victims and patients being treated for intravenous drug addiction, cystic fibrosis, leukemia and organ transplants can die from a *Pseudomonas aeruginosa* infection. It is estimated that *P. aeruginosa* accounts for up to 20 percent of hospital infections. This is a well-known cause of infection acquired in newborn ICUs. A total of forty-nine infants were infected with this organism in 1997 and 1998. Until now, it had only rarely been linked to contaminated hands. In 1999, there were infant deaths in an Oklahoma City's hospital blamed on *P. aeruginosa.* It was found on employees who had long fingernails or artificial nails. (Underlying conditions such as an outer ear infection or nail infections may also be associated with harboring *Pseudomonas.*)

Hygiene Tips for Medical Staff

British researchers found that the transmission of bacteria could be reduced if nurses and therapists routinely wore protective masks while caring for their patients. Most hospitals do not require the routine use of masks even for high-risk patients. The study found that the antibiotic-resistant bacteria thought to be responsible for most hospital outbreaks, *Staphylococcus aureus,* was greatly reduced when masks were worn. Since many people carry this bacterium in their nose and throats, they were not able to spread it to their vulnerable patients. Also, because the workers were not able to touch that part of their face, they did not contaminate their hands with the *S. aureus* bacteria (*J Hosp Infect* 2001) and spread it to others.

Extensive studies of showering and bathing conducted since the 1960s show that these activities increase the dispersal of skin bacteria into the surrounding environment. These studies prompted a change in practice among surgical personnel, who are now generally discouraged from showering immediately before entering the operating room. Staff members should not wear jewelry except wedding bands and wristwatches. Long finger nails and cosmetic nail treatments should not permitted.

Checking In: What You Can Do

So if you are lying defenseless in the hospital, how do you protect yourself from these nasty bugs? Here are a few tips. If a doctor, nurse, aide or any hospital staff arrives to give you a pill, a shot, new linens or an examination, ask them if they have had a chance to wash their hands. People get so busy in the hospital that they may simply forget, but you do not need to share someone else's infection. There needs to be a wash basin in your room that makes it easy for the staff to use. If not, ask them to use the bathroom sink. If the staff member is wearing gloves, ask if they just cared for a patient, and if so, could they put on new gloves.

Be sure to wash your own hands regularly while hospitalized as well, even if you need to ask someone to bring a wash basin over to the bed. Also, if you are sharing a room, do not share your roommate's towel or other personal items. Ask relatives who are sick to stay home. Finally, if you are scheduling elective surgery and are fighting the flu or a cold, postpone your surgery until you are completely well.

You could also consider investigating the hospital's infection control program. Hospitals must have a program that meets certain standards in order to keep their accreditation. Ask whether there is an infection-control professional on staff, particularly if you have some reason to feel uneasy about something you have seen. Hospitals keep track of the number of infections patients get while under their care, even though these figures are not usually disclosed. (Some consumer advocates would like to see this information made public.)

If you are pregnant, you also need to take extra care while in the hospital. Women who deliver their babies by Cesarean section or who have assisted deliveries are more likely to be back in the hospital within two months than women who have uncomplicated natural births. These new moms often return to the hospital for problems such as uterine infection, gallbladder disease, postpartum hemorrhage, obstetrical surgery-wound complications and even appendicitis. Implicated women need to be even more aware of the risks of post-delivery infection.

Ultrasound Hygiene

The incorrect use of lubricant during ultrasound scanning is blamed for an outbreak of antibiotic-resistant *Staphylococcus aureus* infection in a German hospital maternity ward. It was found that the spatula used to apply the sonogram gel was being reused, contrary to hospital policy. (*Infect Control Hosp Epidemiol* 2000).

Water Births and Preterm Babies

Water births, pioneered in the 1960s, are becoming increasingly popular. The problem is that the birthing-pool water may become contaminated with amniotic fluid, blood and fecal material, all of which contain large quantities of maternal bacteria and viruses. A more reasonable approach is to ensure that infection control policies for water births include adequate pool maintenance and decontamination.

At birth, infants are often diffusely covered in blood and amniotic fluid, as well as other birthing fluids. Usually they are bathed to remove these unsightly fluids with total body immersion. This is not recommended, however, especially for preterm babies, since the skin of a newborn is ideal for absorbing unwanted microorganisms. Washing should be restricted initially to the head and neck. To prevent outbreaks of bacterial infection, it is very important to enforce disinfecting hands, limit the use of tap water for handwashing and use sterile water to wash the preterm babies.

Antibiotic Therapy for Hospital Infections

In closed environments such as hospitals, the resident bacteria are exposed to dozens of different kinds of antibiotics simultaneously. Populations of resistant organisms have evolved that are able to survive exposure to almost every known antibiotic, even the most expensive and powerful agents held in reserve. Hospitalized patients who develop infections with these bugs can face very serious trouble.

Sometimes novel combinations of drugs can treat them or the newest experimental drug is tried out, but more and more often there is no available treatment. This is happening all across this country. Patients are dying from hospital-acquired drug-resistant pneumonia, wound or bloodstream infections and meningitis, as their doctors stand by helplessly. We are more powerless against some infections today then before the time of antibiotics.

Health-Care Workers and Respiratory Infections

Having a viral upper respiratory infection has the ability to spread other bacterial infections. These kinds of infections may be behind explosive outbreaks of infection seen in day-care centers, homeless shelters, the military and in hospitals. Outbreaks can occur when certain pathogen bacteria, such as group A *Streptococcus pyogenes* or

Staphylococcus aureus, colonize in the rectum, vagina or on the skin of health-care workers even though they do not show any symptoms of infection. When infected individuals develop an upper respiratory tract infection, the bacteria are spread in the air, called the "cloud phenomenon."

A variety of infectious agents can be transmitted from healthcare workers to patients in this manner in spite of standard infection control measures such as hand washing. While it is well known that healthcare workers can transmit airborn infections such as tuberculosis, chickenpox and influenza, they can also transmit lesser known bacterial pathogens through the air as well. It is thought that *Clostridium diphtheriae, Haemophilus influenzae, Neisseria meningiditis, Streptococcus pneumoniae, Yersinia pestis* and *Bordetela pertussis* can also be spread in this way. It is suspected that nasal colonization of *S. aureus* in healthcare workers is quite common (20 to 90 percent). Since adults have an average of two viral upper respiratory infections each year, "cloud" adults may be working around patients in hospitals all year and putting them at risk for infections.

What if you have a healthcare worker transmitting these pathogens during surgery? They could be the operating room nurse, surgeon, the anesthesiologist or a technician. The mechanism by which the

Hospitals Save, Hospitals Kill

Over two million Americans enter hospitals each year with one ailment and wind up with another. Being in a hospital exposes people to hospital-acquired infections that are fatal to as many as 88,000 Americans a year and untold numbers in other countries. The very technology that can save can also kill. Every piece of equipment and every invasive technique give antibiotic-resistant organisms an opportunity to develop.

Seventy percent of these infections are due to organisms resistant to at least one antimicrobial agent. Although 1.8 million fewer patients were admitted to U.S. hospitals in 1995 than in 1975 (35.9 million versus 37.7 million) and the average length of stay was lower (5.3 days in 1995 versus 7.9 days in 1975), the national hospital infection rate has increased as much as 39 percent. The major resistant pathogens causing these infections are *E. coli, Staphylococcus aureus, Enterococcus spp.* and *Pseudomonas aeruginosa.*

pathogen becomes airborne is not entirely clear and could include increased activity, friction with clothing, or even passing gas if the colonized site is the rectum. When these pathogens are transmitted to someone with compromised immunity, the resulting illness can be serious and even deadly. Plus, it may be hard to locate these bacteria-carrying workers because they are not having symptoms. It may also be difficult to eradicate the bacteria in some patients because of constant reexposure from family members who are also colonized with the same bacteria.

How common is this? It is thought that up to 10 percent of basically healthy people are S. aureus nasal carriers and disperse the organism into the air. Although regular nasal breathing doesn't usually cause this dispersal to happen, coughing, sneezing, snorting and talking increases the chance. When infected individuals move about, large numbers of bacteria are dispersed into the air because of bacteria on skin and clothing. Bacteria can also be spread when making a bed.

In other studies concerning a newborn nursery setting, it was found that infants who were exposed to nurses who had colonized pathogens on their body had a high risk of getting them by airborne transmission. As far back as 1960, the *American Journal of Diseases of Children* presented a brief editorial entitled "The Preposterous Cloud Baby." The first sentence of the introduction stated, "Once in a blue moon a journal is privileged to publish an article which introduces an important revolutionary concept." These researchers discovered that a viral upper respiratory infection was the essential "cloud factor." Up to 75 percent of newborn infants who carried the staph bacteria nasally became cloud babies once they acquired a viral upper respiratory infection. Most importantly, these cloud babies were also capable of causing staph outbreaks. In spite of what was believed to be a revolutionary concept, not much as been written on this subject until recently.

Nursing Home Dangers

If you or a loved one will soon be residing in a nursing home, be sure to observe its cleanliness carefully. Ask to see where the food is prepared and how they wash their linens. Are soap and paper towels readily available so the staff can wash their hands, and do they? Is there a smell of urine when you walk in the door? The elderly are particularly at risk in hospitals and long-term care facilities, or because of home care. It is up to us to use whatever preventive methods necessary to ensure their safety.

Ocean Swimming, Pools and Hot Tubs

SWIMMING LINKED TO INFECTIONS

Have you ever looked forward to going to the beach only to find a sign saying it is closed to swimming when you arrived? Do you know why authorities close beaches? Usually, it is not because of an oil spill or toxic industrial waste, but rather microorganisms. They come from storm water runoff or animal and human waste in sewage spills or overflows. In fact, thousands of beaches are closed each year with nearly 70 percent of them due to high levels of pathogenic bacteria. These disease-causing microorganisms can cause gastrointestinal and upper respiratory infections and skin rashes. Surfers commonly get sinus and ear infections. The consequences can be particularly serious for children, the elderly and anyone with a compromised immune system. It seems to be getting worse each year.

Perhaps the best evidence comes from research led by Robert Haile at the University of Southern California. It involved interviewing 11,000 swimmers in Santa Monica Bay in the summer of 1996. The study found that the closer people swam (with their heads submerged) near a storm drain, the more likely they were to develop gastrointestinal and upper respiratory infections. The illness rate was higher after days when the bacteria and virus counts near the storm drain were high.

Thankfully, since there is better water testing, the public is notified sooner and illness can be prevented. Santa Monica Bay beaches in California now have signs next to storm drains warning swimmers to take a dip elsewhere or risk becoming ill. However, because each state or local agency may have different monitoring programs, if they have any at all, it is hard to be sure that you will have the same protection at a beach in California as you would in New Jersey. The differences are so great that some closed beaches may not be as contaminated as others that are still open. Some beaches aren't monitored at all. To date, the states that do not regularly monitor beach water for your swimming safety are Alabama, Georgia, Louisiana, Oregon and Washington. The states that do not usually notify the public if bacteria counts are high include Mississippi and Texas. The public is not warned In Puerto Rico either.

The states that border the coasts or the Great Lakes and have comprehensive programs to monitor beach water and inform the public of their findings are: Connecticut, Delaware, Illinois, Indiana, New Hampshire, New Jersey, North Carolina and Ohio. Fourteen other states, including California and Florida, monitor some beaches, but not others, even though California was supposed to begin a comprehensive beach-water monitoring program in 1999.

Since water quality is not standardized, the risk to the public remains high. Until a better method is developed to determine the safety of beach water, be cautious when swimming. To find out which beaches are monitored, visit the EPA's website at http://www.epa.gov/ost/beaches. You can also find out if your state or county is monitoring its beaches by checking http://www.nrdc.org.

If you are not able to get information about the safety concerning the beach you are planning to visit, choose a swimming area that is next to open ocean water. You want to avoid beaches with discharge pipes and poor water circulation. Also, do not swim for forty-eight hours after a heavy rainstorm. There could be high concentrations of microorganisms and toxic runoff from the city upstream. This goes for rivers and creeks as well. Moreover, avoid putting your head underwater, and do not let your children splash or swallow the water. It is very important to wash off after your swim as well. It is important to take these safety measures because with the increasing use of coastal areas as a depository for all kinds of waste, the rate of illness related to swimming there can be expected to increase.

HYDROTHERAPY POOL DANGERS

Hydrotherapy pools are used by diverse groups of people and are potentially hazardous. Hydrotherapy has become popular, and many district hospitals have installed pools. Despite careful control of water quality, users still can suffer from pool-related skin, ear, chest and gastrointestinal infections from time to time. Numerous microorganisms have been implicated in these infections, including *Pseudomonas aeruginosa, Legionella spp.* and some viruses.

INDOOR HOT TUBS RISKY FOR LUNGS

What can be the harm of sinking into a bubbly, steaming, indoor hot tub? According to new research, frequent use of indoor hot tubs can raise the risk of a bacterial lung disease. It turns out that a cousin to the tuberculosis-causing bacteria can live in hot tub water and the mist that indoor hot tubs give off. Bubbles rich with the bacteria rise up, burst and disperse bacteria throughout a room. Recently, nine people, including four children, were treated for a lung disease caused by these bacteria. Other organisms have also been found such as *Pseudomonas* and *Candida*. Since diseases due to these organisms do not require notification of public health authorities, it is unknown just how many cases really exist.

Symptoms include fever, fatigue, night sweats, coughing and weight loss. A person with this condition may also find it difficult to breathe or have pain when breathing. However, unlike its relative, tuberculosis, this bacteria is not contagious. Remember though that doctors can misdiagnose this condition by mistaking it for other lung infections. Since indoor hot tubs are becoming more common, you need to know about the increased risk associated with their use.

Schools and Day Care Centers

LUNCHROOM OUTBREAK

Several months ago, nearly two hundred Michigan schoolchildren developed stomach pains and jaundice and were found to have hepatitis A. Their illness was traced back to strawberry shortcake that was served at school. The dessert was made from frozen strawberries grown in Mexico, processed in southern California, and contaminated with the hepatitis A virus somewhere along the line. During the summer months, imported berries sometimes cause outbreak of infectious diarrhea. In one case, raspberries from Guatemala were identified as the vehicle that infected many people who lived in North America with an unusual diarrhea-causing parasite called *Cyclospora cayetanensis*.

DAY CARE DANGERS

Researchers found resistant *Streptococcus pneumonaie* strains in the siblings of kids attending a day-care center. This suggests that the spread of such germs may not be confined to the child-care facility alone. The day-care center worked as an incubator spreading the bacteria throughout the community. High rates of respiratory infections among kids often leads to high use of antibiotics, which is making the bacteria even tougher than before.

Restaurants

Americans are eating out more often, and they may also be exposing themselves to dangerous bacteria. For instance, the plates on which commercial meals are served may become contaminated with bacteria if they are not allowed to dry properly before being piled up after washing. Twenty-four hours after washing, investigators found no apparent difference in bacterial growth between those stacked wet and those fully air-dried. However, after forty-eight hours, a significantly higher amount of various bacteria were evident on the wet-stacked dishes.

This time-temperature-moisture problem sets up an ideal environment for microbial growth. The Food and Drug Administration code specifically recommends air drying of all commercial dishware in order to prevent such food contamination problems. Consumers should pay attention not just to what they eat, but to whether or not what they eat is safely prepared (*Journal of the American Dietetic Association 2001*).

RESTAURANT E. COLI

In August 2000, sixty-four confirmed cases of *E. coli* surfaced at a second Sizzler restaurant. The first Sizzler infected fifty-six people, with sixteen children getting sick. Six other cases of *E. coli* were confirmed in the same town. Twenty-two people required hospitalization as a result of the outbreak, and a three-year-old girl died. Not too long after this incident, contamination at a Wendy's restaurant in Salem, Oregon, made about seventy people sick.

What about eating out at fast-food restaurants? The meat is cooked so fast that it may be left undercooked in the center of the hamburger patty. This can pass live bacteria to your digestive tract. Many cases of foodborne illness have been traced to undercooked ground beef in hamburgers.

Salons and Tattoo Parlors

MANICURES & PEDICURES

Probably the most serious health risk related to nail cosmetics is the threat of contracting an infection from manicure tools and instruments that have not been properly sterilized. Improperly sterilized instruments can transmit a variety of infections to customers. These include not just

---

Can Touching Doors Spread Disease?

Even though some people fear it is possible to contract a bacterial infection from touching a door handle in a public restroom, it is extremely unlikely if you just use good hygiene practices. If there is no other way to open the door, then use a paper towel or tissue when touching the door handle. In order to stay healthy, be sure to wash your hands frequently, particularly when other family members or co-workers are sick.

bacterial infections, but warts, hepatitis B and C, and even HIV. Most salons are beginning to take adequate precautions to prevent contamination, but you should ask about their sanitation practices.

State inspectors have found contagious bacteria at some dirty salons, especially at discount nail salons. Perhaps the economics of discount salons cause them to cut corners. Furthermore, many salons use employees that cannot read English and do not read the labels that tell them how to disinfect their supplies. What puts people at risk are soaking tubs not cleaned after each use, as well as nail buffers and boards used several times when they should only be used once. In some salons, nail clippers were found to be unclean and had fecal bacteria on them.

TATTOOS AND PIERCINGS: THE PRICE OF BEING IN STYLE

Many people will permanently decorate their skin with tattoos or choose to have some part of their body pierced. Although most of them will not have any serious medical problems, body piercing and tattooing do have health risks. These procedures have been implicated in a number of adverse oral and systemic conditions. Unsterilized needles can carry HIV and hepatitis. In fact, as a precaution against the transmission of bloodborne diseases, the U.S. and Canadian Red Cross will not accept blood donations from anyone who has had a body piercing or tattoo within a year. The Centers for Disease Control and Prevention have also deemed nonsterile piercing a serious health risk.

Body piercing is mostly self-taught and self-regulated. The piercing industry is overpopulated with fly-by-night operations and unscrupulous sorts. There is no standardized training, no licensing and no inspections. There are still reputable practitioners that sterilize their instruments and practice safe health measures by wearing sterile gloves and a mask. You need to ask before having any piercing done.

The ear lobe is one of the safest places to pierce because it has a good blood supply, which is crucial in case of infection. One of the highest risk areas to have pierced is the tongue. This is due to the vast amounts of bacteria in the mouth. There is a wide range of concerns about puncturing other body parts of the body as well. This is because most piercing sites have a low blood supply and don't have the ability to fight off an infection.

CHAPTER 8

Other Factors for Bacterial Overgrowth

Good Water, Bad Water

Water is necessary for optimal health, including preventing bacterial overgrowth, but is also implicated in the development of an overgrowth. Various pathogens can get into water increasing our risk of infection, but the chemicals used to remove them may also make us more vulnerable to bacteria in the long run. Recent research has also found a variety of other substances, including pharmaceuticals, contaminating the water supply. Let's take a brief look at the role water plays in our fight against pathogenic bacteria.

The Body's Need for Water

When the water within cells is fairly constant, all goes well. Water has several major functions in the body. First, it prevents toxins and chemicals from accumulating. Second, water must transport all minerals and nutrients necessary for metabolism into the cells and remove substances that damage the cell, as well as protect the protective outer membrane from damage or invasion. Next, it transfers information from one nerve cell to another. Water is involved in every function of the body. People with a greater percent of body fat have less total body water, however, and are more susceptible to fluid imbalances. The body's water percent also decreases with age.

Moreover, adequate water in the body generates negative ions. Studies have reported that ions have a pronounced effect on all life.

Research done on airborne bacteria that cause respiratory illnesses found that only a small amount of negative ions were necessary to kill these bacteria.

The chemistry of our body fluids must be balanced in order for the process of fermentation to function normally. For water to be effective in influencing health, it must contain ionized minerals required to nourish and protect cells. Because of so much contamination from our environment, minerals become depleted, resulting in disturbances in our body, increasing the process of illness and aging.

Water as a Source of Infection

Potential fluid imbalances aren't the only reason for concern. Factors for bacterial overgrowth can also be found in the water we drink. We don't always think about where the water comes from and whether it is contaminated. The following examples are possible ways to pick up harmful bacteria:

- Water is used in vast quantities in health-care premises. Many microorganisms can survive and flourish in this water and can be transferred to vulnerable hospital patients in direct (inhalation, ingestion, surface absorption) and indirect ways (instruments and utensils). Many outbreaks of infection occur because of a lack of preventative measures and ignorance about the source and transmission of opportunistic pathogens. If the main water supply is contaminated with microorganisms, they may recontaminate objects during rinsing.
- Private water supplies may be used solely for domestic purposes or on a larger scale to supply nursing homes, hospitals and houses. This includes water from a well, borehole or spring. Monitoring private supplies can be a problem since water quality can change with the weather and smaller supplies are monitored infrequently.
- Storage tanks should be protected from extraneous contamination, including bird and vermin contaminants, and should be free from bacteria, particularly E. coli. Uncontrolled water supplies are readily contaminated with bacteria.
- Holy water is a potential source of cross-infection with various bacteria. Sterile holy water is one solution.
- A number of outbreaks have been reported implicating contaminated ice machines. Coliform contamination and environmental bacteria were found in the water source.
- An outbreak of Streptococcus bacteria was traced to the communal use of bidets. Decontamination of the water spray nozzle and drain was

necessary to control the outbreak. Routine cleaning might have prevented its occurrence.

Heavy Rainfall

More than two thirds of infectious outbreaks between 1948 and 1994 were preceded by heavy rainfall according to a study (*American Journal of Public Health 2001*). This can overload municipal water systems resulting in contaminants in the drinking water supply. It seems that heavy rainfall is a good pathway for infectious agents from animal feces to be brought to the water supply. If you are in an area of high rainfall levels, it would be better to find a safe source of water during that time. You could also boil the water or use a high quality water filter.

To Drink or Not to Drink?

Just how many Americans drink water that is polluted with fecal matter, parasites, disease-causing microbes and pesticides at levels that violate the Safe Drinking Water Act standards? In *USA Today*, December 1998, it was stated that 9,500 water systems had significant violations of drinking water standards that were characterized by the EPA as serious threats to public health. Only 105 of those violations drew any enforcement action, such as fines or lawsuits, by government regulators.

Literally thousands of tons of drugs and hormones are used by people yearly to treat illnesses and depression, to prevent unwanted pregnancy and regulate PMS and menopause. Italian researchers found many of these therapeutic drugs in their drinking water and rivers, contaminating the environment. How did they get there? Experts theorize that there are drugs contained in human waste that get flushed down the toilet. Drugs may also be improperly disposed of or are part of industrial waste. There is also widespread reliance on drugs in animal farming. In fact, many of the drugs found in this study were not approved for human use.

Improper disposal of expired medications and manufacturing facilities also contribute to this contamination. Since pharmaceutical products can have long half-lives, they can accumulate and reach detectable and biologically active amounts. Many of these drugs end up in our drinking water. Several commonly used medicinal drugs can persist in the environment for more than a year, and some can persist in the environment for over twenty years. I recently asked different pharmacies what they did with expired medications. Many of them said that they flushed them down the drain. Others put them in landfills.

The concentrations of drugs measured in the water may not cause any noticeable symptoms at present, but what will the long-term effects be? Moreover, we may be exposed to medications that we would never want to take. Pregnant women and children are being exposed, as well as those potentially allergic to the medications they are exposed to. People with compromised immune systems can also suffer from exposure. Incompatible medications may be found together in the water supply, or they may be combining with other harmful contamination from pesticides, herbicides, chlorine and other toxic chemicals in our waterways. The water utilities want to add still another toxin, fluoride, to many of our drinking water systems instead of cleaning up our existing water supplies. This may have already occurred in your area. However, this excuse for drinking water can be avoided by buying a reliable water filter system that can filter out most of these substances.

Chlorinated Water

Most of us have grown up using chlorine products to whiten and disinfect. We write on paper made white by chlorine and even drink and bathe in chlorinated water. After all, who wants bacteria-infested water? However, long-term residual effects from chlorine exposure may be a health hazard. The U.S. Environmental Protection Agency (EPA) has found dioxin (a toxic byproduct of chlorine) to be much more toxic than even DDT.

Chlorine is a manufactured substance produced through an industrial process. It does not occur naturally in the environment except as a yellow gas on rare occasions. Many people think that chlorine is basically safe, but the issue is not just how toxic chlorine is, but how the byproducts of chlorine (organochlorines and dioxins) remain in the environment. They do not break down readily and continue to accumulate. One of the largest users of chlorine is the paper industry, which needs chlorine to break down the lignan that holds the wood fibers together and to bleach paper to make it white. The results of this process are in wastewater (that end up in streams and waterways where they come into contact with other organic materials and surfactants. These chemicals combine to form a host of extremely toxic organic chemicals.

The water becomes polluted, the fish become contaminated, animals eat the fish, and people eat the contaminated animals and fish. When we are exposed to these toxins, they accumulate in our fatty tissues. These contaminants are also hormone disrupters because they mimic estrogen. Now they cause hormonal imbalance, suppressed immune systems, reproductive infertility and alter fetal development. It would be hard to find any human who does not have detectable levels of dioxin.

Not only is chlorine a substantial environmental problem caused by the paper industry, it is also in household bleach and cleaners. Chlorine is a respiratory irritant and when mixed with other common household products, it gives off a toxic gas. One example of chlorine's toxicity is the number of calls to the Poison Control Center concerning household cleaners. It is estimated that more than 28 percent of all calls are related to poisonings by chlorine products, and the victims are usually under the age of six. Our bodies can metabolize many things, even many environmental toxic substances that we are exposed to daily. Unfortunately, dioxins and other organochlorine compounds are not some of them. Even low levels of dioxins remain in the body and continue to accumulate.

It is very important that our water is sanitized, but there are alternatives to chlorine. Chlorine is used because it is effective at killing organisms, it is cheap, and it does not break down. There are other substances that are good sanitizers, but they break down quickly. So by the time the water reaches someone's home, it is contaminated. The ultimate solution may be to have home-based water filtration/sanitizing systems, which would eliminate the problem of trying to prevent water contamination caused by hundreds of miles of pipes installed many years ago.

There are other facts about chlorine that you should also be aware of. For instance, when you open the door of your dishwasher after washing, toxic volatized chlorine from dish detergent and tap water is released into the air. Thanks to chlorine pollution, Americans ingest a daily amount of dioxin that is already three to six hundred times greater than the EPA's so-called "safe" dose. Studies also show that 40 to 70 percent of the dioxin in bleached coffee filters is leached into coffee; dioxin found in paper milk cartons also leaches into the milk. Chlorine found in many household products such as coffee filters, disposable diapers, paper towels, and bathroom tissue are also readily absorbed through the skin. Sucralose is suppose to be the safe replacement for Nutrasweet, but Sucralose is basically chlorinated table sugar, and it may have many of the safe risks as chlorine. Chlorinated swimming pools are another way to be exposed to chlorine, especially for those of you who swim regularly.

Hydrogen peroxide is available to both the paper and soap industries as a bleaching agent. Another new technology is the use of ozone. Other non-chlorinated household cleaning products, readily available to the consumer, achieve the same bleaching and disinfecting results as chlorine, but are nontoxic.

Chlorine alternatives such as hydrogen peroxide (Baquacil) and ozone are not toxic. Part of being healthy is cleaning up our environment so we will not be exposed to toxic materials. One way of doing this is to purchase chlorine-free products. We do not need to continue to use harmful substances simply because we have used them up to this point. New technology allows us to make better choices and replace many of these toxic ingredients with products that are nontoxic. Your buying choices make a difference.

Fluoride in the Water

Chlorine isn't the only harmful substance in water, however. For some of us, fluoride has become a part of the water supply as well. Before World War II, there was not any U.S. commercial production of fluorine. What prompted its manufacture was the processing of uranium ores needed for the atomic bomb. Fluorine compounds, or fluorides, are listed by the U.S. Agency for Toxic Substances and Disease Registry as among the top twenty of 275 substances ranked as the most significant threats to human health. In Australia, the National Pollutant Inventory ranked fluoride as high as twenty-seventh out of 208, based on its ability to be a health and environmental hazard.

Fluoride reacts with hydrogen in drinking water to form hydrofluoric acid bonds that are extremely dangerous and can affect the immune system. Much is known about the harmful effects of fluoride, but that has not stopped it from being put into the drinking water of many towns and cities. In India and some other countries, high levels of naturally-occurring water fluoride is linked to a condition called crippling skeletal fluorosis, a bone-deforming arthritic disease. In my book, *Natural Treatments for ADD and Hyperactivity,* I also discuss the link between the use of fluoride and attention deficit/hyperactivity disorder. Anyone who wants to be healthy should avoid fluoride.

What about preventing cavities? One Canadian study found that residents of fluoridated Toronto have double the fluoride in their hipbones compared to residents of non-fluoridated Montreal. (Toronto has been fluoridating for thirty-six years.) Yet Montreal has never fluoridated and has a cavity rate lower than Toronto's. The truth, now becoming increasingly evident, is that fluoridation and the proclaimed benefit of fluoride as a way of preventing dental decay is one of the greatest frauds ever perpetrated upon an unsuspecting public.

Fluorides are cumulative toxins. The fact that fluorides accumulate in the body is the reason that U.S. law requires the Surgeon General to set a maximum contaminant level for fluoride content in public water supplies as determined by the EPA. This requirement is specifically aimed at avoiding the previously mentioned condition known as crippling skeletal fluorosis, a disease thought to progress through three stages. The EPA maximum level is designed to prevent only the third and crippling stage of this disease and is set at 4 ppm or 4 mg per liter. It is assumed that people will retain only half of this amount (2 mg), and therefore 4 mg per liter is considered safe.

In 1998 EPA scientists, whose job and legal duty was to set the maximum contaminant level, declared that this 4 ppm level was set fraudulently by outside forces in a decision that omitted 90 percent of the data showing the mutagenic properties of fluoride.

The truth is that more evidence shows that fluorides and dental fluorosis are actually associated with increased tooth decay. The most comprehensive U.S. review was carried out by the National Institute of Dental Research on 39,000 school children aged five to seventeen years. What it did show was that children who drink fluoridated water had almost 10 percent more decay.

Currently, up to 80 percent of U.S. children suffer from some degree of dental fluorosis, while in Canada the figure is up to 71 percent. Before the push for fluoridation began, the dental profession recognized that fluorides were not beneficial but detrimental to dental health. In 1944, the *Journal of the American Dental Association* reported, "With 1.6 to 4 ppm fluoride in the water, 50 percent or more past age twenty-four have false teeth because of fluoride damage to their own."

Ireland is considering changing its laws that require the fluoridation of all drinking water. This is due to mounting controversy and growing public concern over the possible health risks. If Ireland does decide to change its fluoridation practices, it will not be alone. Sweden, Norway, Denmark and Finland banned water fluoridation during the 1970s and 1980s because not enough was known about the long-term health effects. Germany rejected the practice in 1975 as "foreign to nature, unnecessary, inefficient, irresponsible and harmful to the environment." A year later, the Dutch rewrote their constitution to outlaw fluoridation. Moreover, France's chief of public health declared in 1980 that fluoridation was "too dangerous."

The overuse of fluoride-containing toothpaste or other sources of fluoride in very young children can be quite detrimental and cause a condition known as "dental fluorosis." Dental fluorosis is a condition characterized mainly by an unsightly discoloration of the teeth, which starts as white spots. The bones and virtually every organ might also be affected due to fluoride's ability to accumulate in the body, and its known anti-thyroid characteristics. Dental fluorosis occurs during the stage of enamel formation and is therefore a sign that an overdose of fluoride has occurred in a child during that period.

The condition is particularly a problem in children under age six, whose permanent teeth are developing even though they have not yet erupted through the gums. Children who live in areas with non-fluoridated drinking water can get fluorosis from fluoride supplements or brushing more than once a day with fluoride toothpaste, especially in the first two years of life when their teeth are developing.

One example of this involved a child who had been using fluoride toothpaste since the age of eighteen months. Her mother always observed the tooth washing and never let her daughter use more than the recommended pea-size amount of toothpaste. Yet, at the age of nine, the child began having leg pains, flu-like symptoms and constant headaches. Her condition was not diagnosed until one astute doctor noticed that her teeth were mottled brown. The family lived in an area that did not have fluoridated water, so the condition known as "dental fluorosis" had to come from the toothpaste.

Subsequent tests revealed high levels of fluoride in the child's system. Soon after she stopped using the toothpaste, her symptoms disappeared. Now, she only has these problems when visiting areas where the water is fluoridated. It is important to take serious the warning on fluoridated toothpaste against accidental ingestion. The problem with small children is that they tend to swallow everything that goes into their mouths.

The use of professional dental applications of fluoride may not be providing any benefit to children either, even though they are widely used and generally accepted to reduce the rate of tooth decay. During a period averaging around five years, over 15,000 children were studied along with the treatment provided by 1,500 different dentists. Differences in tooth decay rates were not seen for either baby teeth or permanent teeth. Even the *Journal of the American Dental Association* (2000) stated that fluoride does not reduce cavities. So why do dentists continue to apply fluoride to people's teeth? Financial profits are probably the main reason.

There are already numerous recommendations that dentist-applied topical fluorides should be used only in children with moderate to high rates of decay. It is doubtful that these guidelines are being followed when approximately two-thirds of the children in a study received topical fluoride at every recall visit, nearly two times per year. The American Dental Association still recommends fluoride supplements for children six months to sixteen years old in non- or low-fluoridated communities. They continue to cling to this outmoded idea and are failing to protect our children from fluoride poisoning.

New research shows that swallowed fluoride carries little, if any, benefit. Fluoride's adverse effects occur upon ingestion by getting into every cell of the body. Half of all ingested fluoride remains in the skeletal system and accumulates with age. Several studies have linked fluoridation to an increase in hip fractures. Yet in 1999, the U.S. Center for Disease Control (CDC) released a glowing report on the fluoridation of public water supplies, citing the procedure as one of the century's great public health successes. However, the same report hints that the benefit of fluorides may not be due to ingestion. In fact, the CDC report acknowledges new studies which indicate that the effects are topical rather than systemic. How can the CDC consider the addition of fluoride to public water supplies to be a public health success while admitting at the same time that fluoride's benefits are not systemic, or in other words, are not obtained from drinking it? Other laboratory and epidemiologic research suggests that fluoride prevents dental cavities predominately after eruption of the tooth into the mouth, and its actions primarily are topical for both adults and children.

The relentless promotion of fluoride as a dental benefit does not make the unsuspecting public demand the proper assessment of its toxicity, despite the fact that this substance may be contributing to many diseases—particularly those involving thyroid dysfunction. In the United States, most people are kept entirely ignorant of any adverse effect that might occur from exposure to fluorides, which can come from many different sources:

- Food products and beverages coming from fluoridated cities
- Fluoridated dental products
- Fluoride-containing pesticide residues in food
- Industrial fluoride air emissions
- Some medicines such as Prozac, anesthetics and other medical products
- Showers and humidifiers if using fluoridated water
- Some foods such as tea where it is found naturally
- The interaction of fluoride with aluminum cookware

Decision-makers at 3M Corporation recently announced a phase-out of some Scotchgard products after discovering that the product's primary ingredient was a fluorinated compound. 3M's research showed that the substance had strong tendencies to persist and accumulate in animal and human tissue.

In addition, fluoride content in tea has risen dramatically over the last twenty years due to industry contamination. The aluminum content was also high. The longer a tea bag steeps the more fluoride and aluminum is released. After ten minutes, the measurable amounts of fluoride and aluminum almost double. Next to water, tea is the most widely consumed beverage in the world, and it can be found in almost 80 percent of all U.S. households. On any given day, nearly 127 million Americans drink tea. The high content of both aluminum and fluoride in tea is a cause for great concern as aluminum greatly potentiates fluoride's effects on protein activation, cell communication and thyroid hormone function and regulation.

Every year hundreds and thousands of tons of industry fluorides are also emitted. Industrial emissions of fluoride compounds produce elevated concentrations of the toxin in the atmosphere. Hydrogen fluoride can exist as a particle, dissolving in clouds, fog, rain, dew or snow. In clouds and moist air, it will travel along the air currents until it is deposited as acid rain or acid fog. In waterways, it readily mixes with water.

Even more disturbing is the fact that 90 percent of the fluoride we use to fluoridate U.S. drinking water systems comes directly from the phosphate fertilizer industry. The fluorides used to fluoridate drinking water are mostly silicofluorides, which contain trace amounts of arsenic, mercury and lead and have never been safety tested in humans or animals. Fluoridation supporters claim that these heavy metals are so diluted that they do not pose a threat. However, in 2000, the EPA Assistant Administrator, Charles Fox, said "there are no water quality criteria for fluoride either for the protection of aquatic life or for the protection of human health."

There has been long-held suspicion that fluoride has the ability to act synergistically with other toxic minerals in drinking water such as aluminum. Aluminum sulfate (alum) is used to clarify drinking water. In 1994, the *New York Times* reported a scientific study which revealed that aluminum and fluoride in water could be responsible for the alarming increase in Alzheimer's disease and dementia. In 1999, the U.S. Environmental Protection Agency confirmed kidney and brain damage in rats exposed to less aluminum fluoride than what is added to drinking water.

A report by the National Institutes of Environmental Heath Sciences acknowledged that fluoride has been observed to have synergistic effects on the toxicity of aluminum. Most water treatment systems result in increased levels of aluminum in the finished drinking water. They stated that fluoridation will result in aluminum fluoride complexes that can enhance neurotoxicity, or that fluoride itself will enhance the uptake of aluminum. Other studies have shown that in the presence of fluoride, aluminum leaches out of cookware. Using non-fluoridated water showed almost no leaching from aluminum pans.

The incidence of Alzheimer's disease and Alzheimer's-like dementia is hitting people at much younger ages. The average age used to be sixty-five or older, but now it is affecting more people in their forties. (About 160 million people in the United States drink artificially fluoridated water.)

Several years ago, fluoride was found to induce genetic interference. Could this be implicated in the development of neurological disorders such as autism? While this is unproven, it is biologically possible. A review in *Nature* describes fluoride's potential as "sculpting the developing brain." Fluoride's effects on the brain need to be determined if we allow children to be subjected to the potential risk of water fluoridation (*British Medical Journal* July 2001).

The National Sanitation Foundation International reported that the most common contaminant detected was arsenic, and it occurred five times more frequently than any other contaminant, and well above allowable levels for water treatment chemicals. The EPA's fifty parts per billion (ppb) arsenic standard could account for one cancer in every one hundred people who drink two liters of water a day. The Natural Resources Defense Council wants the levels reduced to 3 ppb. They stated that even at this reduced level, there is still a higher risk than traditionally accepted in drinking water. Yet in an unexpected and disturbing move, President Bush ordered the EPA to rescind the Clinton Administration's decision to lower arsenic levels to the prevailing world standard for safety.

Even if you avoid using fluoride, you still need to practice good dental hygiene. There are excellent non-fluoride toothpaste carried in most health food stores. A healthy diet is still the most important way of preventing cavities. Reducing your intake of sugar and processed foods is also important.

If you are not yet convinced of the need to avoid fluoride, I would suggest doing a little research of your own about its harmful effects. There are literally thousands of pages documenting the problems with fluoride and the reasons to eliminate it. The Fluoride Action Network has great articles about the relationship between fluoride and hip fractures, as well as many other articles from around the world. For more on the cover-up of the source of the materials used to fluoridate drinking water check online at www.fluoridealert.org and www.nrdc.org.

Andreas Schuld is head of Parents of Fluoride Poisoned Children, an organization of parents whose children have been poisoned by excessive fluoride intake. The group includes educators, artists, scientists, journalists, authors, lawyers, researchers and nutritionists. It is active in worldwide efforts to have the toxicity of fluoride properly assessed. For further information, visit their website at www.bruha.com/fluoride.

Bottled Water

To avoid the dangers of tap water, many people have turned to drinking bottle water. However, there is little assurance that this water is any safer than tap water and may even be worse. Approximately 60 to 70 percent of bottled water sold in the U.S. is completely exempt from FDA rules because it is packaged and sold within the same state. Drinking water sold from vending machines commonly found outside supermarkets often contains dramatically higher levels of bacteria than typical tap water, according to a Los Angeles County study. Some of the facts reported include:

- 93 percent of the machines tested had bacterial levels up to 163 times as high as in domestic tap water.
- 38 percent of the machines failed to remove common organic compounds as required by the state.
- 25 to 40 percent of bottled water is derived from tap water sometimes with additional processing, sometimes not.
- One brand labeled "Spring Water" came from an industrial facility near a hazardous waste dump.
- About one-third of bottled water tested contained significant levels of chemical and bacterial contaminants.

Furthermore, a new study by the World Wildlife Fund, a conservation organization, is urging people not to use water from plastic containers for the benefit of the environment. Every year 1.5 million tons of plastic is used to bottle water. According to the study, bottled water may not be safer than tap water in many countries, but sells for up to one thousand times the price. It is the fastest growing drink industry in the world and is estimated to be worth $22 billion each year. Bottled water is portrayed as being drawn from pristine sources and as being healthier than tap water. In many cases, the only difference is that one is put in bottles rather than coming through pipes. Actually there are more standards regulating tap water in Europe and the U.S. than those applied to bottled water.

Additionally, toxic chemicals are released during the manufacture, disposal and transportation of the bottles. Bottled water does not address long-term sustainable solutions concerning healthy drinking water. Clean water should be a major priority. It is important to protect our rivers, streams and wetlands to ensure that tap water is delivered to us in the healthiest form possible at a reasonable price. The best solution is to add a reverse-osmosis water filter that will also remove most of the undesirable chemicals added to drinking water. The next best choice is probably the Culligan filter, which is available at an inexpensive price. For more information on water filters, see my book *The Parasite Menace.*

Heavy Metals

As discussed to some degree in the last section, toxic heavy metals are being found in elevated levels in critical tissues and organs throughout our bodies. We all get too much mercury both from silver amalgam fillings and even from some of the fish we eat. As we age, not only do we accumulate a heavy metal burden, we also become more susceptible to their toxic effects. Despite this, the U.S. does not have any regulations that limit the amount of heavy metals permitted in fertilizers. Industries are using this loophole to recycle these toxic wastes. Fertilizers may contain cadmium, lead, arsenic, dioxins and other waste products that come from mining, smelting, cement kilns, wood product industries and medical and municipal incinerators. This recycling saves money for industry and conserves space in hazardous waste landfills, but at our expense.

Consider the following excerpt from an *Associated Press* articlefrom July 1997: "A dark powder from two Oregon steel mills is poured from rail cars into silos at Bay Zinc Company in the state of Washington under a federal hazardous waste storage permit. Then it is emptied from the silos for use as fertilizer." When it goes into the silo, it is hazardous waste, but when it comes out of the silo, it is no longer regulated. Yet it is exactly the same material. In response to this and other articles, the state of Washington is finally testing fertilizer products for toxicity to crops, livestock and people. Their state legislature is considering stopping toxic metal content in fertilizers, but what about your state?

To combat these potential health hazards, many people are buying organic foods and supplements from health food stores. However, just because a product is sold in a health food store does not mean it is entirely safe. Information obtained from a variety of these so-called "healthy" products reveals that all of the colloidal liquid mineral products tested contained too many toxic minerals. These included mercury, lead, arsenic, cadmium and aluminum. Most of them did not contain enough of the beneficial minerals to offset their toxicity problems. The bottom line? Save your money and do not spend it on overpriced colloidal liquid mineral products with questionable contents.

Although I cannot possibly cover all of the available information on heavy metals, I do want to convey to you their dangers. Heavy metals are linked to immune suppression and bacteria resistance. Many heavy metals also play a role in the overgrowth of intestinal pathogens. In addition, many people have an excess of more than one type of heavy metal in their body. The following is a list of potential heavy metals and just some of the reasons to avoid these substances:

ALUMINUM

There may be widespread contamination of aluminum on commercially grown food, including some organic food. The testing for organic certification is for labeled herbicides and pesticides, not aluminum content. The contamination of our food crops and livestock is spreading throughout this country and into our food system, but the reason for this is still unknown.

Back in 1989, a Texas farmer named Rocky Williams noticed there was something wrong with his land's vegetation and wildlife. He was growing organic grain on his eight hundred acres, but after four to six weeks of growing, the grain sorghum and hay yellowed and became stunted, as if some material had been applied to the crops. What made this even more unusual was that the damage was random and in forty to fifty foot wide strips, as if some material had been sprayed by air.

The Texas Department of Agriculture and USDA officials refused to investigate. So he sent crop samples to a private lab and was told that the problem appeared to be aluminum toxicity. Usually, plants have concentrations of ten to twenty parts per million (ppm) of aluminum in their tissue. Vegetables that Williams tested contained 350–3,500 ppm of aluminum. Crop samples that were taken from areas in New Mexico, central Texas, Oklahoma and Kansas also showed high levels of aluminum that ranged from 350–3500 ppm. Williams claimed to have evidence that this contamination occurred in forty states.

COPPER

Copper toxicity may be the scourge of the century. It is one of the most commonly encountered imbalances found on mineral tests today. Copper directly and indirectly affects virtually every body system with many bodily dysfunctions related in some way to copper toxicity. For instance, copper interferes with adrenal and thyroid gland activity, creating symptoms relating to low thyroid function and adrenal insufficiency. Moreover, it can take six months to several years to correct a copper imbalance depending on the severity of the imbalance.

Zinc is important to maintaining a healthy immune system, but there is a widespread deficiency of this mineral in the U.S. population. Since zinc and copper normally exist in a delicate balance, when zinc is deficient, copper tends to accumulate in various storage organs. Zinc deficiencies are often due to chronic stress and a high sugar and carbohydrate diet. If copper levels continue to elevate, they depress zinc levels even more. Many children today are born deficient in zinc because their mothers are also deficient. Refining foods also removes zinc.

Many diets are high in copper and low in zinc, especially vegetarians eating excessive soybeans, nuts, seeds, tofu, avocados and some grains. Fast food hamburgers and many popular foods are soy-based. Soybean protein is being used in a wider range of foods today. Other high copper foods are organ meats, shellfish, wheat germ and bran, yeast, corn oil, margarine and mushrooms. Individuals with a copper toxicity frequently have an aversion to eating red meat. The irony is that they are likely to become vegetarian and begin eating the very foods that are high in copper. Many such people have an insatiable craving for sweets, fruit and fruit juices.

Copper plumbing is also a source of copper toxicity. It was thought to be a great advance in the 1940s and still exists in many homes today. Water coolers and icemakers in refrigerators often use copper tubing as well. Water sits in these units accumulating toxic levels of copper. Additionally, copper cookware and teakettles can be a source of copper toxicity, if used frequently. Copper is frequently added to vitamin supplements, particularly to prenatal vitamins. This can be harmful for some women who already have elevated copper levels. In fact, one side effect of birth control pills is that they tend to raise copper levels in the body.

Some areas of the U.S. have high amounts of naturally occurring copper in the water supply. Copper sulfate is added to some municipal drinking water supplies to kill yeast and fungi. Copper sulfate is added to swimming pools and may be sprayed on fruits and vegetables to retard algae and fungus.

IRON

There are many disease-causing bacteria that feed on excessive iron in the body. Unfortunately, many people have dangerously elevated levels of iron because they have mistakenly been taking too many vitamin and mineral supplements which contain iron. Having elevated iron levels is as dangerous as having elevated levels of lead. If you are not anemic, you should not be taking iron supplements.

MERCURY

Mercury amalgams influence the immune system and can increase mercury resistance in the bacterial microflora of the mouth. The World

Health Organization reported in 1991 that dental amalgams constitute the major human exposure to mercury. The level of mercury in the blood and urine correlated with the number of amalgam fillings. This was confirmed by a recently published study funded by the National Institutes of Health. However, the dental branch of the FDA stills refuses to investigate the toxic potential of dental mercury. Since mercury is a well-known and potent brain toxin, it is possible that it could cause or make worse neurological disorders, including Parkinson's, ALS (amyotrophic lateral sclerosis), MS (multiple sclerosis) and autism. Mercury toxicity also has the potential to cause kidney dysfunction.

The American Dental Association continues to remain in denial about the toxicity of mercury. But according to the *Associated Press*, a coalition of public interest groups sued the American Dental Association and the California Dental Association recently in Los Angeles Superior Court, claiming they misled the public about the dangers of mercury in tooth fillings. The lawsuit also alleges that these organizations prevent dentists from discussing the dangers of mercury with their patients. They also asked the court to stop them from referring to fillings as silver amalgams when they have equal parts mercury.

There is also a form of mercury that is even more toxic to the nervous system than the vapor or liquid forms. It is called methyl mercury. It requires specific bacteria to convert mercury into methyl mercury. There are many commonly occurring strains of bacteria that can hook methyl groups to mercury in a process called methylation. Where do these bacteria live? There are several species of bacteria in the mouth, as well as a dozen different bacteria in the intestinal tract that can methylate mercury, including *Streptococcus, Staphylococcus, E. coli, Lactobacillus, Bacteroides* and even some yeast. Another interesting thing about these methylating bacteria is that they can both methylate and de-methylate depending on the chemistry of the intestinal contents.

Although the amount of toxic mercury that the body accumulates is more likely to come from amalgams than from fish, caution is still needed when buying and eating fish, especially for pregnant and nursing women and small children. Women who eat a lot of ocean fish during pregnancy or even a small amount of highly contaminated fish can expose their developing fetus to the toxic effects of mercury.

The mercury crosses the placenta to harm the developing nervous system, including the brain. This accumulation of mercury has been linked to an increased risk for nerve damage, birth defects, psychomotor retardation and even cerebral palsy, especially in children whose mothers consumed large amounts of mercury-contaminated fish or grain during pregnancy. Even the government is taking this seriously and has issued warnings for pregnant women. It is thought that about

10 percent of pregnant women (about seven million women) have levels above those considered safe for a developing fetus. If you do eat fish, consider chlorella supplementation to bind the mercury in the fish instead of allowing it to be absorbed into your system.

The mercury that gets into fish is largely due to power plants that burn coal for generating electricity. These plants pollute the air with 80,000 pounds of mercury per year before it is deposited into the ocean where it continues to accumulate in fish that are higher up the food chain. These power plants are the largest man-made source of environmental mercury and are currently completely unregulated. Federal decision-makers should require power plants to significantly reduce their mercury pollution and ultimately move away from polluting sources of power.

There are major variations in mercury contamination across fish species, so it is hard to know just how much mercury exposure there is. During 2001, the FDA came up with its own list of fish that pregnant and nursing women, or women considering pregnancy should avoid, but it may not be totally accurate. This list of fish includes: tuna steaks, sea bass, oysters from the Gulf of Mexico, marlin, halibut, pike, walleye, white croaker, shark, swordfish, tilefish, king mackerel and largemouth bass. Not every serving of any of these fish is contaminated with dangerous levels of methylmercury, but the odds are greater that consumption of a single meal of these fish will expose a fetus to a potentially hazardous amount.

The worst offenders are large predatory fish such as swordfish, shark and large species of tuna that are used mostly for fresh steaks or sushi. Still others are mahi mahi, blue mussels, eastern oyster, Atlantic cod, pollock, salmon from the Great Lakes, blue crab from the Gulf of Mexico, wild channel catfish and lake whitefish. It is impossible to evaluate the risk from every recreational fish caught, but since many of the large predator sport fish are so universally contaminated with mercury, they should be added to the list of fish to avoid during pregnancy. The smaller species of tuna typically used for canning, such as skipjack and albacore, have much lower levels of mercury.

The FDA needs to expand its methylmercury sampling program to include a host of fish where the data indicates that pregnant women and their babies could receive a potentially unsafe exposure from a relatively small amount of fish. These include: orange roughy, bluefish, Pacific cod, bonito, porgy, yellowtail, rockfish, Dover sole, lake trout, grouper, sand perch, red snapper, white perch and flounder.

A major flaw in FDA's system is the agency's own lack of comprehensive data on methylmercury in fish. In January 2001, the FDA recommended that pregnant women avoid consumption of king mackerel based on methylmercury levels from a study published in 1979. There are many other species where the data on methylmercury contamination are similarly outdated, but where the available information indicates a potential problem.

Different government agencies recommend different fish and different amounts to eat. I believe it would be best not to eat more than one meal a month for all species of fish, even though the FDA suggests eating twelve ounces a week of any kind of fish. Those considered safer to eat during pregnancy are: farmed trout, farmed catfish, farmed shrimp, fish sticks, summer flounder, wild Pacific salmon, blue crab from the mid Atlantic, croaker, sardines, freshwater sport fish and haddock. (Exclude shellfish and fish without scales (catfish) if you want an even safer diet.)

Eating farm-raised fish is not necessarily healthier, including farmed salmon. Salmon are usually fed grains such as corn and soy and cannot form the beneficial omega-3 fatty acids so important to our health. Farm-raised fish may also be exposed to high pesticide levels because of agricultural run-off or from grains that are heavily sprayed.

You may be surprised that most of the available salmon and other fish in grocery stores and at restaurants are from fish farms. Fish farmers are beginning to branch out into new species such as sea bass, tuna, cod and halibut. Some grocery stores offer both farmed and wild fish. Usually, the wild variety will be more expensive. The word "Atlantic" on the package of fish does not usually describe where the fish came from, but is instead the variety of fish.

Another source of mercury may surprise you. It has been found in vaccines commonly given to children. Immunizations for *Haemophilus influenzae* type b, hepatitis B, diphtheria, tetanus and pertussis have been a source of controversy in recent years because of the use of thimerosal, a preservative containing mercury. Without us knowing this, thimerosal has been used since the 1930s. At the highest risk from exposure are pregnant women and fetuses. With an increased number of vaccinations combined with a sharp rise in reported autism and ADHD cases, some parents and physicians are finally questioning the safety of the inoculations.

The United Kingdom's *Sunday Times* reported that the World Health Organization has launched an investigation into a possible link between vaccines that contain mercury and a rise in the incidence of autism among children in Britain. The project aims to check for a link between the use of vaccines that contain the preservative thimerosal, which is almost 50 percent mercury (also known as ethylmercury), and a range of neurodevelopmental disorders, including autism. Thimerosal is now hypothesised to carry risks similar to methylmercury. Dr. John

Clements, of the WHO immunization program, is quoted as saying: "We have permitted the use of thimerosal in vaccines for many years as an essential preservative in multi-dose vials. The study is to see if there is any evidence of a negative effect."

The newspaper reported speculations that an accumulation of mercury may damage the brain, central nervous system and gastrointestinal tract, as well as lower the functioning of children's immune systems so they cannot cope with the combination measles, mumps and rubella vaccine, possibly triggering autism. It also said that in 1999 the U.S. Food and Drug Administration revealed that the amount of mercury intake from vaccinations in some babies during their first six months may have exceeded the limit set by the Environmental Protection Agency. As a result, the FDA and the European Agency for the Evaluation of Medicinal Products said thiomersal is being phased out of vaccines.

According to the medical journal *Lancet* (July 2001), persistent concern about the safety of vaccinations prompted the U.S. National Academy of Sciences Institute of Medicine to review the evidence for an association between thimerosal and neurodevelopmental outcomes, particularly autism. In June of 1999, the American Academy of Pediatrics and the U.S. Public Health Service, acknowledging that mercury exposure from vaccinations given in the first six months of life exceeded maximum acceptable levels established in federal guidelines, called for a halt to the manufacture of thimerosal-containing vaccines. Although no longer routinely given in the USA, they are still the norm in many other parts of the world, especially in developing countries where using multi-dose vials is less expensive.

TESTING FOR HEAVY METALS

There are several ways to test for heavy metal toxicity. None of them are one hundred percent conclusive, but some of them can offer valuable information. These tests include hair analysis, red blood cell mineral levels, blood and serum levels, and provocative testing. When evaluating results using hair, however, you need to rule out external contamination.

Ways to Reduce Heavy Metal Toxicity

- Review your diet to make sure that it is rich in minerals and does not contain sources of heavy metals.
- Look at your water source, since water can be contaminated with

heavy metals. It may be time to purchase a water filter system that filters them out.

- Look at your exposure from household products. Review your hobbies, occupational activities, and surroundings to see if they could be hiding heavy metals.
- If you have mercury amalgams, a biologically oriented dentist needs to evaluate the state of the amalgams and the potential for removal. Removing fillings can be a costly procedure. The benefits and risks should be carefully evaluated before taking this step. It is important to consult a dentist who has been trained in this procedure and has the appropriate equipment.

Travel

There are approximately one billion airline trips per year, and nearly fifty million travelers venture from industrialized countries to underdeveloped nations. Many of these travelers will develop some type of illness, and about 1 to 5 percent will seek medical attention. More than half of these travelers will lose three of their average fourteen days of travel because of illness.

In many countries, there are deteriorating public-health infrastructures and higher population densities with unsanitary conditions. There has also been a rise in people living with organ transplants or diseases that compromise their immune systems such as AIDS, cancer and diabetes. This creates an environment for the growth of disease-causing bacteria. With an increase in international travel, these organisms are being brought back home. Plus, more food is being shipped internationally, transporting dangerous organisms around the world.

TRAVELER'S DIARRHEA

The most common cause of travel-related illness worldwide is diarrhea, and the most likely pathogen is *Escherichia coli*, or as we have come to know it, *E. coli*. There are also some important regional differences. For example, *Campylobacter jejuni* diarrhea is an important issue in Southeast Asia, *Vibrio parahaemolyticus* accounts for a significant portion of infectious diarrhea in Japan, and the parasites, giardia and *Cryptosporidium*, are common in Leningrad. Typically, bacterial pathogens causing travel-related diarrhea require a large number of organisms to produce symptoms. Fewer organisms may be required in individuals who use antacids or are immune compromised. The exceptions to this are cysts of parasites, where as few as one to ten organisms are required to produce symptoms. There are also some very virulent strains of bacteria that cause symptoms even in low numbers, such as *Shigella*.

If your diarrhea is persistent, the more likely cause is the bacteria *Clostridium difficile* or the overgrowth of some other bacteria. Of course, it could be parasites. Many of these organisms, such as *Campylobacter* strains in Thailand, are now becoming resistant to drugs. When traveling, I can't stress the importance of one of the most effective preventive strategies: the "boil it, peel it, cook it or forget it" philosophy.

To keep from getting travelers' diarrhea greater precautions need to be taken. In a survey of more than 30,000 short-term visitors to Jamaica, it was found that tourists who decided to have an all-inclusive vacation package that included all meals and beverages, had higher rates of diarrhea than tourists who planned their own agenda and did not use the all-inclusive vacations packages, which include buffets. It is highly probable that meals served buffet style put people at a higher risk for food poisoning.

Diarrhea was also significantly higher during the summer months of May to October. The majority of the people who had symptoms allowed ice cubes made with tap water in their drinks, ate raw foods such as salads, consumed dairy products or tap water, and ate incompletely cooked hamburgers, chicken, lobster or shrimp. Travelers need to be more aware of high-risk foods and drinks. For more information on travelers' diarrhea refer to Section 3.

AIRLINE FOOD POISONING

Some incidents of poisoning occur before travelers even land. During the past, there have been warning letters sent to a number of airlines saying that they need to make some corrections in the way their food is handled. Most airlines serve food prepared by catering services. The FDA says that an inspection at the Sky Chef kitchen at Denver International Airport revealed that employees were observed touching their mouths, foreheads and noses, then continuing to work without washing hands or changing gloves. One example in 1993 involved forty-seven passengers aboard a flight from Charlotte, N.C. who suffered a bout of *E. coli* infection from a contaminated salad prepared by an airline caterer.

There have also been concerns about inadequate refrigeration used on board airplanes. A citation was sent to one airline indicating that chicken filets were being kept at a temperature of about 62°F, nearly twenty degrees above the regulatory limit. The FDA also complained that a turkey sandwich on the same flight was also stored at an unsafe temperature.

DO AIRLINES SPREAD DISEASE?

The death of a thirty-two-year-old woman from tuberculosis a few years ago gave health officials particular cause for alarm. Just weeks before, while highly contagious, she flew on a commercial airliner from Hawaii to Baltimore, via Chicago, and back. Even more worrisome, the woman had a virulent form of TB that cannot be killed by the usual antibiotics.

Six other travelers tested positive soon after the flight. All six of the infected travelers sat near the woman on the last portion of her flight. No one in the front of the plane seemed to have been infected, suggesting that the recirculated air was free of the tuberculosis bacteria. The TB picked up by the passengers presumably lingered in the air around the sick woman long enough to be breathed in by those near her. Measles and influenza germs can also linger in the air this way.

Does this suggest that diseases spread easily aboard airplanes or not? Air quality on planes has improved dramatically since the late 1980s, after smoking was banned. Dr. Jon Jordan, who leads medical programs at the Federal Aviation Administration, says that the air filters on most planes are fine enough to trap bacteria and even clumps of viruses. Cabin air is exchanged completely at least ten times an hour, more than in most office buildings. Ventilation systems also bring in high-altitude air that is cleaner than what we breathe closer to the ground. Intake through the jet engines heats the air to germ-killing temperatures. To save money on cooling, airlines in recent years converted to half-fresh air and half-recirculated air, raising the question of whether germs recirculate too.

If the air in a plane is so clean, why do many of us feel crummy after we fly? Ironically, it is probably because of the very mechanisms that keep the air clean. Although the intake air is very dry, airlines choose not to add moisture, in order to keep the air as free as possible of the microbes that infest the humidifying devices. Prolonged exposure to dry air can make you feel dreadful. You can end up feeling headachy and lightheaded, with burning eyes, dry mouth and a scratchy throat. Even with the frequent air exchanges, a crowded plane also has relatively high levels of carbon dioxide that can make you feel congested.

Compounding the problem are the sudden pressure changes associated with air travel, especially likely to cause ear problems in young children and in adults with colds. Then there is the fatigue, anxiety and general stress associated with the trip. All of this can certainly depress your immune system and make you at risk for the next bug that comes along.

Should you worry about catching an illness as grave as tuberculosis aboard an aircraft? Just to play it safe, take a supplement that enhances

The Military Link

Our military's role in policing the world also makes them susceptible to many diseases. We are beginning to see more diseases being brought back to this country. For instance, there were only 147 U.S. casualties listed from the Gulf War, but over 60,000 of the 700,000 troops deployed have shown up for treatment at the Veteran's hospitals. Our Defense Department has refused to acknowledge Gulf War Syndrome as a disease. Yet how many of these soldiers have families that also became sick with the same illness? There are reports that babies born to these families have many medical problems.

In 1996, 77 percent of the freshman class at the U.S. Merchant Marine Academy was diagnosed with pneumonia caused by a strain of *Mycoplasma*. Four years ago, the USS Arkansas sailed into San Diego harbor with the commanding officer and most of its crew incapacitated by influenza. Ninety-nine percent of them had been vaccinated against the flu, but they encountered a new strain in the South Pacific and brought it back to our shores. With so much close contact, military populations create tremendous opportunity for pathogens. Moreover, clothing worn by veterans of the Gulf War is still being sold in Army/Navy surplus outlets. Could disease-causing bacteria still be affecting people who are wearing these clothes today?

your immune system before, during and for a few days after flying, especially when going long distances. It is not just the air on the plane that is of concern, but being exposed to so many potentially sick people in airports. Drink plenty of water before, during and after the flight as well; avoid alcohol and sugar; and try not to fly if you have an upper respiratory infection or any other illness that is contagious.

Medicines and Supplements

BLUE-GREEN ALGAE

Cyanobacteria have shown up in stool cultures of the people who regularly consume blue-green algae. People with a history of dysbiosis should avoid blue-green algae products. A safer alternative source would be the other various kinds of sea kelp and marine algae.

IRON SUPPLEMENTS ATTRACT BACTERIA

As mentioned earlier, iron is unique among essential minerals because it is hard to get rid of it once absorbed into the body. Whatever iron is absorbed must either be used or stored. Excessive storage of iron in the body promotes the generation of free radicals, which can cause tissue damage. In fact, excessive amounts of dietary iron has been implicated by some scientists as a cause of cancer and heart disease. It also increases the risk of bacterial infection.

Except for lactic acid bacteria, such as the beneficial *Lactobacillus acidophilus*, all microbes require iron for growth. Many of them produce special binding proteins to secure iron from their environments. Humans also produce iron-binding proteins to capture free iron so it will not be available to microbes. An excess of iron overcomes this protective mechanism and increases susceptibility to bacterial infection.

The amount of iron needed for optimal health reflects a delicate balance between deficiency and excess. Many commercial iron pills supply too much iron to the body. It is not necessary to take iron supplements or have it present in a multiple vitamin/mineral supplement unless iron deficiency is present (with the possible exception of pregnant women). Talk to your doctor before taking an iron supplement.

THE HARM OF ANTACIDS

As discussed many times previously, overuse of antacids can make the body more susceptible to bacterial overgrowth and other problems, and they should be avoided. Besides breaking down complex molecules to aid in digestion, stomach acid has the important function of killing the bad bugs so that they do not enter the digestive tract. If stomach acid is reduced, which may be caused by infection or acid-lowering drugs, harmful bacteria, yeast and parasites can get through into the small and large intestines where they multiply, use up valuable nutrients and excrete toxins into the body. They also disrupt the normal and healthy bowel flora. By taking antacids, you may be allowing pathogens to survive, often resulting in acute food poisoning and bacterial overgrowth that causes chronic health problems.

In some antacids, calcium carbonate is the "antacid" portion. It is elemental calcium, inexpensive and usually highly absorbable, but with distinct disadvantages. First identified in 1923, there is a syndrome characterized by high levels of tissue calcium, kidney impairment and too much alkalinity in the body. With the growing use of calcium carbonate antacids, the risk of developing this syndrome is increasing. Since the most inexpensive form of calcium is calcium carbonate, many of the popular formulas today contain this substance. In addition, when taken with other substances, such as adrenal cortical hormones or thiazide diuretics, calcium carbonate can be toxic at much lower doses.

The promotion of antacids as a good source of calcium for bone health has bothered me for years. I have seen it suggested by doctors for the prevention of osteoporosis in women and even for growing children. Television and magazine advertisements continue to misinform the public about the use and overuse of antacids. Since antacids undermine your body's ability to absorb calcium, this may help explain why Americans have one of the highest rates of osteoporosis in the world, even with the high consumption of milk and cheese. There is much more to preventing osteoporosis than loading up on calcium, namely, eating a well-balanced and whole-food diet, along with doing weight-bearing exercise. Although it may be important to choose a calcium supplement for the prevention of bone loss, the most preferred source is microcrystalline hydroxyapatite (MCHC). It has been documented in human studies to regenerate lost bone density. For those people requiring calcium and magnesium for soft tissue needs, calcium citrate is desirable.

There are other side effects from using antacids. Calcium-containing antacids can cause an acid-rebound effect, where the stomach produces even more gastric acid, including heartburn, after the antacid has exhausted itself. As a result, you have to take even more antacids. Taking excessive calcium can also lead to constipation. For this reason, antacid formulas combine calcium with magnesium salts to create a laxative effect. They are often combined with aluminum compounds that also tend to be constipating. Since there may be a link between aluminum and Alzheimer's, you might be putting yourself at a higher risk for this condition by taking antacids or any other aluminum-containing products.

You should also avoid antacids that are magnesium or aluminum based if you have kidney disease. Impaired kidneys can not filter out the magnesium or the aluminum. Also, the long-term use of aluminum antacids can rob the body of calcium and end up weakening the bones. The next time you think of using an antacid, just read the ingredients. You may be surprised. Many of these over-the-counter products contain aluminum, sugar, saccharin, calcium carbonate, aspartame and sodium.

Our bodies were not designed to have stomach acid levels suppressed. If that occurs, the enzymes needed to digest foods are not activated, reducing your ability to fully utilize the food you eat. If you, or anyone you know, take antacids, it would be wise to seek help getting off of these products. It is a major tragedy that high-potency antacids became available over-the-counter a few years ago. It was bad enough physicians were using them inappropriately, but now anyone can abuse them and short-circuit their body's normal protective mechanisms. In fact, I have found that many of the people that I treat with an overgrowth of bacteria, yeast and parasites in their intestinal tract have a history of taking antacids.

If you have excess acid production, it can be cause by several factors, including eating too many acid-producing foods in the diet; a genetic predisposition; cigarette smoking; heavy use of aspirin and other non-steriodal anti-inflammatory drugs; physical trauma and stress. There may be temporary relief with antacids or other drugs, but it is easy to become dependent upon them since the real cause is not being addressed.

Years ago, physicians believed that excess stomach acid was the leading cause of ulcers and inflammation of the stomach. This may have been an occasional reason, but not the most important one. Taking antacids only creates an environment that is receptive to the growth of the pathogen bacteria, *H. pylori* and other organisms that would normally be killed by the normal production of hydrochloric acid. With low stomach acid, intestinal bacteria may move upstream into the small intestine causing an additional burden. You can treat pathogen bacteria in the intestines without lasting success, if the body's digestive system is not working properly.

If you produce too much stomach acid or not enough, the symptoms may be similar. Many people with poor digestion suffer from a lack of digestive enzymes, not from too much. You need to know which one is really happening. When you eat, the acid in your stomach breaks down the food's complex molecules to simpler ones so that they can be absorbed in the small intestine. When the stomach contents reach a certain level of acidity, the valve at the base of the stomach opens, dumping the predigested foods into the small intestines. If there is not enough stomach acid present, the valve does not open and the food sometimes comes up, causing a burning sensation and an acid taste in the back of the throat.

For those with low stomach acid, you can start with a small amount of hydrochloric acid when you eat and increase the number of tablets each day. When you feel a mild burning sensation in your stomach, reduce you dosage by one tablet. Most people need at least one to two pills with a meal. With enough acid in the stomach, the symptoms will go away. You will then digest your foods better and absorb more nutrients. After a while you may find that you do not need to take as many tablets to get the same effect. You may need even less with a light meal. For some people other digestive enzymes beside hydrochloric acid are indicated.

Sex and Hormones

SEX AND SPREADING DISEASE

Sexual intercourse during a woman's menstrual period does not cause diseases, but it may help spread them. If the woman is infected with blood-borne micoorganisms that cause disease, such as hepatitis B or HIV, the male partner's risk of acquiring the infection rises with increased exposure to blood.

Hormonal changes during menses, as well as menstruation itself, cause cervical alterations that apparently weaken the mechanical barrier that prevent bacteria from spreading upward. Also, the cervical mucus has the effect of restraining the development of bacteria, but it is at its lowest at the onset of the menstrual period. Your immune system can handle the ascending of a few bacteria. The problem arises if there are too many disease-causing bacteria such as chlamydia or the bacteria that cause gonorrhea. These are the two most common causes of pelvic inflammatory disease.

HORMONES TIED TO BACTERIAL OVERGROWTH

Female baby-boomers are moving into their menopausal years and reaching more and more for hormone replacement therapy. This therapy is popular in both mainstream and preventive medicine. Doctors like to prescribe hormones because their patients are usually able to notice an immediate and dramatic change in how they feel. It is also an economic boom for both the labs that perform hormone testing and for the pharmacies that market the hormones, whether they are natural or synthetic ones. When you are tested for hormone levels you are not tested for their effect on your immune function. Since it is generally recognized that hormone levels do influence immune function, this discrepancy seemed rather odd and somewhat worrisome.

It appears that beneficial bacterial in the bowel microflora might be influenced by hormone levels. Then these friendly bacteria proceed to have a major impact upon immunity. Bacterial microflora also help to regulate sex and adrenal hormones. With these "hormone-microflora-immune" interactions in mind, it can get complicated. Women with too much estrogen and not enough progesterone are likely to have recurrent vaginal yeast infections. There may also be immune system suppression. This occurs because yeast can produce an estrogen identical to human estrogen, and then bind up the progesterone. Yeast overgrowth can also bind up cortisol from the adrenals.

Could some of the sickest people also be taking hormonal supplements? If you have been ill and your doctor suggests hormonal replacement therapy, you might want to inquire about a baseline measurement of your immune function first, especially if you have not yet reached menopausal years. Some doctors are suggesting hormone supplements even to their thirty-something female patients who have symptoms of hormonal imbalances. By having a baseline immune test, you will have the results to guide you later. You will be able to tell if you have created any new problems or complicated previous ones. Retest your hormone levels a few months after starting hormone therapy, just to be sure that your body is utilizing them appropriately. If you decide to take hormone supplements, consider the most natural methods available. Many compounding pharmacies have these products available with a doctor's prescription.

If you decide to take DHEA, which is readily available over-the-counter in the United States, your body can convert it to estrogen. But if you already have too much estrogen, this could be the beginning of a yeast overgrowth, even if you never had this problem before. Several menopausal women reported that their symptoms began soon after they started a synthetic form of estrogen replacement therapy to prevent hot flashes. Stopping the hormones did not reverse the situation once it was set in motion.

Genetically altered soy is creating estrogen levels even higher than before. One effect of more estrogen in our food supply is the early sexual development in children. Girls now show signs of puberty, such as breast development or pubic hair before the age of three. By the age of eight, over 14 percent of Caucasian girls and more than 48 percent of African-American girls had one or both of these sexual developments. Infants fed soy-based formulas have also been placed at risk. These altered soy products combined with other plant estrogens, and estrogens resulting from pesticides, may provide a synergistic effect that could cause endocrine disrupters and lead to an increase in cancers, thyroid abnormalities, etc. There is suspicion that soy increases the risk of breast cancer in women, affects brain function in men, and causes abnormalities in children.

Is the right kind of testing being done on genetically altered soy to detect adverse health effects? It would appear that soy has only been subject to superficial testing. What additional effects created by genetic modification have gone undetected? According to some FDA scientists: "There exists a significant body of animal data that demonstrates thyroid dysfunction and even carcinogenic effects of soy products." Perhaps, if the government does proper toxicity testing on soy, it could upset the whole multi-billion dollar soy industry.

At present, it is legal in the U.S. to label any kind of soy as beneficial for reducing heart disease risk, but illegal to label it as genetically modified. The new labeling arrangements follow a petition submitted to the FDA by the American Soybean Association (ASA), whose corporate partners include the following biotech and agro-chemical companies: American Cyanamid, Bayer, Dow, Du Pont, Monsanto, Novartis and Zeneca.

Engineered soy and other high estrogen-containing plants are being fed to cows along with bovine growth hormone. All people who drink non-organic milk and dairy products are consuming elevated estrogen levels. In 1994, the FDA approved the use of bovine growth hormone (BGH), a genetically engineered hormone. Dairy farmers supply this hormone to increase milk production by 10 to 25 percent. Recent studies found that this increase in estrogen found in milk also significantly increased the risk of women getting breast cancer and men getting prostate cancer.

BGH is banned in both Canada and Europe. Cows treated with BGH are also more likely to contract mastitis, a persistent bacterial infection of the cow's udders. These cows are then treated with antibiotics and sulfa drugs. Trace amounts of these drugs are still found in their milk and passed along to consumers when they use non-organic dairy products. This keeps our intestinal microflora in a state of imbalance. It is important to look at the relationship of hormones, intestinal microflora, immunity and antibiotics, and to see how they are related to the overgrowth of bacteria in the intestinal tract.

Root Canals

Inside dead teeth, anaerobic bacteria exist that are a constant source of toxins that flood into the bloodstream every time a person chews. The only solution is to remove the source of the infection. X-rays do not always reveal the problem. The infection from dead teeth can now cause systemic symptoms in the body that are frequently overlooked. It is thought that 70 to 75 percent of root canal teeth are infected.

Global Warming Spreads Infectious Disease

Climate change associated with global warming is already increasing the spread of infectious diseases, according to researchers at the New York University School of Medicine, and is likely to cause increasing threats to public health if not reversed. An article in the *American Journal of Industrial Medicine* (2001) notes that global warming brings with it changes in vegetation and distribution of disease vectors, which leads to increases in microbial populations, while atmospheric ozone depletion has been linked to increased host susceptibility.

Diseases & Their Links to Bacterial Overgrowth

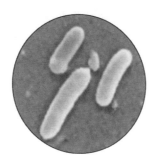

CHAPTER 9

Introduction to the Disease-Bacteria Link

DESPITE THE PREVAILING medical theories about many "mystery" conditions, there is mounting evidence to support the belief that bacteria play an integral role in many chronic diseases, including cancer. Bacterial infections have been linked to ulcers, Alzheimer's, heart disease, kidney stones and gallstones, fibromyalgia and Crohn's disease, to name just a few. It has also been theorized that arthritis, schizophrenia and autoimmune diseases like lupus and multiple sclerosis are also linked to microbial infection.

In fact, although doctors and scientists have been quick to identify the infectious nature of many acute illnesses (like childhood diseases) as far back as the nineteenth century, resistance to emerging theories about the role of infection in chronic disease still persists today. Why? Part of the reason is probably due to the nature of the disease itself. Acute illnesses show obvious and distinctive symptoms closely after infection. Many chronic illnesses (like hepatitis and several sexually transmitted diseases) which have been solidly linked to microbial infection also have a distinctive acute phase before they become chronic. Compare that with ulcers or heart disease, which do not have identifiable acute symptoms and may have extended incubation periods. These covert infections are better able to avoid detection and often thrive as a result.

Another complication is mainstream medicine's refusal to believe that the causes of disease can be the result of a combination of infection and other factors (like genetics). Cancer research, for instance, was stymied in the 1960s and 1970s because researchers believed it was either caused by microbial infection or it wasn't. As a result, when cancer-causing genes and environmental links to cancer were discovered, infectious links were dismissed or forgotten, and research to uncover such links lost funding. Still, infectious links to cancer have and continue to be made. For instance, cervical, head and neck cancers have been linked to the papillomavirus, liver cancer to hepatitis viruses, and stomach cancer to *Helicobacter pylori*. In fact, it is now estimated that at least 15 percent of all cancers can be linked to microbial infection, and amazingly, less than 5 percent are known to have no involvement from an infectious organism. (Seventy-five percent of cancers currently remain unexplained.)

The influence of bacteria can be seen in less serious conditions as well. Chronic indigestion, acne, gingivitis, chronic fatigue and even bad breath are linked to infectious bacteria. And researchers are beginning to see how some of these destructive infections are systemic (develop within) instead of communicable (travelling from person to person). Although modern medicine has been slow to see the existence and dangers of bacterial overgrowth, possible links between bacteria and chronic illnesses are not difficult to make. Plus, understanding about the diversity and ingenuity of infectious diseases is growing daily.

Microorganisms have a phenomenal ability to transform and adapt to ever-changing environments, in order to avoid detection and survive. It has been discovered, for example, that *Streptococcus pyogenes* may damage the heart because its proteins are able to disguise themselves as proteins of the heart. These mutations and adaptations stand in stark opposition to the prevailing germ theory of disease (one germ-one disease) proposed by Pasteur. Instead, scientists are finding that one pathogen can be responsible for a number of conditions. For instance, the bacteria associated with gingivitis (*Porphyromonas gingivalis*) and the bacteria that cause pneumonia (*Chlamydia pneumoniae*) have both been linked to atherosclerosis. *Chlamydia pneumoniae* has also been linked with multiple sclerosis and Alzheimer's, though there is still a great deal of scientific debate over these links.

The Way Bacteria Change

Ordinary bacteria and fungi, including the yeast *Candida albicans*, are capable of mutating to a form that does not have a surrounding cell wall (called a "cell wall deficient form"). Sometimes, but not always, they can also revert back to their original form again. This transformative ability allows these organisms to hide out inside other cells, making them hard to find. They are called "L-forms," named for the Lister

Institute where they were first discovered. According to Professor Lida Mattman, Ph.D., in her book *Cell Wall Deficient Forms: Stealth Pathogens*, these pathogens are not familiar to most practicing physicians. Only a few laboratories test for L-forms, and university research centers spend very little time exploring these organisms.

Below are some pertinent facts about L-forms:

• When bacteria change into the L-form, they are more likely to cause disease than bacteria in their original form.

• L-form bacteria outnumber original-form bacteria by as much as ten-fold. If the original form is cultured from the blood, the L-form will be there as well, but usually in greater numbers. The L-form may be present even if the original form is not.

• The L-form and the original form of the same species of bacteria can be resistant to different antibiotics. It will take antibiotic combinations to eradicate both forms. The antibiotic, penicillin, may be the most effective inducer of L-forms.

What does all of this mean? Well, it might explain why you have the symptoms of bacterial overgrowth but your lab cultures come back negative—the L-form cannot be detected. How will we be able to detect these L-form variants if laboratories cannot recognize them? One prime example is the unexplained negative lab cultures, which sometimes occur when diagnosing urinary tract infections (cystitis). If there is blood in the urine from an unknown cause, it may be caused by an L-form organism, and sometimes by L-forms of two species acting together. The L-form is not in the urine, but inside the red blood cells in the urine. If you have chronic urinary infections and your routine urine cultures come back negative, you may need to consider L-forms as the cause. Otherwise, you will continue to have this problem and not receive proper treatment.

Another chronic condition that could be the results of L-forms is sinusitis. Routine cultures taken from the sinuses are usually inadequate for diagnosing this common, almost untreatable condition. Uveitus (inflammation of the uvea of the eye) may also be caused by L-form pathogens, as may the autoimmune disease, rheumatoid arthritis. L-forms are even suspected of crossing the placenta where they might enter the fetus during early stages of fetal development.

Dr. Mattman says to look for L-forms everywhere, in even the most unsuspected conditions, because they can almost always be found if the right laboratory techniques are used. Our drinking water may harbor L-form bacteria. As long as we lack adequate methods of detection, we will never know what other environments L-forms thrive in. They may even be causing hospital-acquired infections since detection of these organisms is not routine, even in large diagnostic labs. Hopefully, as new technology provides better ways of recognizing them, we will be able to pinpoint the illnesses affected by L-form pathogens.

The Pathogen Switch

Of course, L-form theories aren't the only ones that have been developed to explain bacterial overgrowth and disease. Researchers at the University of California at Santa Barbara have found a gene "switch" in bacteria that may trigger infection. For example, a gene in the bacterium *Salmonella*, called DAM, can create a protein that activates other genes to begin infection. However, this process appears to occur only after *Salmonella* enters the intestines of a human or animal. Outside a host, the DAM gene is inactive and unable to cause infection. Findings like these could lead to treatments designed to turn off these gene switches, thereby preventing illness.

Genes: Jumping the Species Barrier

Genes can also be dangerous in other ways. Genetically modified genes can jump the species barrier. There is evidence that genes used to modify crops may cause bacteria to mutate. In a four-year study performed by German zoologist Professor Hans-Hinrich Kaatz, researchers found that a gene used to modify rapeseed (canola oil) could be transferred to bacteria living inside the guts of honeybees. Britain's agriculture minister suggested that any farmer growing these rapeseed crops should rip them out of the ground. This lends more credence to the claims that such technology could pose serious health risks.

Research suggests that genes used in genetic modification technology could contaminate many types of bacteria, including those living inside the human digestive system. It could have an impact on the vital role of beneficial bacteria in fighting disease, aiding digestion, facilitating blood clotting, and other beneficial functions. Nevertheless, Professor Kaatz has been reluctant to talk about his research, because he fears a backlash from the scientific community similar to the one faced by Dr. Arpad Pustzai, who claimed that genetically modified potatoes damaged the stomach lining of rats. He was fired and had his work discredited.

Dr. Mae-Wan Ho, a British geneticist and a critic of genetically modified technology commented on Kaatz's findings saying, "These findings are very worrying and provide the first real evidence of what many have feared. Everybody is keen to exploit genetically modified technology, but nobody is looking at the risk of gene transfer. We are playing about with genetic structures that existed for millions of years and the experiment is running out of control. One of the biggest concerns is that the antibiotic-resistant gene used in some of these crops will cross over to bacteria, and leave us unable to treat serious illnesses like meningitis and E coli."

An Escape Route

Even if bacteria aren't resistant to a particular antibiotic, they have developed other ways to avoid them. Scientists have found that bacteria can hijack certain cellular structures to get into immune cells and hide from the body's own defenses. It also allows them to avoid antibiotics or other bodily defenses. According to an issue of *Science*, the bacteria *E. coli* use this escape route. There is some evidence that HIV may also use this pathway to avoid the immune system.

The Bottom Line: What Your Doctor Doesn't Know May Keep You Sick

Mainstream medicine has certainly improved our quality of life, advanced healthcare and broadened our understanding of how the body works. Nevertheless, medical research is big business. The biggest foundations are entrenched bureaucracies with close ties to pharmaceutical companies, hospitals, universities, and government agencies. These organizations, which include the American Cancer Society, the American Heart Association and many others, have a vested interest in the conventional treatment of medicine, not alternative or complementary ones. Therefore, moneys collected are given to research projects with the greatest potential for maximum profit.

Unfortunately, quite often, conventional medicine finds one-size-fits-all treatments more profitable than finding cures for many medical conditions. Physicians of this type of medicine are taught how to cut the body with surgery, poison the body with drugs, and injure the body with radiation. This approach to medicine violates the first principle of medicine, which is to "first do no harm."

The successes of modern medicine are matched with its failures, particularly with patients suffering from life-threatening or chronic illnesses like cancer and heart disease. A holistic approach used by someone well trained in alternative or complementary medicine may be the answer to these failures. The approach of complementary medicine takes into account the patient and their environment, and it uses methods to fortify, detoxify and balance the body's systems so that it is better able to heal itself. This approach moves you from "sick care" to "health care" by focusing on prevention. It also may change a patient's perspective about what is causing their illness and how they can fix it. You may find that a different approach may be exactly what you need to finally overcome your illness.

Is It All in Your Head?

Many medical doctors prefer not to deal with chronic illness, especially chronic fatigue and chronic yeast problems, because they are not quite sure how to combat them. "Time is money." Most doctors simply do not want to waste time trying to treat these health conditions while fighting with HMOs over coverage. HMOs are for-profit organizations that must answer to the interests of their corporate stock holders. As a result, they may be more interested in holding down costs than providing adequate health care. HMOs often establish firm policies that discourage doctors from recognizing and treating conditions that are going to require too many office visits.

A consequence of this medical bureaucracy is the dismissal of legitimate health problems as being "all in the patient's head." In fact, both PMS and fibromyalgia were initially considered to be problems of psychiatric origin without physical cause, despite evidence to the contrary. Even with all the evidence linking infectious microorganisms to chronic diseases, your doctor may not take the time to find out what is really the matter with you. If they do not keep up-to-date on the latest medical research, they may not even believe in bacteria overgrowth in the digestive tract, and therefore, will not perform the necessary tests to check for it.

In response to these lapses in conventional medical care, you may need to take more responsibility for your health care by doing your own research and perhaps switching healthcare providers. Your answers may be only a library visit away, and with the availability of the internet, medical information is much more accessible. (Of course, not all internet sites are created equal, so it is imperative that you check the credibility of each health site you visit.) There are also quality publications about complementary medicine you may want to subscribe to. Once you are armed with scientific research about your condition, your doctor is much more likely to listen.

To help get you started, the next chapter gives an alphabetical listing of some major bacteria that are potentially dangerous, followed by a chapter of conditions which have already been linked to infectious pathogens and bacterial overgrowth.

CHAPTER 10

Types of Bacteria

A Crash Course in Bacteria

Hundreds of varieties of bacteria live in the environment of the intestinal tract. Some of them are beneficial, some may become dangerous, and others are harmful only when found in great numbers. As previously mentioned, there is a profound relationship between the microflora in the digestive tract and our overall health. Altered bowel microflora can lead to chronic bacterial overgrowth, resulting in various chronic or systemic health problems.

Most testing to determine the overall health of the resident bowel microflora measures three frequently found organisms: *Lactobacillus acidophilus*, *Lactobacillus bifidus* and human *E. coli*. Many researchers believe that these three organisms have intrinsic benefits, aiding digestion while helping to prevent the overgrowth of harmful organisms. Bacterial lab cultures also identify potential pathogens. The reason the word "potential" is used is because most of these organisms are opportunistic, meaning they only overgrow if they are given the opportunity to do so. When they are kept in check and the internal terrain of the body is healthy, they do not cause disease.

It is also possible to harbor dangerous pathogens and appear healthy. Other people may have major gastrointestinal complaints or other illnesses, but only test positive for weak or questionable pathogens. Some types of bacteria do not cause acute intestinal disturbances but may cause various chronic or systemic problems, including species of *Bacillus*, *Citrobacter*, *Klebsiella*, *Mycoplasma*, *Proteus* and *Pseudomonas*.

Bacteria are also distinguished from one another by their size, shape and staining characteristics, as well as other factors. (For instance, a spherical bacterium such as *Staphylococcus* is a coccus; a rod-shaped bacterium such as *Escherichia coli* is a bacillus.) The Gram stain allows clinicians to distinguish between the two major classes of bacteria: gram-positive and gram-negative. Gram-positive and gram-negative bacteria have similar internal but very different external structures. Bacteria that cannot be classified by Gram stain include *Mycobacterium, Mycoplasma* and *Chlamydia*. They have very different structures from bacteria tested using Gram stain, and so they have to be detected using other methods. Knowing which class a bacterium belongs to is very important because many antibiotics, herbs and other treatments used to treat bacterial infections work best on one specific class.

Another classification for bacteria is whether they are aerobic or anaerobic. Aerobic bacteria live in oxygen-rich environments, and anaerobic bacteria live where the oxygen content is low or absent. This classification may become important when trying to diagnose a bacterium and prescribe a treatment.

The following is a list of gram-positive bacterium discussed in this book: *Bacillus, Clostridium, Enterococcus, Listeria, Staphyloccus* and *Streptococcus*.

The book also discusses gram-negative bacterium, which are listed here: *Aeromonas, Bacteroides, Brucella, Burkholderia, Campylobacter, Citrobacter, Enterobacter, Escherichia, Helicobacter, Klebsiella, Lactobacillus, Leptospira, Neisseria, Plesiomonas, Proteus, Pseudomonas, Rickettsia, Salmonella, Shigella, Vibrio* and *Yersinia*.

Let's discuss some of the major bacteria in more detail. (For information on specific bacteria linked to food poisoning, see Appendix A).

Bacillus cereus

This gram-positive bacterium has recently been turning up in the intestinal tract of some of my patients, even though it is usually implicated in cases of food poisoning. I suspect that some of these bacteria remain in the digestive tract even after the initial food poisoning has resolved. They establish themselves and overgrow when the opportunity presents itself.

Bacillus cereus is usually of low virulence and is widespread in air, soil, water, dust and animal products. Even though this bacterium is considered a weak pathogen, it deserves special mention because it is the species most likely to cause an opportunistic infection and is considered a pathogen in any amount. Furthermore, it will not always cause symptoms and is usually a transient visitor. A *Bacillus* specie may be isolated from the stool in 15 percent of healthy individuals. See the section on food poisoning for more information.

Bacteroides fragilis

This bacterium is another opportunistic pathogen, and despite its name, it is far from fragile. It is actually one of the hardier and more easily grown bacteria. *Bacteroides* gain access to tissues through trauma or a breakdown in normal host defenses. Members of the *Bacteroides fragilis* group are the most commonly isolated gram-negative, anaerobic pathogens in humans. In fact, wound infections caused by these bacteria have been increasing in the last decade.

Most overgrowths in the intestinal tract start out in areas of microflora imbalance. *Bacteroides fragilis* constitutes less than 10 percent of the *Bacteroides* species in the normal intestinal microflora, but it is the most likely one to cause problems. When there is putrefaction in the digestive tract from diets high in fat and meat, and low in insoluble fiber, you will often find increased concentrations of *Bacteroides* species. As a result, it is often implicated in cases of diarrhea, presumably due to its toxin production.

In susceptible individuals, *Bacteroides fragilis* may be involved in ulcerative colitis. It is thought to release enzymes that may stimulate the production of cancer cells. It is important to remember that like any possible pathogen, the presence of *Bacteroides fragilis* does not guarantee disease or automatically warrant treatment. Its presence should be weighed along with the levels of beneficial bacteria, particularly the bifidobacteria, as well as immune function and symptoms.

Bacteroides fragilis is usually resistant to penicillin and is almost always resistant to cephalosporins and clindamycin. It also has the ability to become antibiotic-resistant. In fact, according to *Emerging Infectious Diseases* 2001, the antibiotic metronidazole has been the drug of choice for preventing and treating such infections for the last forty years, but resistance to the antibiotic is developing in India. The precise incidence of resistance to metronidazole is difficult to estimate since most laboratories in the world are not doing routine antimicrobial sensitivity testing of anaerobes. There has also been a possible increase in the incidence of metronidazole-resistance *Bacteroides spp.* in the United Kingdom. However, since antimicrobial resistance of anaerobes varies from one hospital to another and between different geographic locations, it is unknown how often this is happening.

Chlamydia pneumoniae

Members of this group were once thought to be large viruses, but now are classified as bacteria, including the specie *Chlamydia pneumoniae*. This is a "stealth" pathogen because it can hide inside human tissue cells, thereby evading detection by the immune system. Only recently has *Chlamydia pneumoniae* become known as the cause of chronic health problems. Therefore, it is usually not suspected. Moreover, it may be hard to distinguish from another stealth pathogen, *Mycoplasma pneumoniae*, which can also cause pneumonia. Some people think that they have the flu and blame their symptoms on a virus instead of considering *Chlamydia*.

Chlamydia pneumoniae has been recognized as the cause of acute and chronic respiratory illness and accounts for up to 19 percent of community-acquired pneumonia. It is spread by person-to-person transmission through the air with an incubation period of seven to twenty-one days. Outbreaks have been reported in schools, military barracks, nursing homes and among family members. However, not everyone with *Chlamydia* has symptoms.

Because our understanding of the bacterium has grown, *Chlamydia* is now making news as a suspected culprit in a number of chronic illnesses, including coronary heart disease. In fact, these intracellular bacteria are thought to cause a wide spectrum of diseases including ear infections, chronic fatigue and fibromyalgia, among others. It is also theorized that when *Chlamydia* is present in an individual with asthma, their symptoms worsen. Recently published reports implicate *Chlamydia* as one cause of multiple sclerosis and perhaps Alzheimer's disease, Guillain-Barré syndrome, and other degenerative motor diseases. There is some evidence that ulcerative colitis is caused by these bacteria as well. There has not been any association with Crohn's disease so far, but it seems possible that this bacterium may be implicated in that also. Why this pathogen selects one site over another is unclear. It may select receptive tissues based on some genetically determined typing.

Chlamydia pneumoniae is a suspected participant in the development of arterial plaques and atherosclerosis. It is theorized that the bacteria become lodged in the walls of blood vessels for years, where they induce inflammation as a response to the infection. This leads to a build-up of arterial plaque that restricts the flow of blood and may eventually lead to heart attacks and strokes.

Since *Chlamydia* is a foreign protein, it is capable of producing chronic inflammation. It can also cause organ damage through the production of free radicals. When attacked, these bacteria change to a dormant, but infectious form. Because of this ability to hide, they are not easily detected by ordinary lab diagnosis methods. It has taken new sophisticated technology to change that. Still, even the best lab can fail to detect stealth bacteria on the first try. Moreover, short-term antibiotics will not work, so long-term antibiotics will probably be necessary. However, because of *Chlamydia's* ability to develop antibiotic resistance, antibiotics may not be the final answer anyway. In fact, an overgrowth of the yeast *Candida albicans* in the intestines may also be somehow related to systemic *Chlamydia* and should be considered when determining treatment. (This may also be true for another stealth bacteria, *Mycoplasma*.)

Chlamydia trachomatis, the specie known to cause the sexually transmitted disease, chlamydia, is also found in the blood of 20 percent of the people diagnosed with fibromyalgia (*Journal of Infectious Disease* 2000). As a sexually transmitted disease, chlamydia continues to be the most commonly reported infection in the United States. There are an estimated three million new cases each year. Up to 40 percent of women infected with this species of chlamydia will develop pelvic inflammatory disease, if not treated. In the United Kingdom, nearly 11 percent of young women are thought to have infection with this bacteria, and half of them are without symptoms (*British Journal of General Practice* 2001).

Citrobacter freundii

This gram-negative bacteria is found in mammals, birds, reptiles and amphibians, as well as in soil and water. It is an opportunistic pathogen in humans, which can contaminate the throat, urine, sputum, blood, wounds and the digestive tract. It possesses toxins similar to some strains of *Salmonella* or the more pathogenic *E. coli*. *Citrobacter freundii* may appear among the normal intestinal microflora, but they can cause health problems when they overgrow. Consider this microbe a pathogen in any amount.

This particular specie of *Citrobacter* is one of the most common causes of intestinal bacterial overgrowth I have seen since beginning stool testing in my patients. They can invade the intestinal lining and cause irritation. The symptoms vary, but there is usually a sense of unwellness, along with various digestive symptoms. As with any bacterial overgrowth, symptoms may appear vague since the infection is not acute. Over time, an overgrowth of these bacteria can produce low levels of toxins that are able to get into the general blood circulation and produce symptoms far from where the bacteria are living.

Clostridium difficile

This organism has a profound effect on the medical care system and is the most common cause of outbreaks of diarrhea and colitis in adults who are hospitalized or in nursing homes. *Clostridium difficile* occurs when antibiotics or other factors disrupt the normal colon microflora, allowing an overgrowth to produce disease. Taking almost any antibiotic can lead to *Clostridium difficile* infection, but clindamycin, broad-spectrum penicillins and cephalosporins are most often implicated. Hospitalized patients who are taking antibiotics and have bowel surgery, uremia or intestinal ischemia, or those who have undergone chemotherapy or bone marrow transplantation, are also at high risk for getting this pathogen.

The spread of *Clostridium difficile* is not limited to hospitals and nursing home facilities, though is most easily spread in these places. *Clostridium difficile* has the ability to form spores that are easily transferred on the hands and in the stool of hospital staff working around patients. In one study, 21 percent of the patients that tested negative for this bacteria before being admitted to the hospital later tested positive after spending time there.

The onset of symptoms may be rapid, occurring within forty-eight hours after beginning antibiotic use, or they can be delayed as long as six to eight weeks after antibiotics have been discontinued. People can also develop a *Clostridium difficile* infection that persists for months to years despite repeated antibiotic treatments. In the beginning, people usually experience an explosive type of diarrhea of a watery consistency. Other symptoms may include constipation, reactions to food, intestinal pain, rectal bleeding, rashes, depression, unprovoked anger, irrational behavior, general fatigue, joint and tissue pain, and even weight loss. There can be severe complications, such as intestinal perforation, as well.

In mild cases, there may be only minimal inflammation or edema in the colon. Most of the time symptoms consist of uncomplicated diarrhea with some abdominal cramping. About 20 to 30 percent of the time, infection involves colitis (abdominal pain, nausea and fever). In these severe cases, the colon can resemble other conditions like ulcerative colitis.

Diagnosis is confirmed by detecting the bacterial toxin in the stool. Standard antibiotic therapy with vancomycin or metronidazole is effective 80 percent of the time. However, these bacteria may be resistant to antibiotics, so in the remaining 20 percent, sufferers may experience further episodes of diarrhea or colitis as long as a month after the antibiotic has been discontinued. Once standard antibiotics fail to work, these bacteria are likely to recur. Most antibiotics share the risk of further disturbing the protective normal microflora in the colon and making a person even more susceptible to recurrences. Drugs that are effective against these bacteria will not work when it is forming spores. Spore production will usually continue until the antibiotic being used is stopped.

As you can see, it is difficult to maintain balance in the intestinal microflora while giving antibiotics to kill this organism. Oral *Lactobacillus acidophilus* may be helpful, but in one study, the non-pathogenic yeast, *Saccharomyces boulardii*, was found to have a better protective effect. In the study, nineteen children with the average age of eight months were given *Saccharomyces boulardii* (250 mg) two to four times a day (depending on their age) for fifteen days. In the majority of the children, diarrhea ceased by the end of the first week, and there were not any adverse reactions to the yeast. *Lactobacillus casei* (subspecies rhamnosus) is another beneficial bacterium that may prove helpful against *Clostridium difficile*. The adult dosage is ten to 100 billion colony-forming units per day (cfu); infant dosage is 500 million cfu per day.

In hospital patients with another type of infection, it is common to find concurrent infections with *Clostridium difficile*. For instance, the bacterium may be present in people who are also infected with the vancomycin-resistant bacteria, *Enterococcus* (*Am J Gastroenterol* 2000). In addition, antibiotic-resistant *Staphylococcus aureus* is commonly found in individuals who also have *Clostridium*. When coinfections are present, they can be more dangerous and harder to treat.

Escherichia coli (E. coli)

The *E. coli* normally found in our intestinal tract has been unfairly maligned. It is not the same deadly strain mentioned in several recent news reports. This strain of *E. coli*, like other beneficial bacteria, is responsible for producing the body's own natural antibiotics. Taking oral antibiotics wipe out our friendly populations of *E. coli*, as well as other beneficial bacteria in the gut, creating an imbalance in the intestinal tract. Under these circumstances, even intestine-friendly bacteria can cause problems.

An overgrowth only usually results in a minor bout of diarrhea or vomiting, but in young children, the elderly and those with weakened or underdeveloped immune systems it can be problematic. These bacteria can be transmitted between people, especially among infants in diapers or people changing those diapers. It can also be transmitted during sexual intercourse. And in women, the bacteria can easily spread to the bladder.

In fact, an overgrowth of *E. coli* is the most common cause of bladder and kidney infections. These bacteria grow rapidly in urine and are responsible for more than 90 percent of urinary tract infections that develop outside of hospitals. Mild urinary tract infections may have no symptoms, and severe ones can involve the entire urinary tract and the kidneys. The most common symptoms are pain on urination and increased urine frequency. When the kidneys are involved, fever and flank pain is common. The duration of symptoms varies considerably, depending on the severity of the infection and what methods of treatment are being used. People with urinary catheters or enlarged prostate glands are also more likely to be infected by this strain of *E. coli*.

E. coli mutates in the presence of antibiotics or antiseptics just like all microorganisms do. *E. coli* has mutated into one of six known virulent strains, the most common one is known as *E. coli* 0157:H7. This is the one often mentioned in the news. The proper disposal of feces from infected people, good hygiene and careful hand washing with soap, helps limit the spread of infection. See the sections on food poisoning in Chapter 11 and Appendix A for more information.

Helicobacter pylori (H. pylori)

Since it was found in 1982, *Helicobacter pylori* (*H. pylori*) has been the topic of extensive research. *H. pylori* is a gram-negative bacterium that infects the stomachs and intestinal tracts of more than 50 percent of the population worldwide. It is mostly acquired during childhood and, if not treated, persists chronically, causing chronic gastritis, peptic ulcer disease, and in some individuals, gastric cancer and gastric lymphoma (tumor). Once acquired, *H. pylori* is persistent and can inhabit the human stomach for years, for decades, or possibly for life, without proper treatment.

It is believed that 90 to 100 percent of people with duodenal ulcers, 70 percent with gastric ulcers, and about 50 percent of the people over the age of fifty will test positive for *H. pylori*. Despite its prevalence, most people remain uninformed about the dangers of this bacterium and are unaware that *H. pylori* is responsible for nine out of every ten stomach ulcers in the U.S.

For years it was believed that stress and spicy foods caused ulcers. Although both may worsen the symptoms and pain of an ulcer, they are not the cause. The prevalence of this bacterium is believed to be partially due to the acidic nature of the American diet and the subsequent overuse of antacids that reduce the production of hydrochloric acid in the stomach. *H. pylori* finds an ideal environment in people who already produce a reduction of stomach acid, either by medication, the natural aging process, antacids or some other reason.

The job of stomach cells is to secrete hydrochloric acid (HCl). Low output of HCl appears to predispose people to the overgrowth of *H. pylori* and other pathogens. When this happens, the stomach will become more alkaline. Our stomachs were not designed to handle reduced acid levels because they prohibit us from fully utilizing the foods we eat. Since *H. pylori* is quite sensitive to an acid pH, it produces a thin acid-neutralizing layer around itself that protects it from the harsh stomach environment until it is able to damage the acid-producing cells. If the bacteria are present in the stomach long enough, they can cause improper digestion and ulcers, which interfere with nutrient absorption and the proper breakdown of proteins. Reduced nutrient uptake decreases the body's ability to repair itself, and the other changes increase risks for food allergies, yeast overgrowth and autoimmune disorders like rheumatoid arthritis. Overall, this process has an extremely detrimental effect on immune function and overall health.

However, these bacteria cannot thrive in an environment that stays too acidic. They like a pH of about 5.0. They will migrate to areas where the pH is comfortable and will avoid a pH of less than 2.5. In fact, they have difficulty colonizing in a pH of less than 3. So altering the pH of the stomach's environment will help to get rid of the bacteria and repair tissue damage caused by them.

In fact, it is now believed that certain bacteria, such as *H. pylori,* cause a wide variety of diseases in the body. There is evidence that one strain may increase the risk of heart disease by triggering a low-grade inflammatory process that can persist for years, creating a steady, long-term strain on the cardiovascular system. It is not known for sure if *H. pylori* actually causes or merely contributes to heart disease, but the end result is the same—and serious. One study in the *British Medical Journal* (Oct. 2000) reported that heart attacks were twice as common among people infected with *H. pylori* than those not infected by this bacterium.

In a recent report from physicians at an Italian hospital/university, a forty-two-year-old man with angina-like chest pain was diagnosed with changes in his coronary arteries. Conventional drugs for angina did not relieve the condition, but after further testing, a virulent strain of *Helicobacter pylori* was found. It is believed that his condition was triggered by inflammation due to a chronic bacterial infection.

This bacterium may also be responsible for extreme morning sickness, according to a recent study. Researchers at the University of Vienna in Austria found that over 90 percent of pregnant women with severe nausea and vomiting were infected with *H. pylori*. Early in pregnancy a woman's body undergoes changes that affect the acidity (pH) of the stomach. This in turn may activate latent *H. pylori* residing there. Women with this condition may vomit three or more times each day, experience weight loss and have electrolyte imbalances. This condition can continue throughout pregnancy.

H. pylori has also been linked to an increased risk of other chronic inflammatory conditions including systemic lupus erythematosus, Sjogren's syndrome, rosacea, psoriasis, allergies and different types of cancers, including stomach cancer. Chronic inflammation is a complex process that sometimes causes cells to change in response to invading pathogens. If the process continues over a sustained period of time, it can lead to severe tissue damage or even cancer. Dental plaque can also harbor *H. pylori* and may act as a source of re-infection. This organism only flourishes when local conditions are favorable. When *H. pylori* is eliminated, a person often returns to a state of health.

The bacterium may also cause B vitamin deficiencies. For instance, one study detected *H. pylori* in 56 percent of 138 people with vitamin B12 anemia. Detection and eradication of these bacteria produced a significant improvement of B12 statue in 40 percent of the infected patients.

Available studies suggest that for the general population, the most likely mode of transmission is person to person, either by the fecal-oral route or oral-oral route (through vomit or possibly saliva). There is a higher incidence of infection among institutionalized children and adults, as well as clustering of infections within families. This supports the person to person route of infection.

H. pylori has also been known to be transmitted following endoscopy by doctors looking for esophageal reflux. There is some speculation that *H. pylori* may even be the cause of reflux disease. Waterborne transmission, probably due to fecal contamination, may be an important source of infection, especially in parts of the world where untreated water is common. Recent studies in the United States have linked infection with consumption of *H. pylori* contaminated well water.

It may also come from a common environmental source, the housefly. *H. pylori* is well adapted to living in the stomach of flies. Because houseflies frequently come into contact with human food and fecal matter, it is very possible that they act as one source for spreading *H. pylori*. However, evidence is lacking. Nevertheless, the hypothesis is appealing since flies are known to carry many other infectious diseases.

Animals may also be a source for the bacteria. Although *H. pylori* has been isolated in domestic cats, additional research has suggested that this bacterium is probably uncommon and should not be a major concern for cat owners. However, several studies have suggested sheep as a possible source of transmission, a hypothesis that deserves additional investigation.

Some genetic factors may make some people more susceptible to infection as well. It appears that people with an "O" blood type are more at risk for developing ulcers. At first it would seem that it is because these individuals make more stomach acid. Although this may be true, experts believe it is probably due to the tendency of *H. pylori* to attach more efficiently to the blood cells of people with "O" blood type. Research has also shown a higher occurrence of *H. pylori* in males. However, the majority of these infections seem to be due more to lifestyle than genes.

You can compare *H. pylori* to flies on garbage. The flies do not cause the garbage. *H. pylori* has only been given an environment where it can thrive. Conventional medicine is obsessed with killing the infective agent rather than addressing the underlying cause. They do not seem to understand that the internal terrain (or the host's susceptibility to infection) is more important than the germ. We must do whatever is necessary to make our body an inhospitable place for disease to flourish. Using drugs to eradicate *H. pylori* will work occasionally, but if you do not treat the underlying cause you will usually repeat the treatment.

How do we beef up our internal terrain? Adequate nutritional status, especially frequent consumption of fruits and vegetables and of vitamin C, appears to protect against infection with *H. pylori*. When food is prepared under less than ideal conditions or exposed to contaminated water or soil, the risk increases. Poor hygiene and crowded conditions may facilitate transmission of infection as well.

If you suspect that you have *H. pylori* but tested negative for this organism in the past, there is a new test recently okayed by the FDA. It is an IgA enzyme immunoassay (EIA) kit used to detect IgA antibodies. There are also tests that are supposed to detect IgG antibodies which may help your physician by providing a more complete picture of antibody response. With previous testing methods, some patients remained undiagnosed and untreated. The company, Enteric, based in Westbury, New York, said that it would first market the test in the U.S. and then in Europe through Sigma Diagnostics and Alexon-Trend. Kyowa Medex Co. will market the test in Japan following regulatory approval in that country.

Another test that may be more accurate is the urea breath test. For more information, visit www.gsdl.com/assessments/heliobacter. An Israeli medical device maker, Oridion Systems Ltd., has also received clearance from the USDA to market a noninvasive testing device called BreathID. As soon as the FDA clears the test, it will be available for doctors to detect *Helicobacter pylori* in a single office visit.

Klebsiella pneumoniae

Klebsiella is widely distributed in nature, occurring in soil, water and grain. A certain amount is even present among the normal bowel microflora. The *Klebsiella* group includes a few opportunistic pathogens that cause problems in hospitals, including infections in the lungs or the urinary tract. Moreover, *Klebsiella* is very resistant to antibiotics and is usually acquired in hospitals among patients with weakened immune systems. Outbreaks particularly occur in urological patients and in neonatal and intensive care units. The bacteria are usually spread from the hands of the clinical staff to susceptible individuals.

In large amounts, these bacteria are considered pathogenic and may indicate a bowel microflora imbalance. An overgrowth of this bacteria will often present gastrointestinal symptoms and may lead to increased intestinal wall permeability and subsequent autoimmune syndromes, as well as malabsorption and opportunistic infections. I see this organism frequently in patients with chronic digestive symptoms. *Klebsiella* may be the cause of cystitis, pneumonia and prostatitis also. It has been linked to the autoimmune diseases, rheumatoid arthritis and ankylosing spondylitis. In the intestine, *Klebsiella* may not cause any symptoms at all.

Mycoplasma fermentans (incognitus)

Mycoplasma is a unique bacterium in that it is the smallest free-living organism currently known. The main difference between *Mycoplasma* and other bacteria is that most bacteria have a solid cell wall structure and can grow in the simplest culture media. *Mycoplasma* does not have a cell wall, and like tiny jellyfish with a pliable membrane, they can take on many different shapes. This makes them difficult to identify as the cause of disease. *Mycoplasma*, unlike viruses, can grow in tissue fluids (blood, joint, heart, chest and spinal fluids), and unlike most normal bacteria and viruses, they can dwell undetected inside any living tissue cell without killing it.

In some people *Mycoplasma* acts like a living thorn—mycoplasma-adhesion proteins are very similar to human proteins and can completely mimic the protein cell of the host. Once they attach to a host cell, their unique plasma and protein coating mimics the host's cell wall, and the immune system cannot differentiate *Mycoplasma* from the body's own cells. Once attached to a human cell, it competes for nutrients with its host. As nutrients are depleted, these host cells begin to malfunction (which is thought to be the cause of some cancers).

Mycoplasma causes its host to wage war against seemingly healthy cells; an event common to all autoimmune diseases. This allergy-induced inflammation often results in heated, swollen and painful inflamed tissues like those found in rheumatoid diseases, fibromyalgia and many other autoimmune disorders such as lupus and MS.

Today, there are over 100 species of *Mycoplasma*, but most of them do not cause disease in humans. However, at least five species are now linked as direct causes or significant co-factors for many chronic diseases including rheumatoid arthritis, Alzheimer's, multiple sclerosis, fibromyalgia, chronic fatigue, diabetes, Crohn's disease, ALS, asthma, lupus, infertility, AIDS, Gulf War Syndrome, and certain cancers and leukemia. Slow-growing infections may cause or promote a host of other chronic illnesses. *Mycoplasma* also is believed to infect females four times more often than males.

The first connection between *Mycoplasma* and rheumatoid diseases was made in 1939. Unfortunately, *Mycoplasma* did not become part of the medical school curriculum until the late 1950s when one specific strain was identified, proven to be the cause of atypical pneumonia and named *Mycoplasma pneumonia*. The association between autoimmune disorders and *Mycoplasma* was first reported in the mid 1970s after four species of the bacteria were localized in joint tissue. Since that time, testing methods have progressed and more *Mycoplasma* species have been identified. These bacteria are good examples of how a hidden pathogen can reside in one part of the body and then move out of its typical environment and into other parts of the body, causing other diseases.

Mycoplasma fermentans may also be associated with other forms of arthritis besides rheumatoid arthritis. It was detected in 88 percent of both rheumatoid and non-rheumatoid arthritis patients, including four different strains found in those with gout, reactive arthritis, juvenile chronic arthritis, ankylosing spondylitis, and psoriatic arthritis. However, it was not detected in any osteoarthritis patients.

Over the last twenty years, more reports reveal that diseases caused by *Mycoplasma* have increased. There have been symptoms from the skin, central nervous system, heart and other organs. It has also been found in the oral and genito-urinary tract, as well as in the cerebrospinal fluid of people with meningitis and seizures and in the bone marrow of children with leukemia. In fact, one company, International Molecular Diagnostics, Inc., in Huntington Beach, California, (714-799-7177) has found *Mycoplasma fermentans* (incognitus) in many people diagnosed with chronic fatigue syndrome.

It is amazing that these bacteria can cause so many seemingly unrelated diseases in humans. As with all *Mycoplasma* species, it all depends on where the bacteria reside in the body and which cells they invade. *Mycoplasma* is highly adaptable to changing environments and can move anywhere in the body, invading virtually any type of cell.

Many people came back from the Gulf War suffering from undiagnosed illnesses now thought to be *Mycoplasma fermentans* (incognitus). Symptoms often resemble those of chronic fatigue and fibromyalgia. Despite the connection, the military found nothing wrong and often prescribed antidepressants for the symptoms. If you have these symptoms and served in the Gulf War (or have had any connection to persons who served there), please explore the possibility of a *Mycoplasma* infection.

How would these servicemen have been exposed to the bacterium? During the 1991 Gulf War, Iraq fired off a number of scud missiles that exploded in the air near their intended targets, but did little physical damage. Some theorize that these missiles could have delivered biological warfare agents such as the *Mycoplasma* bacteria. Consider that these servicemen were healthy enough to pass their physicals prior to the war; however, just a few years later, these same men were dying of congestive heart failure or other unusual illnesses. In fact, it is estimated that somewhere between 50,000 and 100,000 Gulf War veterans and their close family members became ill since that war ended. There is also a high incidence of deaths among that population. *Mycoplasma fermentans* (incognitus) was identified in many of the returning veterans who had the classic symptoms of Gulf War syndrome and may explain the drastic health changes in affected service men.

In fact, the first report about *Mycoplasma fermentans* (incognitus) came out of a biological warfare center where it was considered a contaminant in a weapons-grade culture. The incognitus strain may be a new one, bio-engineered in a laboratory in order to make it more pathogenic and invasive. Today, when strange diseases begin showing up, you cannot help but wonder if they are a natural phenomenon or something that came out of some government's germ warfare department. See Chapter 12 for more information about the use of *Mycoplasma* in bioterrorism.

Mycoplasma infections are airborne, which means they may be picked up without contact from an infected individual, and they can have a long latency and slow onset. They can also be transmitted to immediate family members after prolonged contact. Research indicates that infection from these bacteria may be carried in the blood and saliva. It may also be acquired through blood transfusions since *Mycoplasma* testing is currently not required. *Mycoplasma* can even pass through the mother's placenta into newborns, where it can cause serious illness.

The symptoms of this bacteria include (in descending order of frequency): aching joints, chronic fatigue, memory loss, night sweats, headaches, skin rashes, concentration loss, depression, muscle spasms, nervousness, diarrhea, blurred vision, anxiety, breathing problems, chest pain, dizziness, nausea, stomach pain, vision problems, light sensitivity, loss of balance, hives, sexual disorders, urination problems, hair loss, chemical sensitivities, frequent coughing, bleeding gums, eye redness and eye pain.

To further complicate things, *Mycoplasma* is not easily detected by ordinary lab diagnostic methods; however, new sophisticated technology is starting to change that. Only a very few specialty labs, such as the one mentioned above, are testing for *Mycoplasma* by means of forensic "gene-tracking" PCR (polymerase chain reaction). The diagnostic test for *Mycoplasma* is much more affordable now than it used to be. The cost for testing is now in the $250 range; it used to be more like $2,500. Careful blood handling and accurate results go hand in hand. This should be considered when choosing a lab to perform *Mycoplasma* detection. According to the *Mycoplasma Registry*, blood shipped at room temperature loses 50 percent of the DNA within six hours and 100 percent after seventy-two hours. There may be value in using live blood analysis to detect *Mycoplasma*.

The good news is that *Mycoplasma* is usually treatable with multiple courses of antibiotics over a long period of time. It is more successful if treatment is started as soon as possible after the symptoms begin. The bad news is that many people cannot take a long course of antibiotics, and it is unknown at this time what alternative treatments would be effective. I have hope that a new homeopathic nosode therapy will prove helpful, as well as a treatment plan that includes boosting the immune system. Many people are probably exposed to *Mycoplasma*, but only some succumb to their debilitating effects. This is why strengthening and aiding the immune system becomes so important.

Proteus mirabilis

There are four species of *Proteus*, but *Proteus mirabilis* causes most human infections. These organisms are normally found in soil and water, but *Proteus* is also an opportunistic pathogen living among the normal intestinal microflora. *Proteus mirabilis* is often cultured from superficial wounds, ear drainage and sputum, particularly in people whose normal microflora has been compromised by antibiotic therapy.

There may also be deep-seated *Proteus* infections in the sinuses and urinary tracts of people with chronic problems (or kidney or bladder stones). Once established in the urinary tract, *Proteus* strains appear to be particularly virulent. They seem to possess the ability to adhere to the lining of the kidney and therefore cause disease. In large enough numbers, *Proteus* bacteria may cause diarrhea and intestinal distress and can be a factor in rheumatoid arthritis. I often find overgrowths of this organism in the intestinal tract when stool samples are checked.

Pseudomonas aeruginosa

Infections with this potential pathogen are usually found in the urinary tract, ears and other areas in debilitated people with diminished immune function. Those being treated with an indwelling catheter are also vulnerable. The organism usually plugs the catheter with mucus, resulting in an infection in the urethra. *Pseudomonas* breeds in moist places, such as sinks, respiratory equipment, incubators and even hand lotion. Infants, burn victims, patients being treated for intravenous drug addiction, cystic fibrosis or leukemia, and those with organ transplants may even die from a *Pseudomonas* infection. This bacterium can also cause a serious ear infection called malignant external otitis, as well as blood poisoning and eye or heart inflammation. In fact, it is estimated that this pathogen is involved in up to 20 percent of all hospital infections.

In August 1998, there was an investigation as to why *Pseudomonas aeruginosa* infections were increasing in the neonatal ICU units of several hospitals. Checking common environmental sources such as tap water, sinks, respiratory equipment and environmental surfaces in the neonatal ICU failed to disclose a common source of infection. However, when healthcare workers were evaluated, 5 percent of the clinicians and 10 percent of the nurses were found to have *Pseudomonas aeruginosa* on their hands. Some of them continued to harbor this pathogen on an ongoing basis. A common denominator was the presence of artificial fingernails, nail wraps and long, natural fingernails. Underlying nail infections may also be associated with persistent hand colonization of these bacteria. Older healthcare workers, because of age-related skin changes, may also be more likely to have positive hand cultures.

Another report about *Pseudomonas* and newborn infections in an Oklahoma City hospital had similar findings. This bacterium was transferred from under the long nails of three nurses who handled these high-risk babies. Precautions should be taken in all hospitals, but particularly in neonatal intensive care units, where outbreaks have occurred.

Recently, Canadian physicians also reported what they believe to be the first outbreak of "*Pseudomonas* hot-foot syndrome." According to the *New England Journal of Medicine* 2001, investigators reviewed medical records of forty children between the ages of two and fifteen with intense pain in the soles of their feet within forty hours after using the same municipal wading pool between March and May 1998. Almost all of the children were healthy, but developed symptoms of severe swelling, redness and burning, incapacitating pain in their feet between ten to forty hours after using the pool. Pain was so severe as to make walking or even wearing socks unbearable. Some severely ill patients had mild fever, malaise and nausea. After several days, the children's feet appeared bruised, and the skin began to peel. A stronger chlorine solution did not prevent further cases until an ammonium compound and ozone were used. The outbreak ceased when the pool was chlorinated, pool filters were replaced, and the pool bottom was sanded to eliminate rough spots. Cases have also developed on the extremities after the use of a hot tub. This new syndrome is probably more common than currently recognized, and doctors should be alerted to its possibility in both children and adults who may have recently scraped their feet while swimming.

Several cancer patients being treated at the University of Iowa Hospitals and Clinics also developed serious *Pseudomonas aeruginosa* infections that were traced to a contaminated drain in a whirlpool bathtub. Researchers found that the design of the drain, which closed about one inch below the drain's strainer, allowed water to become contaminated as the tub was filled. A survey revealed that seventeen bathtubs in sixteen nursing homes were contaminated in the same way. Evidently, such tubs are used in many hospitals and may be an unrecognized source of infections as well. Using whirlpool bathtubs with drains that seal at the top would eliminate this potential source of infection.

Pseudomonas is commonly isolated from stool and may be acquired through exposure to contaminated water, including bottled drinking water. In large concentrations, it may lead to diarrhea and intestinal distress. I find *Pseudomonas* frequently in the stool samples of people with chronic digestive problems. Often, antibiotics will not control this organism. Most doctors are unaware of the intestinal overgrowth of *Pseudomonas* and its link to chronic health problems, and thereby are unable to adequately treat this problem.

Staphylococcus aureus

Hospitalized individuals are particularly susceptible to this gram-positive organism. If this bacterium gets into the bloodstream through an open cut or wound, it can infect internal organs and cause life-threatening infections. Staph infections can attack any part of the body—skin, eyes, nails, and even the inner lining of the heart. They can also cause blood poisoning, surgical infections and pneumonia. In fact, staph infections are some of the most common bacterial and surgical wound infections.

Staphylococcus aureus is usually harmless to humans and is often found in the nostrils and on the skin. In a susceptible person, however, these bacteria can overgrow in the intestinal tract, causing chronic irritation and other systemic health problems. One young woman became infected with *Staphylococcus aureus* after a splinter remained in her finger for a period of time. Later, there was an overgrowth of this same organism in her intestinal tract. She had not felt well for a year, but no one had thought to culture her stool to find out what was making her sick. Even if lab tests are performed in cases like these, it does not guarantee that doctors will find the bacterium. Often, conventional lab tests do not show overgrowths with this pathogen. Using a specialty lab, several times in the recent past I have found *Staphylococcus aureus* overgrowing in patients' intestinal tract in sufficient amounts to cause illness.

As with most bacteria, they are opportunistic and grow wherever the internal terrain is no longer healthy. Symptoms vary, depending on where the infection develops. People with a chronic illness, such as cancer, chronic liver or kidney disease, or those who inject illegal drugs (cocaine, heroin, etc.), are particularly susceptible to severe staph infections and overgrowths. Infections can also be spread on the skin. Eczema can cause a person to scratch, often leading to secondary trauma and/or infections.

Furthermore, it is becoming increasingly difficult to treat bacterial infections caused by *Staphylococcus aureus* because the bacterium is growing more resistant to antibiotics. In fact, many authorities now know that this bacteria has the ability to send mobile antibiotic-resistant genes through host populations to be transferred to strains that have not even been exposed to the antibiotic (*Proc Natl Acad Sci USA* 2001). For instance, investigators from the National Institutes of Health evaluated thirty-six strains of *Staphylococcus aureus* obtained from four continents, some from as early as the 1960s. Eleven were resistant to the antibiotic methicillin.

There is also a recent case of the new antibiotic linezolid not working against *Staphylococcus aureus*. Except for vancomycin, it is the only other drug that can be used to treat methicillin-resistant staph infections (*Lancet* 2001). This finding comes at a time when the U.S. Centers for Disease Control and Prevention have launched an initiative to reduce the use of vancomycin among hospitalized patients.

Although investigators believe that new antibiotics will solve the problem, the main reason that this bacterium has mutated in the first place is because of the unwarranted and dangerous misuse of antibiotics. Staph infection could perhaps become an even greater threat than *E. coli* 0157:H7 in the future.

CHAPTER 11

Alphabetical Listing of Disease-Bacteria Links

Acne

The presence of acne is often a sign of an imbalance in the microflora of the intestinal tract. The responsible bacteria overgrow in the intestines, and the toxins that leak through can get into the body and may aggravate the skin. Balancing the intestinal microflora may aid in resolving acne.

ADD/ADHD

According to research, a prior infection with the *Streptococcus* bacteria may contribute to the development of attention deficit/hyperactivity disorder (ADHD). This is the same bacterium that causes strep throat. In one study, children with ADHD had higher blood levels of two types of anti-strep antibodies than other people in the study. The results also show an association between a prior strep infection and the enlargement of the basal ganglia, a small structure inside the brain that helps to regulate thought and behavior. A *Streptococcus* infection may set up an immune response that injures the basal ganglia in susceptible people, causing these structures to malfunction. It is important that an infected person receive the correct treatment.

The diets of affected children should also be examined. Many of these children could be eating diets high in sugar and simple carbohydrates, which feed bacteria and depress the immune system. Suppressed immunity may make them more susceptible to infection. I seldom see a child diagnosed with ADD/ADHD that eats a healthy diet. For more information about this condition read my book, *Natural Treatments for ADD and Hyperactivity*.

Another theory is that ADHD is caused by a fungus, since fungal metabolites are often found in the urine of these individuals. Some children's symptoms often decrease dramatically after taking antifungal agents. One thing I know is that ADD/ADHD may have many different causes but none of them are due to a Ritalin deficiency.

Alzheimer's Disease

Although the causes of Alzheimer's still remain a mystery, Pennsylvania scientists have discovered *Chlamydia pneumoniae* in the brains of people suffering with the disease. There is also new evidence that the bacterium *Mycoplasma* may be a factor for many types of degenerative diseases, including Alzheimer's. Of course, there may be other factors that cause the disease, but it is definitely worth exploring the possibility of an infectious agent.

Arthritis

A vast amount of research supports the involvement of intestinal bacteria in the development of reactive arthritis, and bacterial overgrowth has been frequently proposed as the cause of other rheumatic diseases. It is thought that a bacterial overgrowth from pathogens such as *Shigella*, *Campylobacter* or *Klebsiella* can cause an immune response that results in arthritic conditions. In some cases, toxins from the bacteria may enter the blood causing other types of inflammatory joint diseases.

Another microbe linked with reactive arthritis is *Yersinia enterocolitica*. This triggering microbe can persist in a rather passive state in the host cells, but when the opportunity is right, then it can become invasive. Several other microbes share this same feature, such as *Chlamydia*. If you have arthritic pain, consider these stealth pathogens as probable causes. Getting rid of these bacteria is necessary for effective and long-term results.

Rheumatoid arthritis may have an infectious cause as well. In fact, a number of studies found that using low-dose, long-term (but intermittent) antibiotic therapy was effective. This certainly suggests that there are bacteria causing this condition in some people. Most rheumatology investigators believe that an infectious agent causes rheumatoid arthritis. There is little agreement as to the involved organism since there are probably several different culprits. *Proteus mirabilis* is found in high amounts in many people with this condition. In a study of two hundred people with rheumatoid arthritis, 25 percent tested positive for another microbe, *Chlamydia*. The culprit could also be an intracellular bacterium that replicates very slowly called *Mycoplasma*. Unfortunately, most people do not respond to low-dose antibiotic therapy when the cause is *Mycoplasma*, unless treatment is started very early in the disease process.

But there is evidence supporting the hypothesis that *Mycoplasma* is a common cause of rheumatoid arthritis. As far back as 1939, Dr. Sabin, the discoverer of the polio vaccine, first reported a chronic arthritis in mice caused by *Mycoplasma*. He suggested this agent might be the cause in humans with rheumatoid arthritis. Dr. Thomas Brown, a rheumatologist who worked with Dr. Sabin, was also a strong advocate of the *Mycoplasma* theory for over fifty years of his life.

Even as far back as 1970, four different strains of *Mycoplasma fermentans* were implicated in other forms of arthritis (*Journal of Clinical Microbiology* January 2000), including gout, reactive arthritis, juvenile chronic arthritis, ankylosing spondylitis and psoriatic arthritis. (However, it was not detected in any of the patients who had osteoarthritis.)

There is also evidence that *Klebsiella pneumoniae* may cause ankylosing spondylitis. People with this condition often have high starch diets and high levels of *Klebsiella* in their stools. Starch is the perfect diet for concentrations of *Klebsiella* in the intestinal tract.

Moreover, there are some forms of arthritis caused by the Lyme disease tick that appear in untreated people for months or even years after being infected. The problem with the blood test for Lyme disease is that it only detects *Borrelia burgdorferi*. It does not detect other species such as *Borrelia garinii* or *Borrelia afzelii*. Even the conventional Western blot test may be negative (*Arthritis Rheum* 2001). Beside blood tests, it may be necessary to have urine tests or other types of testing, and to repeat these tests several times before they detect the correct organism. If *Borrelia* is suspected and the tests remain negative, it may be wise to treat for this organism anyway. See the entry on "Lyme Disease" later in this chapter for more information.

Asthma

Over the past twenty years, the prevalence of asthma has steadily climbed in the U.S. and worldwide. One theory about this dramatic rise in asthma sufferers comes from studies which found that infants who have more colds and other infections have lower asthma rates later in life. When babies are exposed to germs early in life, they may be better able to cope with infections, thereby decreasing the tendency of the immune system to overreact to normally benign substances like dust and mold. The modern phenomenon of placing children in sterile environments and giving them antibiotics for every sniffle may actually have helped make them more susceptible to asthma. There is even some speculation that this overactive immune system begins in the first months of life.

Another theory about the causes of asthma has to do with certain by-products of bacteria called endotoxins, which are found in household dust. Endotoxins appear to block certain processes in the immune system, potentially leading to asthma. Many homes tested positive for high levels of endotoxins after dust samples were collected from the living room, kitchen, bedroom floors, couches and children's beds. Endotoxins are also found in soil and in the excrement of humans and animals, including household pets.

There is also evidence that *Chlamydia pneumoniae* may play an important role in asthma. Blood tests showed evidence that many asthmatics not only had past bacterial infections, but continue to suffer from chronic infection (*Am J Respir Crit Care Med* 2001). Another study found that a substantial number of people with chronic stable asthma were infected with *Mycoplasma* and/or *Chlamydia* in their airways. If these finding are correct, it could mark a drastic change in asthma treatment (*J Allergy Clin Immunol* 2001).

One experimental treatment that has been getting some notice is probiotic therapy. There is evidence that it may be helpful to give beneficial bacteria to expectant mothers with newborns that are predisposed to asthma. The researchers recruited near-term pregnant women who had a family history of allergic diseases and gave some of them the probiotic *Lactobacillus rhamnosus* with good results.

Atopic Dermatitis (Eczema)

Probiotic therapy may also be useful for expectant mothers with babies predisposed to eczema, according to a new Finnish study. The researchers recruited pregnant women who were close to delivery and had a family history of allergic diseases. They gave some of them *Lactobacillus GG* with promising results. There is some speculation that the alarming increase in eczema may be due to an overactive immune system in the first months of life. This same Finnish group claims that infants taking probiotics have decreased milk allergies and skin complications.

There is also evidence of intestinal imbalances and malabsorption in the majority of people with eczema. Treatment with antibacterial herbs (like echinacea) often produces major improvement in the gastrointestinal symptoms as well as improvement in the severity of the eczema. Of course, there may be multiple underlying causes for eczema.

Perhaps one of the most dangerous habits of the eczema sufferer is "scratching the itch," which can result in the skin being heavy colonized by bacteria, especially *Staphylococcus aureus*. In fact, ninety percent of the people with eczema will end up with staph infections if they continue to scratch their skins with their fingernails.

Autism

Children with autism often have frequent ear infections that are treated with antibiotics. The problem with this treatment method is that pathogens find favorable growth conditions if the protective intestinal microflora is disrupted by the regular use of broad-spectrum antibiotics. These pathogens may begin producing toxins that affect the brain. Some research in this area came from Dr. William Shaw, Ph.D., who spent the last several years measuring urinary organic acid levels in autistic children and in other children with severe developmental delays or other neurological abnormalities. Early in the testing, certain compounds were identified in the urine that were not of human origin. They were assumed to be unimportant at the time because they were considered to be the metabolites of microbes. Later, Dr. Shaw began to believe that this finding was indeed important.

One compound that was found in autistic children may be the result of a mixture of different members of the *Clostridia* family, not just *Clostridium difficile*. This mix is also found in many schizophrenics. It is thought that this compound may inhibit the enzyme that converts dopa to dopamine, an important neurotransmitter. This pathway requires a vitamin B6 derivative and could possibly explain why vitamin B6 in large doses is useful in reducing some symptoms of autism. (Consider using the pyridoxal-5-phosphate form of vitamin B6 in case the enzyme that is required to convert B6 is not present.) *Clostridium* is not susceptible to the majority of commonly used broad-spectrum antibiotics, and so it is not killed by them.

However, one successful treatment involved an autistic child with severe chronic constipation who was treated with a protocol using beneficial bowel bacteria. Within a few days after beginning treatment, the autistic child began making eye contact and speaking a few words. There was another case of full recovery from autism after the mother gave her child a quart and a half of breast milk daily for four months to build up the child's immune system. Breast milk promotes the growth of the beneficial bacteria bifidobacteria in infants. This in turn may have eliminated the pathogenic organisms from the child's intestines.

A characteristic pattern of intestinal inflammation has been discovered in some children with autism. These children typically have long-standing intestinal symptoms that start around the same time as the behavioral changes. The other consistent feature is mild-to-moderate colitis that lacks the specific diagnostic features of either Crohn's disease or ulcerative colitis. It appears that some forms of autism may arise from the toxic effects of intestinal products on the developing brain.

In one study, autistic children had intestinal symptoms consisting of abdominal pain, constipation, diarrhea (or alternating constipation and diarrhea), and bloating. They were consistently picky in their eating habits, with a diet limited largely to carbohydrates such as cereals, potato crisps, and bread. Moreover, certain foodstuffs such as dairy products were reported by parents to produce deterioration in behavior. Withholding such foods apparently produced behavioral improvement, especially in aggression levels, amount of eye contact, and sleep patterns. According to the parents, undigested food was often seen in the stools. It appears that a gut-brain interaction may be responsible for some of the behavioral features.

Yeast may also be linked to autism because it produces enzymes that digest proteins and fats in order to attach themselves to the gut lining. As the yeast become more invasive, symptoms of leaky gut syndrome develop. This can lead to gluten sensitivity and food allergies, common in autistic children. A diet that restricts grains, especially gluten-containing ones, as well as sugar and milk casein, may be helpful because these foods are required for the yeast's survival. A diet high in vegetables (which contains yeast-fighting phytochemicals) may also decrease yeast growth.

For example, consider the following case: After several courses of antibiotics for ear infections, a three-year-old child develops a severe case of thrush (yeast). He subsequently loses all language skills, stops making eye contact, and became very hyperactive. Upon testing, doctors find a yeast overgrowth in the intestines. Within twenty-four hours of using an appropriate antifungal agent, the child begins having eye contact for the first time in six months, and his other symptoms improve. Some of these same symptoms are found in children with autism, and this case shows that having a pathogenic overgrowth may cause long-term problems such as autism. Many times the problem is not bacteria or yeast, but a mix of pathogens.

A link between autism and vaccinations has also been proposed. In

April 2000, a congressional panel called on the Department of Health and Human Services to begin an investigation into claims that childhood vaccines are linked to autism. One theory is that the immune systems of children who get the MMR (measles, mumps and rubella) vaccine make an immune response not only to the three diseases, but also to their own nervous system. Another theory is that the child's immune system is simply overwhelmed by being hit by so many viruses at the same time. It could be that all of the vaccines given to children in the first two years of their life are just too much for an underdeveloped immune system to handle. Still another theory is that early childhood vaccinations cause the depletion of thymus cells, which puts the child at risk for a depressed immune system, leading to an overgrowth of pathogens in the intestinal tract. Any or all of these theories could be correct and cause or contribute to autism. In too many cases, there is a period of initial normal development before vaccines are given, followed by developmental regression and loss of acquired skills, sometimes occurring over a period of days to weeks.

Autoimmune Diseases

As previously mentioned, there may be a link between autoimmune diseases, such as lupus, and altered gut microflora in the digestive tract. Up until now, the relationship between bacteria overgrowth in the intestinal tract and chronic illnesses has been poorly understood. The main reason for this has been the lack of adequate lab testing and identification of organisms, such as *Mycoplasma* and other cell wall-deficient organisms. This may explain why some cases of antibiotic therapy for lupus have had amazing results. And lupus is not the only autoimmune condition that has been relieved with antibiotic therapy. People with several different types of autoimmune conditions have reported improvement after using specific antibiotics; however, antibiotics are not the only answer. Later in this book I will discuss a number of drugless treatments that work against these harmful bacteria.

Cancer

Bacterial links to cancer may be some of the most controversial, but that doesn't mean they don't exist. A severe imbalance in bowel microflora (dysbiosis) has been implicated in some forms of cancer, such as breast cancer. One theory is that when there are high levels of pathogenic bacteria in the gut, there is also an increase in various bacterial enzymes that cause bile acids to promote the increase of circulating estrogen. This causes an increase in estrogen levels in the blood and urine, possibly contributing to the development of breast cancer. It is also thought that the prevalence of colon cancer is proportional to the concentration in the stool of these bile acids, because they are toxic to the lining of the colon. Other metabolites from microbes also appear to contribute to the development of cancer. They may contribute to inflammatory bowel diseases such as ulcerative colitis.

Normal bowel flora contains a harmless human bacteria called *E. coli*, but certain strains of this bacterium have become more dangerous. Scientists at Humboldt University in Berlin studied the intestines of 125 people with pre-cancer or cancer diagnoses. In many of them, disease-causing strains of *E. coli* were found in the large intestine where they had penetrated the intestinal lining. Researchers were unable to rule out the possibility, however, that these strains of *E. coli* were a secondary effect of the cancer, not the cause of it.

One cancer treatment may also promote bacterial overgrowth. Chemotherapy is a known predisposing factor for anaerobic bacteria infections in cancer patients because it causes gastrointestinal ulceration, which permits anaerobes to enter circulation. Infection by anaerobic bacteria is usually caused by more than one type of bacteria and presents a high risk to the patient.

Cardiac Device Infections

The incidence of infection of implanted pacemakers or cardioverter-defibrillators among patients with *Staphylococcus aureus* may be higher than previously thought (*Circulation* 2001). Researchers estimate that about 70 percent of patients with *Staphylococcus aureus* who have an implanted cardiac device may also have a bacterial infection. Other studies have shown that the incidence ranges up to about 20 percent. Sixty percent of the patients with confirmed device infection showed no "clinically detectable signs" of the infection, researchers noted.

Cardiovascular Disease

You eat a healthy diet, exercise regularly, and keep an eye on your blood pressure and cholesterol. You are doing all you can to prevent a heart attack, or are you? There is growing evidence that pathogenic organisms may play a role in the development of coronary artery disease. It has been known for more than a century that some viruses and bacteria can infect the heart muscle and valves and cause serious illness. Rheumatic fever, for example, is caused by a strep infection that affects both the throat and the heart.

Another prime suspect is a type of pneumonia-causing bacteria *Chlamydia*. Studies have shown an increased incidence of coronary artery disease in people who test positive for *Chlamydia*. This bacterium has been found lurking in the arterial plaque, but researchers aren't sure if the organism injures the arteries or just happens to be there. However, a study published in *Science* found that the presence of *Chlamydia* in some mice triggered such a strong immune response that it caused heart damage. Moreover, recent studies found that people with coronary artery disease who are given *Chlamydia*-killing antibiotics have fewer heart attacks and infections.

Infection with a particular strain of *Heliobacter pylori* may also increase the risk of heart disease. Without proper treatment, *H. pylori* can trigger a low-grade inflammatory illness that persists for years. Chronic infections like these may place a subtle but steady strain on the body's cardiovascular system. Recent studies found that one particular strain of *H. pylori* was most related to heart disease, but it is unknown at this time if it causes or merely contributes to the problem.

Bacteria lurking in dental plaque and on diseased gums could trigger a heart attack, according to a recent study in rabbits. Bacteria found in the plaque promote clumping of platelets, one of the first steps in clot formation that could lead to a heart attack. The bacteria also cause abnormalities in heart function. Two bacteria were looked at in the study, *Streptococcus sanguis* and *Porphyromonas gingivalis*. Over time, both could easily enter diseased gums and then the bloodstream, resulting in infection. Could this also occur in humans? Researchers claim that 60 percent of *Streptococcus sanguis* strains found in the human mouth contain similar components. Removing plaque and keeping your gums healthy may be an important part of decreasing your risk of heart disease.

Cardiovascular conditions have also been linked to the gram-positive, pleiomorphic bacterium *Rothia dentocariosa*, which is commonly found as part of the normal microflora of the mouth, throat and nose. Before now, it was rarely thought to cause disease. Now it is suspected of causing some cardiovascular changes including brain abscesses, aneurysms of cerebral arteries and the abdominal aorta. *Rothia dentocariosa* should be considered as a possible cause of subacute endocarditis, especially in people with periodontal disease and underlying valvular heart disease.

Chronic bacterial infections, including lung and urinary tract infections, as well as gum disease, may also increase the risk of atherosclerosis, a build-up of fatty plaques in the arteries. Previous research has suggested a link between infections and heart attacks, but few studies have examined the relationship between infections and atherosclerosis. People who have chronic infections are more likely to develop new plaque than people who do not have any infections. A study found that it was bacterial infections, not viruses, causing atherosclerosis.

As mentioned, recent treatments for heart disease have begun to include antibiotics, based on findings like the above. Even if antibiotics do prevent heart attacks, however, no one really knows which drugs should be used, at what dose, or how often. For instance, it is quite possible that someone might be harboring several organisms, so choosing the right antibiotic, or a combination of them, would be crucial. Also, some bacteria are easily acquired, so the same person may be infected repeatedly if they have a weakened immune system. Furthermore, antibiotic overuse may encourage bacterial resistance and leave the person more vulnerable to infection. I believe that antibiotics should be used with care and, if at all possible, should be reserved for people who have a known bacterial infection or when there is not an alternative treatment.

Moreover, some people who had symptoms suggesting a heart attack actually were found to have Lyme disease instead. The symptoms included a severe feeling of indigestion in the chest along with a grabbing pain in the lower throat, nausea and lower abdominal pain. After being tested for cardiac problems, all results were negative. Tests were then run to rule out the bacteria *H. pylori,* which also came back negative. There was, however, inflammation in the stomach lining, as well as in the small intestine. Researchers knew to test for Lyme disease because in previous studies, this same inflammation was found in children with Lyme disease who were experiencing gastrointestinal symptoms.

Another possible explanation is that bacterial infections or overgrowths may trigger the immune system to turn against itself. This so-called autoimmune response may damage vessels, making it easier for fatty deposits to accumulate. This bacterial growth may be a powerful mechanism of disease. Remember, a weakened immune system and an unhealthy terrain open the door for these infections to manifest themselves in the first place.

Chronic Fatigue Syndrome (CFIDS)

Mycoplasma fermentans (incognitus) has been found in many people diagnosed with chronic fatigue. The sicker the person is, the more likely it is that they have a *Mycoplasma* infection. When *Mycoplasma* is eliminated, many cases of chronic fatigue also resolve. In one study, it was found that around 70 percent of chronic fatigue syndrome patients had *Mycoplasma* DNA in their bloodstream, indicating the presence of this organism. In contrast, only 9 percent of seventy healthy individuals carried such signs. However, very little federal research money has been granted to independent researchers for finding the cause of this illness. The official government position is that CFIDS is not infectious, but how can we be sure without more research into the cause?

Crohn's Disease

Crohn's is a potentially devastating disease that affects the digestive tract. It is often looked at as incurable because it is viewed as an immune system malfunction that wreaks havoc on the intestines. However, the symptoms of cramping and bloody diarrhea may simply be the immune system's attempt to spew out a pathogen such as bacteria. This contradicts the popular notion of intractable autoimmune diseases.

In fact, one piece of research strongly links Crohn's disease to the bacteria *Mycoplasma pneumoniae*. I usually find an overgrowth of some pathogenic bacteria in the intestines of people with Crohn's disease. The ones I find most often are *Citrobacter, Proteus, Pseudomonas* and *Klebsiella*. However, a new Italian study suggests that some cases of inflammatory bowel disease, including Crohn's disease, may be cause by cytomegalovirus (CMV), especially in those cases that do not respond to steroids.

In Japan, the elimination of possible food allergens is the first treatment used for people with active Crohn's disease. Approximately 80 percent of the people who use this type of diet experience a remission of their symptoms in about three or four weeks. Evidence of remission is apparent on radiographic and endoscopic exam in about eight weeks after beginning treatment. What this means is that food allergies may be a major contributing factor in Crohn's disease. It is possible that food allergies depress the immune system, making the host susceptible to bacterial overgrowth or organisms such as *Mycoplasma*. Anyone with an inflammatory bowel disease should have a comprehensive bacteria, yeast and parasite test. *Mycoplasma* is not easy to detect and specialized lab tests may be necessary.

Moreover, a faulty gene has been found in some people with Crohn's disease. This gene usually triggers a reaction to bacteria invading the gut, but in some people with Crohn's disease, this gene is damaged. Therefore, it cannot respond the way it is supposed to when harmful bacteria invade the intestinal tract. Both American and European research groups have been working to prove that this gene, called Nod2, is acting as a guardian that protects the body against bacteria that invade the intestines. For more information refer to the May 2001 issue of *Nature*.

Cystic Fibrosis

Pseudomonas aeruginosa is a major pathogen found in children with cystic fibrosis. It is unknown at what point these children acquire this organism; however one study indicated that children are likely to be colonized or infected very early in life. Therapy to prevent infection with *Pseudomonas aeruginosa* will have to be applied early and in such a manner as to avoid resistant types (*J Infect Dis.* 2001).

Two reports published in the *Lancet* (2001) indicate that a cross-infection can occur with a transmissible strain of *Pseudomonas*, meaning that people in the study were doubly infected after contact with colonized individuals during hospital stays. It may be worrisome for people with cystic fibrosis to attend school or social events where other people with cystic fibrosis may transmit to them other strains of this bacterium.

Dental Disease

The amount of people who become ill after having a root canal is alarming. This problem appears to be infinitely more serious than the mercury amalgam issue ever was. Apparently, there are bacteria harbored in root canals no matter how perfectly they are done. These bacteria can mutate and become toxin factories, spreading these toxins into the bloodstream and causing degenerative diseases. In fact, it has been reported that only 20 to 25 percent of root canals are not infected with anaerobic bacteria and/or *Mycoplasma*. If you had an increase in symptoms following a root canal, you might be suffering from this type of infection.

Many people can handle having a root canal for many years without any difficulty. Individuals with good genetic backgrounds and strong immune systems, who practice good nutrition and are in good health can take care of potentially destructive bacteria quite adequately, but in susceptible individuals, it can be quite dangerous. Even healthy individuals who have had a severe accident, contracted a bad case of the flu or have been under extreme stress may be vulnerable. Their immune systems, which were previously able to cope with these bacteria, have become overwhelmed, and these individuals now develop diseases in the liver, kidneys, eyes, etc. The infection that came from the tooth has traveled to some other area of the body and manifested itself as a new infection. For more information, read *Root Canal CoverUp, Exposed!* which is available from Price-Pottenger Nutrition Foundation (PPNF) at P.O. box 2614, La Mesa, CA 91943 or by calling (800) FOODS-4-U.

An infected root canal isn't the only potentially dangerous dental condition. The same bacteria that causes gum disease can enter your bloodstream and damage other parts of your body. Researchers from the University at Buffalo, New York, reported that people with severe gum disease are twice as likely as those with healthy gums to have a stroke caused by blocked arteries. Furthermore, researchers at the University of Alabama at Birmingham reported preliminary results of a study suggesting that pregnant women with severe periodontal disease may be more likely to give birth prematurely.

According to the American Dental Association, three out of four adults over the age of thirty-five have some form of gum disease. Plaque, the film of bacteria that sticks to teeth, is the chief culprit. Smoking, alcohol, stress and poor diet can contribute to this problem. Early warning signs of gum disease include: gums that bleed easily; red, swollen or tender gums; gums that have pulled away from the teeth; persistent bad breath or a chronic bad taste in the mouth; and permanent teeth that are loose or separating. Treatment ranges from thorough plaque removal to antibiotic therapy. In severe cases, surgery may be needed to repair and rebuild damaged tissue.

Depression, Chronic

Studies have shown that immune dysfunction may precede the development of depression. This suggests that depression may be indirectly related to immune activation and not merely a psychological reaction. Toxins found in the urine of individuals with depression may come from pathogenic bacteria and fungus. Following treatment with oral antifungal agents and antibiotics, depressive symptoms in case studies lessened, often dramatically. Remember, without identifying the actual organism, the correct treatment may not be found, and therefore, symptoms will not improve.

How could immune activation affect mood? During a physical illness, the immune system serves as a sensory organ, communicating with the brain through the secretion of intercellular mediators called cytokines. An association exists between high cytokine levels and psychological disturbances, particularly depression, as well as other psychological disturbances.

Another theory involves a natural antidepressant, called phenylalanine, that is produced in the cell walls of the beneficial bowel bacteria *Lactobacillus acidophilus* and other gram-positive bacteria. It is believed that increasing beneficial bacteria in the intestinal tract may relieve mild depression. This means that supplementing with a probiotic may be an important tool for many individuals.

Diarrhea

Diarrhea is the occurrence of loose, watery stools more than three times in one day. It is a common problem that usually lasts a day or two and goes away on its own without any special treatment. However, prolonged diarrhea can be a sign of other problems and has dangerous side effects. Diarrhea can cause dehydration, which is particularly dangerous in children, the elderly, and anyone with a compromised immune system. If the diarrhea continues for more than two days, it must be treated to avoid serious health problems.

In fact, diarrhea is the second most common health problem in the U.S. after respiratory infections. Approximately 200,000 children are hospitalized each year with this condition, most under the age of five. In the elderly and critically ill patients, diarrhea can result in electrolyte losses and changes in nutritional status. It can even contribute to their death.

In small children, severe diarrhea lasting just a day or two can lead to dehydration. Because a child can die from dehydration within a few days, the main treatment for diarrhea in children is rehydration. Take your child to the doctor if any of the following symptoms appear:

- Stools containing blood or pus, or black stools.
- A temperature above 101.4°F.
- No improvement after twenty-four hours.
- Signs of dehydration that include the following: In children, a dry mouth and tongue; crying that does not produce tears; three hours or more without a wet diaper; sunken eyes, cheeks or abdomen; a high fever, listlessness or irritability; and skin that does not flatten when pinched and released. Adults often have increased thirst, less frequent urination, dry skin, fatigue, headache and light-headedness.

For the various types of diarrhea, one of the most successful treatments has been the use of beneficial living organisms (probiotics) that help balance the microflora and prevent harmful bacteria from taking over. Using probiotics can reduce the need for antibiotics, and they cost less and are better tolerated than drugs. One of the simplest and most effective ways to combat diarrhea is to take the probiotics *Lactobacillus acidophilus* and bifidobacteria every hour. Probiotics are incredible healing agents and seem to work to resolve most cases of acute infectious diarrhea relatively quickly.

For instance, hospitalized infants are at especially high risk for acquiring intestinal microbes that can cause diarrhea. However, in one study, when infants were given a formula containing *Lactobacillus GG* bacteria, it helped to ward off intestinal problems. In one study reported in the *Journal of Pediatrics* 2001, there was an 80 percent reduction in the risk of developing diarrhea after using probiotics. Also, there were no adverse side effects reported from the treatment.

There are several theories about how *Lactobacillus GG* or any probiotic might help prevent intestinal disorders. They may compete with harmful microbes for nutrients in the body or synthesize microbe-fighting compounds. The recommended dose is one capsule or one-fourth teaspoon of the powder every thirty to sixty minutes until the diarrhea stops. It usually resolves in about four hours.

Saccharomyces boulardii is another probiotic effective in treating diarrhea in the elderly and critically ill patients. Individuals with AIDS (or who are HIV positive) and suffer with chronic diarrhea may find this probiotic useful in preventing the typical symptoms of malabsorption and weight loss. Often, these individuals do not respond to traditional antibiotic therapy due to their compromised immune systems and debilitated state. However, in one study, when AIDS patients received *Saccharomyces boulardii* for two to four weeks, they experienced a significant decrease or total cessation in diarrhea. (Patients experienced little change after the first week, so it is important to continue treatment for multiple weeks.) *Saccharomyces boulardii* is especially helpful for diarrhea caused by poor diet, stress, travel and antibiotics; however, it may take a high dose of *S. boulardii* to be effective, in the range of two to three grams a day. Despite these high doses, no side effects have been observed.

Traveler's diarrhea is a common complaint among tourists and other travelers visiting developing countries, people on cruise ships, or military personnel overseas. The frequency of traveler's diarrhea affects approximately twelve million people each year. Symptoms may occur several days after exposure and last for three to four days if untreated. Some cases may last a month with symptoms including abdominal cramping, malaise, nausea, fever or pain. Usually traveler's diarrhea is a self-limiting disease without complications, but it can be hazardous to children when it causes dehydration. It is advisable to drink additional water or beverages that include electrolytes.

Antibiotics, such as ciprofloxacin, are commonly prescribed to travelers. This antibiotic often induces another form of diarrhea caused by *Clostridium difficile*, which is not killed by the antibiotic. *Saccharomyces boulardii* has been effective against diarrhea caused by *Clostridium difficile*. Taking *Saccharomyces boulardii* instead of an antibiotic for diarrhea may shorten its course while discouraging *Clostridium* overgrowth.

When antibiotic use is absolutely necessary, be sure to supplement with the beneficial bacteria, *Lactobacillus acidophilus* and bifidobacteria to prevent antibiotic-induced diarrhea. To be effective, be sure to take a supplement containing at least fifteen to twenty billion organisms. It is also important to take the supplement as far away from the time you take the antibiotic as possible.

You can take the following precautions to prevent traveler's diarrhea when you go abroad:

- Do not drink any tap water, not even when brushing your teeth.
- Do not drink unpasteurized milk or dairy products.
- Do not use ice made from tap water.
- Avoid all raw fruits and vegetables (including lettuce and fruit salad) unless they can be peeled and you peel them yourself after proper washing.
- Do not eat raw or rare meat and fish.
- Do not eat meat or shellfish that is not hot when served to you.
- Do not eat food from street vendors.
- Drink only bottled water or bottled carbonated soft drinks. Do not let anyone else break the seal.

Although usually not harmful, diarrhea can become dangerous or signal a more serious problem. You should see the doctor if you have the following:

- Diarrhea for more than three days.
- Severe pain in the abdomen or rectum.
- A fever of 102°F or higher.
- Blood in the stool or black, tar-like stools.
- Signs of dehydration.

Until diarrhea subsides, try to avoid milk products and foods that are greasy or very sweet. These foods tend to aggravate diarrhea. As you improve, you can add soft, bland foods to your diet, including bananas, plain rice, boiled potatoes, toast, crackers, cooked carrots and baked chicken without the skin or fat. For children, the pediatrician may recommend what is called the BRAT diet: bananas, rice, applesauce and toast.

Ear Infections

Every year millions of children receive antibiotics for middle ear (otitis media) infections. The antibiotics kill not only the "bad" bacteria, but also the beneficial ones that form a part of the body's natural defense system. Moreover, the infection often reappears many times over the next few years and is treated with more antibiotics. However, therapies that boost beneficial bacteria may help keep the harmful bacteria from returning, thereby reducing recurrences and complications of this common childhood infection.

In fact, a new British study looked at normal bowel flora as a defense against recurrent otitis media infection. All of the children in the study received a ten-day course of antibiotics to treat the infection. After completing the antibiotic treatment, half of the children received a nasal spray for ten days containing beneficial bacteria. About two months later, these children received another ten-day course of the spray. Almost twice as many children treated with the beneficial bacterial did not develop another ear infection during the next three months compared with children who were not given the nasal spray (*British Medical Journal* January 2001).

I believe that the long-term solution for recurrent ear infections is to never use antibiotics in the first place. This method just starts a child down the road of bacterial imbalance, which almost ensures that there will be more ear infections. If an antibiotic must be used, then put the child on a probiotic as well. The best approach to ear infections is to find out what is causing the problem in the first place. A common cause is eating and drinking foods such as dairy or other foods that produce too much mucus.

Fibromyalgia

There seems to be a link between fibromyalgia and some inflammatory conditions. As far back as a decade ago, doctors in Ireland found that many people who had fibromyalgia also had inflammatory bowel disease (IBD), irritable bowel syndrome (IBS), or inflammatory arthritis. A common pathogen was thought to be a possibility for all of these health problems.

In 1999, Israeli researchers investigated fibromyalgia patients with IBS, Crohn's disease and ulcerative colitis. Fibromyalgia was documented in 30 percent of IBD patients, 49 percent of patients with Crohn's disease and in 19 percent of the people diagnosed with ulcerative colitis. Doctors are also beginning to study the relationship between bacterial overgrowth in the bowels and fibromyalgia at Cedars Sinai Medical Center in Los Angeles. They use a hydrogen breath test to detect the bacteria overgrowth in the intestinal tract.

Some people with fibromyalgia have reported a temporary reprieve from symptoms whenever they are given short-term antibiotics for other seemingly unrelated condition, such as sinusitis or bronchitis. Several of these people also run low-grade fevers every day, which may signify some kind of underlying bacterial infection. In fact, one lab found *Chlamydia trachomatis* in the blood of 20 percent of fibromyalgia patients by using PCR (polymerase chain reaction), an advanced laboratory detection method. Another bacteria suspected of causing fibromyalgia is *Mycoplasma fermentans* (incognitus). The spirochete that causes Lyme disease, *Borrelia burgdorferi,* has also been found in many people with fibromyalgia.

Microscopic examination has shown an abnormal infiltration of specialized immune cells called macrophages surrounding muscle tissue. Macrophages are a type of immune cell that is important for swallowing and destroying microorganisms. They also assist other immune cells in responding to invading organisms. The muscle cells in some fibromyalgics appear to be minimally damaged by the macrophages. Muscle pain and tenderness are the most frequent symptoms, but often there is also joint pain, muscle weakness, fatigue and fever.

Moreover, many people suffer fibromyalgia-type pains after receiving vaccines. One of the compounds frequently used in vaccines is aluminum hydroxide. It was detected in people who had symptoms of fibromyalgia. According to a 2001 issue of a well-respected journal called *Brain,* medical history analysis of patients revealed that all fifty had received vaccines of either hepatitis B virus (86 percent), hepatitis A virus (19 percent) or tetanus toxoid (58 percent) three to ninety-six months before biopsy. It is suspected that the unidentified causes of many diseases may be the result of vaccines affecting our bodies in adverse ways.

Fevers

People often treat fevers as though they are a problem in and of themselves. A fever is actually a symptom of an illness, not the illness itself. Fevers often cause anxiety for parents, because they are not completely sure what to do when their child has one. However, for most children under the age of eight and especially for infants, the severity of a fever is an unreliable indicator of the severity of the child's illness. In fact, infants and toddlers can be very sick with a low or even subnormal temperature, and older children can be quite cheerful with a fairly high fever. The important thing is usually how your child is acting, not the thermometer reading. Body temperature also varies during the course of the day. Fevers usually hit their highest point in the late afternoon and are lowest early in the morning.

When surveyed, most parents thought that a mild to moderate fever could cause harmful effects in their children, along with other misconceptions. In reality, a fever is the body's backup immune mechanism and should not be suppressed unless absolutely necessary. It is one way that the body kills off pathogens such as bacteria and viruses. Unless the fever is over 103°F and climbing, or your child is miserable, avoid giving them anti-fever medication. Fevers that get too high (above 106°F), however, can harm the heart and brain—even in a previously healthy child. But a mild or moderate fever is not dangerous, and taking medication will only suppress beneficial immune responses. In fact, in surveys almost 15 percent of caregivers gave acetaminophen and 44 percent gave ibuprofen to their fevered children too frequently. If you feel that you need to give anti-fever medication, consider non-drug homeopathic remedies or herbal medications.

Moreover, many people do not have a "normal" body temperature of 98.6°F. Do your know what your basal body temperature is? One way to find out is to take your temperature on first waking in the morning for a week when you are feeling healthy. (Women should not do this during ovulation, however.) Then calculate your average temperature by adding all the readings and dividing by seven. Also, remember that children tend to run slightly hotter temperatures than adults. Anything between 97.4°F and 99.4°F could be considered normal. Remember that eating hot food, physical activity, overbundling, hot weather, or an overheated room can drive body temperature up a degree or two, as can ovulation.

Infections are the most common cause of fever, especially in children. Other triggers include juvenile rheumatoid arthritis, tumors and inflammatory reactions caused by trauma. Immunizations, dehydration and some medications, including antihistamines and antibiotics, can also cause fever, as can an overdose of aspirin. Some children will even have a fever when teething.

Any time body temperature increases, salt and water are lost through sweating, and so are vitamins, especially water-soluble ones. It is important to compensate for these losses by drinking an adequate amount of fluids. Small, frequent sips are often best, especially if there is nausea. It is also important to eat nutritious foods or take vitamin supplements during this time. Replacing water-soluble vitamins (chiefly C and Bs) makes sense, but during fevers, the body makes some minerals unavailable such as iron for a good reason. Bacteria need them to thrive.

Don't make your children eat during a fever if they don't feel hungry, however. People with fevers generally do not have much of an appetite. A few days of poor appetite are probably adaptive. Let your child determine when and what she eats. Just bear in mind that the consumption of sugary foods could delay natural immune response. You do need to encourage your child to drink plenty of fluids, however, because dehydration can drive up a fever.

Food Allergies

Food allergies or sensitivities are quite common today and may be connected to intestinal microflora imbalances. Some of the symptoms of a food allergy include gastrointestinal upset, frequent bruising, dark circles under the eyes called "allergic shiners," puffiness around the eyes, muscle pain, fatigue, and even some forms of depression. Exposure to antibiotics or a diet low in soluble fiber may create a deficiency of normal bowel flora. When this deficiency is present, bowel symptoms and food intolerances are more likely to occur.

If you are experiencing food allergies, the answer may be supplementation with a probiotic such as *Lactobacillus acidophilus* and *bifidus*. When beneficial bacteria increase in the stool, most people report a reduction of their gastrointestinal symptoms, including food allergies.

In all the years that I have been testing for food allergies and intolerances, milk is probably the number one food problem I see. Milk products are full of potential allergens. Besides causing allergies, dairy products are acid-forming and mucus-producing substances that provide an ideal environment for the growth of bacteria and fungus. There are also a host of other problems associated with consuming milk and dairy products. Some of the symptoms you can expect are diarrhea, digestive symptoms, skin rashes, diabetes, colic, ear infections, sinus problems, asthma and osteoporosis. Nevertheless, the public is generally not aware that there are many other ways for them to get adequate amount of calcium from their diet besides milk.

No one disputes that cow's milk contains calcium, but how much will be absorbed by the average milk drinker? Consider the following fact: The United States holds the honor of being the highest consumer of dairy products in the world, but also has the highest incidence of bone fractures and osteoporosis. Also, a *Streptococcus* infection that causes pharyngitis is more likely to occur in a milk drinker. (For a list of alternatives to milk as a source of calcium, read my book, *Allergies and Holistic Healing*.)

Still, the dairy industry has been convincing the public for years that the calcium in milk is necessary for the healthy growth of children's bones. The dairy industry has advertised milk so successfully and influenced congress for so long that every child in the public school system receives milk every day, even if they cannot pay for it. This is possible because the Department of Agriculture donates a large sum of money to America's dairy farmers. (In 1999, the sum was $200 million!)

What many Americans may not know is that dairy cows are now being fed high-protein, soy-based feeds instead of the fresh green grass that is natural to a cow's digestive system. Because these cows are also being fed hormones and other unnatural substances, they now produce three times more milk than before, but they need antibiotics to keep them well.

Furthermore, the milk of mammals is animal-specific. It is designed to nourish and protect a specific type of baby. Pasteurization, sterilization and the addition of hormones and chemicals destroy the very protection that milk is meant to provide. Cow's milk has a different composition than human milk and is poorly assimilated by humans. In fact, when animals have been given pasteurized milk for any extended period of time, they deteriorate rapidly.

If you are still drinking milk or serving it to your children, I would suggest that you find something healthier. The high rate of allergies associated with dairy products and the addition of growth hormones and antibiotics to milk should be very good reasons not to put this substance into your body. Also, nearly all dairy cows are raised on grains, not pesticide-free grass, creating an environment of pathogenic overgrowth in their intestinal tracts.

Food Poisoning

At a country fair in upstate New York, an *Escherichia coli* (*E. coli*) outbreak killed a little girl and an elderly man while making hundreds of people sick, and all they did was drink some water. It is believed that cow feces contaminated the water supply. In fact, it is estimated that seventy-six million Americans suffer some sort of illness from the food or water they consume, and the numbers are increasing. Tainted meat and poultry outbreaks still dominate the headlines, and reports of illness from fresh produce are on the rise. The bacterium *Salmonella* alone is responsible for over one million cases and around 5,000 deaths. The very young, the elderly, and those with compromised immune systems are the most vulnerable.

According to the Centers for Disease Control and Prevention (CDC), 325,000 people are hospitalized because of foodborne diseases in the

United States every year. The CDC gets its figures from a precise tracking system called PulseNet, which uses DNA fingerprinting at more than thirty-five laboratories to quickly detect foodborne illnesses. Researchers also used other surveillance systems, death certificates and published studies from academic institutions. Furthermore, the CDC said the number of known causes of food poisoning has increased more than five-fold since 1942.

The increase in food and water poisonings may depend on a number of factors, including an increase in produce from around the world entering the U.S. market, more widespread use of packaged and processed foods, and better technology for tracking outbreaks. The chance of contamination through food-handling errors has also risen as more people eat out and eat processed food.

Contaminated water used to irrigate the plants or unsterilized fertilizer spread on the ground where the plants grew may also contribute to the problem. Even the contaminated hands of field workers could be an issue. Food may also be contaminated while it is being processed or shipped. Once contaminated, the food can grow whole colonies of microbes on the food's surface, eventually ending up on your dinner plate. Why are so many cases of food poisoning happening? It is because of inadequate meat inspection, poor food handling, unsanitary food preparation and improper food storage. Even with this in mind, there are rules for preventing you from getting ill.

One way to avoid food poisoning is to take extra precautions around high-risk foods. The majority of food items that cause foodborne diseases are raw or undercooked foods from animal sources, such as meat, milk, eggs, cheese, fish or shellfish. Food poisoning can also occur in other foods when they are left out for long periods, allowing bacteria to grow and produce toxins. Although animal products are the primary offenders, more fruits and vegetables are being contaminated than ever before because of sloppy agricultural practices which allow contamination. So always wash your fruits and veggies thoroughly before eating them. Of course, processes such as pasteurizing juice and adding antioxidants to beef may help to some extent, but there are techniques you should be practicing on your own. Refer to the treatment section for more information on preventing food poisoning.

Identifying and treating food poisoning can also be difficult because foodborne outbreaks may appear quite different. After all, they involve different kinds of organisms (viruses, bacteria and parasites) contaminating a wide variety of foods grown in different parts of the world. They are also processed or prepared in many different ways.

Symptoms may appear similar to stomach flu and usually include abdominal pain with bloating, diarrhea, fever, nausea, vomiting, headaches, chills, malaise and aching joints. The onset of symptoms can occur a few or many hours later, making diagnosis difficult. The symptoms may resolve, but leave a person weak and dehydrated with electrolyte imbalances. Often, the most serious symptom is dehydration, especially in children, since repeated episodes of vomiting and diarrhea can bring body fluids to dangerously low levels.

Some of the symptoms of dehydration in children are crying without producing tears, dry mouth or tongue, decreased or no saliva under the tongue, sunken eyes, a fever without sweat, dizziness or lightheadedness, decreased urination and increased thirst. To counter dehydration, a doctor may prescribe antidiarrhea medications or drugs that prevent vomiting. Symptoms can become so serious that it may be necessary to pay a visit to the hospital to receive fluids intravenously.

In adults the body resolves most episodes of food poisoning without the aid of any treatment. The vomiting and diarrhea gets rid of most of the offending substance and your immune system takes care of the rest. By the time the stool culture comes back from the lab verifying that you had food poisoning, you are already feeling better and back at work. However, some serious signs require medical attention, including severe stomach pain, a fever higher than 102°F, uncontrollable vomiting or diarrhea, confusion and severe dizziness. Death is rare except in cases of some dangerous bacteria, such as botulism, where there is a 10 to 15 percent death rate. However, we are seeing many more deaths due to a dangerous strain of E. coli than ever before, especially in small children.

It is also a good idea to check with your doctor if the symptoms go beyond ordinary vomiting and diarrhea, such as the presence of blood in your diarrhea or vomit. The color of the blood usually is not bright red, but the color of coffee grounds. Bacteria such as *Shigella, Campylobacter, Salmonella* or certain strains of E. coli can cause this to occur. The correct bacteria can usually be pinpointed by a stool culture or culturing the vomit. Unfortunately, waiting for the results of the lab test may take too long when treatment needs to begin immediately.

The long-term effects of food poisoning may be more difficult to recognize. These symptoms form because the toxins cause disruption of normal gastrointestinal and liver function, nervous function, as well as the effects left on body tissues and organs. After being food poisoned, the body will usually go through a series of responses. First, there will be an attempt by the body to rid itself of the toxins, usually through vomiting and diarrhea. What the body cannot get rid of will end up being deposited into tissues. Then the tissue changes in an attempt to accommodate the toxic substances. This can end up causing colon problems, constipation and other functional changes. In some cases, there may be organ damage, such as toxicity to the liver, pancreas and gallbladder. Intestinal polyps or hemorrhoids may also develop. As damage progresses, it can lead to liver cirrhosis, scar tissue formation and stones. In the most severe cases of food poisoning, especially if the bacterium is botulism or the potentially deadly *E. coli*, it can lead to organ failure.

Most people with healthy immune systems can handle a touch of food poisoning. All you need to do is get some fluids and rest, and you should recover quickly. In some cases, it is a good idea to call your doctor's office and ask if you need additional treatment, depending on how severe and persistent your symptoms are. If you have other medical conditions, you may be at increased risk for more serious forms of food poisoning. People with diabetes, AIDS, liver disease, and cancer (especially during treatments of chemotherapy and radiation) are at a higher risk than people with a healthy functioning immune system. Other risks include chronic alcohol use, lymphoma, leukemia, Hodgkin's disease, and chronic kidney disease, as well as those taking immune suppressive drugs and anyone with reduced normal stomach acidity. The elderly, young children and other people who have weak immune systems are especially vulnerable to foodborne pathogens. If you are pregnant, the consequences of food poisoning can be very serious. You may be included in this high-risk group if you frequently take antacids because stomach acid has the ability to kill many of the organisms that cause food poisoning. Antacids reduce the acidity of the stomach and allow harmful bacteria to survive potentially causing acute food poisoning. Antacids also disrupt the normal and healthy bowel flora, which can contribute to chronic health conditions.

If you do seek professional treatment, remember that some forms of food poisoning cannot be treated with antibiotics. Viruses, for which there are no effective drug treatments, cause some types of food poisoning. Also, antibiotics often do not rid your body of all bacteria including *Salmonella, Shigella* and *E. coli*. On the other hand, there may be cases where an antibiotic can shorten the duration of illness or prevent damage to a fetus, including those caused by the parasite *Cyclospora* or the bacteria *Campylobacter*. There are also homeopathic remedies and botanical medications that have been helpful in the treatment of many kinds of food poisoning. Keep in mind also that antibiotics will most likely kill friendly bacteria in the gastrointestinal tract as well. Without the competition from beneficial bacteria, the pathogens multiply rapidly and begin secreting nasty toxins. This creates the ideal breeding ground for pathogens to reproduce. It would serve you better to increase the intestinal competition against harmful bacteria. This can be accomplished by taking a probiotic such as *Saccharymyces boulardii* or *Lactobacillus acidophilus* and bifidobacteria. For more information, see the entries on diarrhea and seafood poisoning.

Foodborne illness is a common, distressing and sometimes life-threatening problem for millions of people in the United States and around the world. People infected with foodborne organisms may be symptom-free or may develop symptoms ranging from mild intestinal discomfort to severe dehydration or bloody diarrhea. In more serious and untreated cases, death can occur. Foodborne illness is also extremely costly with an estimated yearly total of five to six billion dollars in direct medical expenditures and lost productivity. (Two common forms of bacteria, *Salmonella* and *Campylobacter,* account for one billion dollars in medical costs just by themselves.)

Researchers from the CDC say that too many people are becoming sick and dying from food poisoning. According to recent figures 76 million people become sick from food poisoning each year, 325,000 people are hospitalized, and 5,000 people die. These numbers confirm that the number of illnesses and deaths from contaminated food in the U.S. is unacceptably high. For more information on specific types of bacteria linked to food poisoning, see entries on diarrhea and probiotics, and Appendix A.

Gallstones

Multiple factors contribute to gallstone disease including, but not limited to, obesity, diet, ethnicity, genetics, environmental pollution, gender and metabolic disorders. The use of some drugs may also put some individuals at risk for gallstone formation, such as contraceptives, estrogen replacement therapy and blood cholesterol drugs used to treat cardiovascular disease. People who are dehydrated are more prone to gallbladder stone formation as well.

One side effect of gallstones is the effect they have on friendly intestinal bacteria. Several different types of friendly bacteria, like *Lactobacillus acidophilus* and bifidobacteria, help break down bile acids coming from the gallbladder. Large concentrations of fecal bile acids alter the growth and survival of these same beneficial bacteria. Bifidobacteria, necessary for health and longevity, are particularly sensitive to fluctuations in fecal bile acid amounts. An increase in the dietary intake of fat increases fecal bile acids and causes the bifidobacteria to be inhibited. The growth of bifidobacteria in the colon is also altered by factors in the diet such as indigestible carbohydrates.

A reduction in beneficial bacteria makes way for bacterial overgrowth. The presence of harmful bacteria (especially *Clostridium*) is more likely the result, not a cause, of such a toxic and unbalanced state. In response, anyone suffering with gallstones should consider adding probiotics to their management program. Even if it does not "cure" the gallstones, it will help to bring the intestinal tract into a more balanced state of health.

Gas

Differences in the amount of healthy bowel flora may also account for variations in gas production. Methane is produced by bacterial metabolism in the colon and is only minimally influenced by the foods you eat. Carbon dioxide may also be produced by bacterial metabolism of unabsorbed carbohydrates in the intestines. Some people consistently produce large quantities of methane, others little or none. Symptoms are also very diverse, ranging from mild bloating to intolerable distention.

Gulf War Syndrome

The Gulf War syndrome has sparked a lot of controversy since the diagnosis was first proposed in the late '90s. Among 3,700 soldiers surveyed in 1995, the most common complaints were weakness, fatigue, memory loss, depression, joint pain and multiple chemical sensitivities. One theory about the syndrome is that the bacterium *Mycoplasma* may be the culprit behind these symptoms. Many individuals with Gulf War syndrome tested positive for the infection. In fact, sufferers were seven times more likely to test positive than individuals without the syndrome.

Two federal efforts are underway to determine whether antibiotics can cure this chronic illness. One study, conducted at Walter Reed Army Medical Center, looked at the blood of Gulf War veterans for signs of *Mycoplasma*. The other, conducted at Veterans Affairs Medical Centers nationwide, involved giving antibiotics to some *Mycoplasma*-positive patients. I believe that an impaired immune system is more likely responsible for the infection in the first place. Restoring the integrity of the immune system may allow the affected individual to fully recover from the illness, since they are better able to fight the infection.

Infertility

Some cases of male infertility may also be caused by pathogenic bacteria. One possible explanation for this phenomenon is that the bacteria create toxic by-products that inhibit sperm count. The bacteria may also physically interfere with the motion of sperm tails. Moreover, the bacteria compete for the same foods that sperm need for energy, which may present problems as well. These findings could mean that some cases of male infertility might benefit from an antibacterial treatment.

Inflammatory Bowel Diseases

Twenty years ago, it was proposed that imbalances in the bowel microflora could cause inflammatory bowel diseases. However, conventional medicine has made little progress investigating this theory, despite statistics showing bacterial overgrowth in the small intestines of 20 percent of patients hospitalized with Crohn's disease. In this investigation, both diarrhea and malabsorption were attributed to the presence of these bacteria. I also believe that toxins produced by the responsible bacteria could enter circulating blood, causing systemic symptoms.

In my opinion, gut dysbiosis plays a major role in inflammatory bowel disease, with small and large bowel fermentation being a key component. This may explain why many people with inflammatory bowel diseases improve when given antibiotics. One successful treatment tested was a two-day course of multiple broad-spectrum antibiotics to decontaminate the gut. This was followed by strains of beneficial bacteria, such as *Lactobacillus acidophilus* and *L. bifidus*, to help restore balance to the intestinal tract.

These beneficial bacteria that line the intestinal tract may help to prevent inflammation by actually blocking the inflammatory response. They appear to do this so they will not be attacked by the immune system. By serving themselves, they also serve us.

Influenza

A report from Japan stated that mice given a nasal spray containing the beneficial bacteria *Lactobacillus casei* showed fewer problems from the influenza virus. This probiotic was given to the animals for three days prior to inoculation with the virus. The mice that had received the probiotics had a 90 percent lower viral level compared with those not treated. Even more amazing was the fact that 69 percent of the nasal-spray mice survived their bout with the flu, while only 15 percent of the untreated animals were able to survive (*Clinical and Diagnostic Laboratory Immunology* May 2001). It is unknown if other beneficial bacteria would be just as effective or what the effects would be in humans, but it would definitely be worth trying.

Interstitial Cystitis

Interstitial cystitis, sometimes called irritable bladder syndrome, is becoming a more frequent problem in the United States, but conventional medicine seems clueless to what causes the illness. In one case, a woman suffered constant pain for almost ten years before a bacterium *Enterococcus* was found to be the cause and eliminated.

The discovery of the link between the bacteria and irritable bladder was made by Dr. Paul Fugazotto who has developed a test using a special soy broth culture of the urine to detect if the gram-positive *Enterococcus* is present. He says that most labs culture gram-negative bacteria, which are contaminants only, instead of the true causative organism. That is why other treatments fail. However, gram-positive bacteria are more difficult to culture from urine, which is why such cultures were rarely used in the past. (The lab that follows Dr. Fugazotto's exact specialized broth culturing techniques is United Medical Laboratory in McLean Virginia at 703-356-4422. And if you live in New York, you may have to travel to a neighboring state in order to obtain this special test. New York State law does not permit certain laboratories outside the state to report their results unless they pay an annual fee for a special licensure.)

Another link to irritable bladder was made in 1997, when urologists at Temple University in Philadelphia questioned individuals with interstitial cystitis and determined that they were 100 times more likely to have irritable bowel syndrome and thirty times more likely to have lupus than the general population. They also found that they were more likely to have allergies, sensitive skin and fibromyalgia. Their conclusion was that interstitial cystitis was likely to be associated with certain other chronic diseases.

Fungus may also be a culprit. Fungal metabolites have been found in the urine of people with this condition, and sufferers improve significantly when treated with the antifungal, diflucan, combined with dietary changes. I would also recommend checking for any food allergies or intolerances that could be contributing to bladder irritation.

Irritable Bowel Syndrome (IBS)

A staggering one-third of the U.S. population experiences recurrent, non-specific gastrointestinal complaints or IBS. A diagnosis of IBS is often used when doctors cannot find the underlying cause of digestive and intestinal symptoms. They often consider anxiety or stress to be the primary causal factors for IBS. Even though anxiety and stress may aggravate any condition, I do not believe they are the primary causes, however.

Treatment aimed at reducing bacterial overgrowth in the intestinal tract improves symptoms in many patients, as reported in the *American Journal of Gastroenterology*. It showed that a course of antibiotics can reduce bloating, diarrhea and pain associated with IBS. Although pathogenic bacteria may be at the root of IBS and using antibiotics may make you feel better initially, it will not correct an internal terrain that puts you at risk in the first place.

Developing healthy digestion requires adequate nutrition and possibly taking digestive enzymes. It is also essential to remove other possible irritants, including intestinal parasites, yeast, food allergies and bacteria (and their toxins) to reduce the inflammation. Lactose intolerance and a deficiency of hydrochloric acid or other digestive enzymes have been linked to IBS. Foods such as wheat, milk and sugar often irritate the gut as well. A bacterial overgrowth, reported in as many as 40 percent of IBS cases, may also cause carbohydrate malabsorption, while exposure to antibiotics or a diet depleted in soluble fiber may create a deficiency of beneficial bowel flora. A fiber deficiency and dysbiosis both contribute to IBS and often occur together, so if you suffer from chronic unexplained digestive problems, consider these two conditions as possible sources of your distress and treat them first.

Kidney Infections

Kidney infections occur when infectious organisms, usually bacteria, enter the body and travel to the kidneys where they cause swelling and inflammation. A kidney infection can come on suddenly or recur periodically over the course of many years. Kidney infections are very serious. Left untreated, they can permanently damage the kidneys and result in chronic kidney disease. The infection can also spread to the blood, causing poisoning. Moreover, the bacteria that often cause kidney infections in women have developed resistance to many of the widely used antibiotics.

Anyone can develop a kidney infection, but pregnant women have an increased risk, in part because fetal pressure on the bladder makes it more difficult to empty the bladder completely. Urine left in the bladder is a potential medium for bacterial growth. Symptoms include a rapidly rising fever, frequent urge to urinate even though the bladder seems empty, cloudy or bloody urine, severe nausea or vomiting, and continuous pain that usually begins in the back above the waist and spreads down into the groin.

Another related condition, pyelonephritis, is a serious infection of the upper urinary tract and kidneys that causes more serious symptoms of fever, nausea and painful, frequent urination. In one study, *E. coli* caused more than 90 percent of these cases. Interesting enough, this bacteria has different rates of resistance in different parts of the United States. Among people from Western states the resistance rate was 32 percent; 7 percent in the East; and 14 percent in the Midwest.

Kidney Stones

A biochemist at a university in Finland found tiny bacteria in the urine with an affinity for the kidneys. They believe that these bacteria use calcium and other minerals to form shells around themselves, thereby causing kidney stones. Upon examination of thirty human kidney stones, they found evidence of these bacteria in every stone. In response to these findings, it has been suggested that antibiotics should be given to people with recurrent kidney stones, but since these bacteria can resist many antibiotics, I believe another solution is needed.

Leaky Gut Syndrome (Intestinal Permeability)

The small intestine contains billions of human cells packed tightly together to keep bacteria, viruses and other toxins out of the body's tissues. When this protective barrier is damaged, it is called "leaky gut." Toxins of intestinal pathogens are believed to pass through the permeable intestinal lining and enter the bloodstream. This triggers a reaction by the immune system leading to tissue inflammation, destruction of joint cartilage and joint pain, among other symptoms. People with Crohn's disease and ulcerative colitis are known to have an abnormal increase in intestinal permeability.

Still, despite supporting evidence, many doctors refuse to accept the diagnosis of intestinal permeability as the cause or aggravation of many illnesses including lupus, scleroderma and rheumatoid arthritis. I believe that people with chronic fatigue, fibromyalgia, allergies, musculoskeletal discomforts, and the above autoimmune diseases should be tested for intestinal permeability.

Liver Sclerosis

The lesions of alcoholic sclerosis of the liver may be the result of an increase in gram-negative pathogenic bacteria. It is believed that toxins produced by these pathogens overwhelm the liver's detoxification capacity. Alcohol kills gram-positive organisms (including the friendly *Lactobacillus acidophilus*), but gram-negative pathogens thrive in the alcohol-intoxicated gut.

Lyme Disease

Lyme disease is a tick-borne illness usually caused by the spirochete *Borrelia burgdorferi*. Lyme disease was first recognized in the U.S. in 1975, after a mysterious outbreak of arthritis near Lyme, Connecticut. It took several years before the spirochete was identified. I include some information about this condition because of its ability to mimic many other chronic illnesses. Some people diagnosed with multiple sclerosis, fibromyalgia, chronic fatigue syndrome and other degenerative diseases may actually have Lyme disease.

Ticks that transmit Lyme disease must remain attached and feeding for at least twenty-four hours for the spirochete to be transmitted, but daily removal of ticks will not always prevent Lyme disease. It is also possible to be infected by more than one type of Lyme-causing spirochete carried in the same tick, especially if the tick remains on a person for an extended period of time.

Moreover, it is not as rare in some areas as people think. For instance, many doctors believe that Lyme disease cannot be acquired in Florida, but the Florida Department of Health has issued reports saying differently. And the incidence of the disease in Sweden rose 200 percent between 1992 and 1997, due partly to an increase in the numbers of tick-carrying deer.

Furthermore, it is a misconception to believe that ticks are the only carriers of the disease. It can also be transmitted by fleas, gnats, mosquitoes and mites, and by human-to-human contact. There have also been reported cases where children who have been breast-fed by infected mothers have subsequently developed Lyme disease. It can also be transmitted through the placenta of developing fetuses or via semen during sex, so it is important to treat any sexual partner of an infected individual. Otherwise this organism can pass back and forth. Transmission may also occur through blood transfusion and possibly from drinking unpasteurized goat or cow milk.

Lyme disease begins with flu-like symptoms, along with a headache, stiff neck, low-grade fever, muscle aches and pains, and fatigue. A unique, enlarging rash appears at the bite site days to weeks after the bite occurs, but only if there is a bite and then, only in about 30 to 40 percent of cases (and fewer than 10 percent of infected children). The rash is usually more or less circular, but painless at the bite site. Many people do not even notice the rash. If left untreated, the infection can lurk for months or years and re-emerge to cause a long list of frightening complications, including arthritis-like joint pain, swelling and personality changes. Some people have chronic inflammation or symptoms of indigestion. There may be cognitive disorders such as trouble concentrating and memory problems.

There are several reasons why Lyme disease is so difficult to test for and treat. First, as mentioned, the bull's eye rash that is supposed to appear after being bitten does not show up in everyone. Also, the disease can move through the body very quickly. It can travel through blood vessel walls and through connective tissue even better than in blood. Animal studies show that in less than a week after being infected, the spirochete can deeply embed itself inside tendons, muscles and even the heart or brain. Unfortunately, Lyme disease is also notoriously difficult to diagnose because blood tests are not always accurate. Most of the standard tests used (like ELISA and Western Blot) are unreliable. These tests will not show positives immediately after exposure, and only 60 to 70 percent of infected people ever develop antibodies to the spirochete, so it might be a good idea to be retested with newer methods if you suspect that you may have Lyme disease. For women, it is best to get tested around the time of menses since the decline of estrogen and progesterone at the end of the menstrual cycle are associated with the worsening of Lyme symptoms.

What makes this organism so hard to detect and treat is that it is pleiomorphic, meaning that it can change its form radically from an organism with a cell wall to one without a wall. When it is present without a cell wall, the Lyme organism lacks the membrane information necessary for the immune system and antibiotics to recognize and attack it (and for most current lab tests to detect it). Not only can it change form, but it can also revert back into the original form. For example, after examining more than eight hundred people clinically diagnosed with Lyme disease by using the RIBb test, most tested positive for the cell wall-deficient form. Because of this ability to change shape at will, it is suspected that any one antibiotic will not be effective all the time. And because bacteria share genetic material with each other, the offspring may develop a resistance to the antibiotic.

As a result of these and other difficulties, Lyme disease may be seriously underreported. If you have arthritis and chronic fatigue, it may be worthwhile to be tested for Lyme disease. There are new DNA tests for spirochete infections, but it is important to find laboratories that specialize in the particular type of test you are seeking, or your results may not be correct. Two new tests are waiting on FDA approval and may be available by this printing. One of the tests is called the Rapid

Identification of *Borrelia burgdorferi* test or RIBb test. It provides results in twenty to thirty minutes. The other is a culture test and staining that allows viewing under a fluorescent microscope in order to detect live cultures that cannot be seen in blood tests. These new tests do not look for antibodies, but for the organism itself.

There is also a possibility of developing a co-infection from the Lyme-carrying tick and other pathogens such as the protozoan, *Babesia microti*. In the western United States, this newly recognized species has been documented to cause disease. Transmission usually occurs via the tick vector *Ixodes dammini*. There are three stages of development (larva, nymph and adult); each is capable of infecting humans.

The symptoms of *Babesia* are gradual and include anorexia, abdominal pain and dark urine. The fever is not typically cyclical, as it is with malaria. Patients may or may not recall any tick bites, but most often, there is a history of outdoor activity or travel to an area where the disease is endemic (in coastal regions of the northeastern United States, such as Nantucket, Martha's Vineyard and Cape Cod, Mass; Block Island, RI; and Shelter Island and eastern Long Island, NY). Other areas where infection is likely include Connecticut, Wisconsin and California. Most cases occur between June and August. Lyme disease is endemic in the same geographic locations as *Babesia,* since the same vector can transmit both diseases.

Treatment of Lyme disease is further complicated by government restrictions. Some physicians are threatened with a loss of licensure if they treat Lyme disease in ways other than the established standard of care. This means that they must prescribe a course of antibiotics lasting no more than thirty days. In fact, fifty physicians in Texas, New York, Oregon, Rhode Island, New Jersey, Connecticut and Michigan have reportedly been investigated, disciplined and/or stripped of their licenses over the past three years because of their approach to healing Lyme disease. Moreover, in most cases, effective alternative/complementary treatments require more doctor time per patient and often include a broad range of medicines and supplements consumed over a longer period of time. This costs more money than the current standard of care accepted by most medical insurers.

The Lyme disease vaccine (Lymerix), approved in 1998, may also cause problems. At the time of approval, there was concern that the vaccine was capable of producing an autoimmune reaction that could lead to arthritis. Also of concern was the possibility that the vaccine could cause a resurgence of symptoms in people previously infected with the Lyme spirochete. In fact, severe arthritis and Lyme disease may be associated with the vaccine. Physicians in areas where Lyme disease is endemic report that they suspect at least 170 cases of severe arthritis and/or Lyme disease may be linked to the vaccine. Most of the reports of reactions come from Connecticut, Delaware, Massachusetts, New Jersey, New York, Pennsylvania and Wisconsin. Even though the developer of the vaccine, Smith Kline Beecham, maintains that the vaccine is safe, susceptible people may still produce adverse reactions and caution should be taken by anyone considering this vaccine.

Lymphoma

Helicobacter pylori (*H. pylori*) is a gram-negative bacterium, most likely acquired during childhood, that infects the stomachs of more than 50 percent of the population worldwide. If it is not treated, these bacteria can cause chronic gastritis and peptic ulcer disease, In some individuals *H. pylori* can eventually lead to gastric cancer and gastric lymphoma (tumors).

In fact, when *H. pylori* is eradicated in people with gastric lymphoma, there is complete remission in approximately 75 percent of the cases. The studies have been small but encouraging in proving that *H. pylori* may be a primary factor in causing lymphoma in the stomach. While a close association between gastric lymphoma and *H. pylori* infection has been established, there are still cases that do not respond to treatment. It seems that there is a significant difference between tumors restricted to tissue near the surface and those that have invaded deeply into the underlying tissue or beyond. Sometimes cells change in response to invading pathogens. These cells are turned off when the causative stimulus is eliminated. However, if the process is sustained for a long time, it can lead to severe tissue damage or even cancer. Consider checking for *H. pylori* if you are diagnosed with lymphoma.

Malabsorption

Harmful bacteria can also cause transient malabsorption, probably the result of superficial damage to the areas where absorption takes place in the intestinal tract. The overgrowth of these bacteria in the intestinal tract is more common than previously thought. Moreover, these bacteria consume much of the dietary vitamin B12 and perhaps interfere with enzyme systems. In some cases, even more severe and long-term damage may occur. If you suffer from chronic malabsorption, ask your doctor to check for pathogenic bacteria in the intestines.

Morning Sickness

An infection with *Helicobacter pylori* (*H. pylori*), the same bacteria that causes stomach ulcers, may cause a severe form of morning sickness during pregnancy. Experts theorize that the early phase of pregnancy causes changes in a woman's body fluid concentration, which affects the acidity of the stomach. A low-acid environment activates latent *H. pylori* residing there. Women with this condition may vomit three or more times each day and experience weight loss of more than 6.5 pounds, along with electrolyte imbalances. This can continue throughout pregnancy unless treated.

Multiple Sclerosis (MS)

Chlamydia, which causes respiratory infections such as pneumonia and is linked to heart disease, was suspected as a possible cause of MS after a team of scientists reported last year they found this bacteria in the spinal fluid of seventeen MS patients. (This particular bacterium is not the same strain of *Chlamydia* that causes the sexually transmitted disease of the same name.) However, another study found no link between MS and *Chlamydia*. Still, it may be worthwhile to test for this bacterium if you suffer from multiple sclerosis, and if present, have it eliminated.

Another theory has been proposed by a Texas A&M University pathologist, Luther E. Lindner, M.D., Ph.D. He found a cell wall-deficient (CWD) variant of a common bacterium in the blood of MS patients but is not naming the organism until he performs more research. It still may be worth considering an infectious organism as a possibility in MS, even without knowing the name of the possible offenders.

In addition, according to a report in an issue of the *Journal of Clinical Investigation* (July 2001), mice deliberately infected with an engineered virus developed severe clinical signs of multiple sclerosis within seven to ten days after being infected. This is the first demonstration that a virus could induce a central nervous system autoimmune disease. If a virus could do this, the same thing could be possible with bacteria.

Musculoskeletal Problems

For many years, it has been thought that a wide variety of musculoskeletal problems begin in the digestive tract. It is thought that the circulating toxins produced from an overgrowth of pathogenic bacteria in the digestive tract could be the culprits behind all those aches and pains. Sufferers may want to discuss this connection with their health-care provider.

Pancreatic Cancer

Helicobacter pylori (*H. pylori*) infections may play a role in the development of some forms of pancreatic cancer (*Journal of the National Cancer Institute* 2001). Although the connection between this bacterium and peptic ulcer disease and gastric cancer is well-known, its connection to pancreatic cancer is still speculative. Moreover, the subjects in the 2001 study were male smokers, and so these finding may not necessarily apply equally to the general (nonsmoking) public. However, this study does raise questions about unexplainable cancers and possible bacterial causes.

Polyps

It seems that the bacterium *Helicobacter pylori* is also associated with polyps. These stomach polyps often disappear after treatment for *H. pylori,* but it can take anywhere from twelve to fifteen months. Untreated, these small growths on the stomach lining can cause stomach pain and bleeding, and may be a precursor to gastric cancer.

Pouchitis

Pouchitis is inflammation of the small intestine common in people with inflammatory bowel disease. Symptoms include frequent and urgent bowel movements, abdominal cramping, bleeding and fever. As many as 50 percent of patients who undergo surgery for ulcerative colitis, subsequently develop pouchitis. Most cases respond temporarily to antibiotics, but the condition recurs in two out of every three cases.

Pouchitis has been linked to reduced levels of some types of beneficial bacteria normally found in the intestinal tract. In one study where probiotics were used to treat pouchitis for nine months, 85 percent of the probiotic group remained symptom free, whereas, all of the non-probiotic group relapsed. The probiotic preparation used in the study contained five hundred billion organisms per gram, including four strains of *Lactobacillus*, three strains of bifidobacteria, and one strain of

Streptococcus salivarius, subspecie *thermophilus*. Patients each received six grams daily of these beneficial organisms. Within four months after stopping the probiotics, all of the people involved in this study experienced a relapse. If you suffer from this condition, probiotics may be helpful, and long-term use of beneficial bacteria is considered safe.

Premature Births

Bacterial vaginosis is common among pregnant women and increases the risk of premature delivery. It affects about 800,000 pregnant women in the United States every year, but many women are unaware they have the condition. If successfully treated for bacterial vaginosis, as many as 80,000 mothers could avoid pre-term births. Similarly, 4,000 infant deaths and 4,000 cases of nervous system damage resulting from premature births could also be avoided.

Psoriasis

An abnormal immune response to components of the microflora in the intestinal tract may contribute to the cause of skin conditions such as psoriasis. The responsible bacteria have not been identified, but they are thought to produce a toxin that causes or contributes to this skin disorder. Psoriasis sufferers should consider treating intestinal pathogens if they also suffer from digestive conditions.

Psychiatric Disorders

Many people diagnosed with psychiatric disorders have food sensitivities and typically less than 5 percent have normal levels of *Lactobacillus acidophilus* in their digestive tract. When their levels of beneficial bacteria increase, many have reported a reduction of digestive symptoms, and the signs and symptoms associated with food allergy decreased.

Plus, *Lactobacillus acidophilus* is often deficient or absent in the digestive tract of schizophrenics. These beneficial bacteria do not seem to easily colonize in people with schizophrenia, so they need to take higher doses than normal. This phenomenon raises questions about a possible link between psychiatric conditions and the digestive system.

Reiter's Syndrome

There is a major association between the overgrowth of pathogenic bacteria and Reiter's syndrome (reactive arthritis). Intestinal overgrowths of *Shigella, Salmonella, Yersinia* and *Campylobacter* are known to cause this type of disorder. It is suggested that the arthritis caused by these organisms may be due to toxins depositing in the tissues. Since joint diseases can be triggered by what is happening in the digestive system, this may explain why fasting often leads to improvement in some forms of arthritis.

Seafood Poisoning

It is possible to be exposed to naturally occurring toxins by consuming contaminated seafood and their products. This can result in a wide variety of symptoms, depending upon the toxin(s) present, their concentrations and the amount of contaminated food consumed. The most significant public health problems are reviewed in this section. Each of these syndromes occurs in various coastal waters of the U.S. and the world. With the increased transport of seafood, as well as international travel by seafood consumers, virtually no one is free of risk.

Records are incomplete because reporting to the Centers for Disease Control (CDC) is voluntary, but the information that is available indicates that ciguatera (pronounced *si gwah the' rah*) fish poisoning is responsible for about half of all seafood intoxifications. A growing body of evidence indicates that incidents of the other types of poisoning may be on the increase since the causative organisms inhabit the temperate coastal waters of the United States. Moreover, cases are frequently misdiagnosed and infrequently reported.

Seafood poisoning is a category that covers a broad range of poisonings caused by a variety of toxins from many different sources, including scombroid fish poisoning, ciguatera fish poisoning, paralytic shellfish poisoning, puffer fish poisoning, amnesic shellfish poisoning, diarrhetic shellfish poisoning and neurotoxic shellfish poisoning.

Although the CDC attributes at least half of all seafood poisoning cases to ciguatera, it is probably underreported and underdiagnosed, so it is hard to know just how common poisoning from this marine toxin occurs. Worldwide, it is estimated that there are between 50,000 and one million cases a year. It is not known how often people in the U.S. are affected, since the problem has only recently become known to the general medical community. The estimate is about 3,000 cases yearly, most of them in Hawaii, Florida, or in people who eat fish imported from tropical pacific waters.

According to the National Center for Environmental Research, the toxins are produced by a bacterial vector, *Ostreopsis lenticularis*, which is present in dinoflagellates (primarily *Gambierdiscus toxicus*). Dinoflagellates are usually attached to larger algae in coral reef environments or in the shallow waters of tropical areas around the world. They are swallowed by small fish that are, in turn, eaten by large predatory reef fish. The fish appear unharmed by the toxin. Since the larger predatory fish consume many of the smaller fish, the toxin becomes concentrated as it moves up the food chain. It is for this reason that large carnivore tropical reef fish are considered to have the highest risk of toxicity.

Recreational fishing in the Caribbean and Pacific Islands causes eighty percent of all cases of ciguatera poisoning, although a few outbreaks have been reported in southern Florida. The areas most affected are Puerto Rico, Hawaii, Australia, Indonesia and Micronesia. Become familiar with local species that pose potential risk when fishing in tropical waters. More than two hundred species of fish have been implicated, the most common being grouper, red snapper and barracuda. Other possibilities include the Spanish mackerel, dog tooth tuna, skipjack tuna, Pacific kingfish, various species of cod, sea bass, barramundi, reef shark, moray eel, coral trout, dolphin fish, trevally, sea perch, parrotfish, surgeon fish, yellowtail, mullet, pigeye shark, amberjack and triggerfish. Listen to official warnings before eating fish from these areas, since high-risk fish imported from these areas could contain the poison.

Toxin production is more likely to occur with recent disturbances in the reef, such as a hurricane, heavy rains, algae bloom, dredging or wharf construction. Dead coral formations provide an ideal environment for the growth of *Gambierdiscus toxicus*. Tropical reefs around the world are being attacked with silt, alien algae, pollution and chemical killers including pesticides, hydrocarbons and heavy metals. Increasing damage to coral reefs correlates with an increasing rate of ciguatera outbreaks. It is also thought that global warming may also be increasing the incidence of poisonings.

The toxin is fat-soluble and cannot be destroyed by cooking, freezing, drying, salting, smoking or gastric juice. The toxins also cannot be detected in the meat by appearance, smell or taste. Everything appears normal. Selecting fish that are not at high risk for carrying ciguatera poisoning may minimize your risk. You should only eat fish smaller than twenty pounds. Smaller fish are less likely to have strayed from areas where ciguatera is a problem. None of the deep-sea fish such as ahi, marlin, mahimahi and ono (wahoo) have been known to carry this toxin. People do not have to avoid all groupers, a popular fish in Southern states.

Just how serious is ciguartera poisoning? Consider the following case: In 1997, an outbreak occurred on a cargo ship that ate a freshly caught barracuda in the Bahamas. All seventeen men who ate the fish became ill three to five hours later. Most began having nausea, vomiting, abdominal cramps and diarrhea. Within two days all of them suffered from neurological symptoms. These included muscle pain and weakness, dizziness, confusion of hot-cold sensations, blurred vision, and numb or itchy feet, hands and mouth. Some of them experienced a metallic taste in the mouth. These somewhat unique features are one way to differentiate ciguatera poisoning from other types of poisoning, although organophosphate pesticides and botulism toxin can produce similar symptoms. They all recovered in about a week, although some had lingering neurological symptoms for months.

The onset of ciguatera poisoning may be slow and insidious if small amounts of the contaminated fish are eaten over several days. It has been known to take up to thirty hours for symptoms to develop. Although nausea, vomiting, abdominal cramps, generalized weakness and diarrhea are most common, neurological symptoms often follow. These include numbness of the lips, tongue, throat and extremities; pain in the teeth or on urination; blurred vision; severe itching; sharp, shooting nerve pain in the legs; profound weakness; and one of the strangest symptoms, the reversal of cold and heat sensations. However, not all people have all of these symptoms. Less commonly, affected individuals may experience chills, sweating, headaches, dizziness and taste disturbances, such as a metallic taste or fuzzy sensation on the tongue. The nausea, vomiting and other gastrointestinal symptoms last for approximately one to two days, but the weakness may last up to a week. Neurological symptoms such as tingling or temperature reversal also generally persist for a week.

In severe cases, there can be low blood pressure, slow heart beat, arrhythmia, heart block and respiratory paralysis. In fact, ciguatera victims can suffer for weeks to months with debilitating neurological symptoms and other intermittent symptoms. In some cases, people have experienced neurological symptoms that lingered on for several years. Such relapses are most often associated with changes in dietary habits or with consumption of alcohol. There have been some deaths resulting from respiratory and cardiovascular failure often after ingestion of the most toxic parts of the fish such as the head, liver, viscera or roe.

The symptoms of ciguatera poisoning can also mimic other illnesses. Prolonged itching can present as a skin disease. Mild poisoning may also be mistaken for general malaise, depression, headaches and muscular aches. In some cases, people have been misdiagnosed with chronic fatigue syndrome because they were suffering with low energy and depression.

Once poisoned, it is also possible to have recurrences of symptoms. Other substances can also trigger symptoms such as ethanol, caffeine and nuts, as long as three to six months after eating the poisoned fish. Pregnant women should be especially cautious since premature labor and spontaneous abortion have been reported, as well as effects on the fetus and newborn child through placental and breast milk transmission.

Moreover, there appears to be sensitivity to certain foods and these should be avoided for at least three to six months after being poisoned. It is also possible develop an extreme sensitivity to other foods and suffer relapses following the consumption of seemingly innocent substances:

- fresh, canned, dried, etc. marine products including fish sauces and shellfish
- beer, wine or any type of alcohol
- tobacco products
- sugar, caffeine, spicy foods and raw vegetables
- fatty or oily foods such as nuts, peanut products, etc.

It has been reported that 75 to 100 percent of the people that eat these contaminated fish will have symptoms, and the symptoms can vary among individuals even eating the same poisoned food. Symptoms can also vary among ethnic groups and locations. It also appears that ciguatera poisoning may be more toxic to humans after eating carnivore species of fish than after eating herbivores.

The only way to be sure that you will not be poisoned is to totally avoid eating any tropical reef fish. If you choose to eat tropical reef fish, talk to locals about fish to avoid. Don't eat the internal organs or viscera of such fish. And remember that the bigger and older the fish, the more concentrated the possible toxin. If you suspect ciguatera poisoning, seek medical care promptly. Freeze any uneaten portions of fish and contact local health officials.

Medical treatment includes a variety of agents, including vitamins, antihistamines, steroids and tricyclic antidepressants. Gut emptying and decontamination with charcoal is recommended during acute symptoms. Other drugs may be necessary to try if symptoms are severe. It is recommended that opiates and barbiturates be avoided since they may cause low blood pressure and interact with the toxins. During the first six days or so, some people have been helped with mannitol infusion carried out in a physician's office or emergency unit of the hospital. This is not a cure or antidote, but relieves many of the more severe symptoms of poisoning, except for the diarrhea. Mannitol appears to be most effective in completely relieving symptoms when given within the first forty-eight to seventy-two hours after ingestion of the poisoned fish. See the web site www.rehablink.com/ciguatera more information about administrating IV mannitol and ciguatera poisoning.

Antidepressants such as amitriptyline and similar medications do seem to have some success in relieving the symptoms such as fatigue and nerve pain. It is possible that nifedipine may be appropriate as a calcium channel blocker to counteract some of the effects. Tocainide has been given orally for several weeks to help nerve cells. Treatment with cholestyramine has been successful in correcting some of the visual symptoms, though it can take twelve weeks for it to work. Some people who were poisoned with ciguatera after eating dusky grouper in the Dominican Republic were treated successfully with an antiepileptic drug. There are also over sixty-four different local herbal remedies, including medicinal teas, used in both the Indo-Pacific and West Indies regions. Other treatments that are sometimes helpful include:

- Megadoses of vitamin B12 in the active form of methylcobalamin have been helpful for the neurological symptoms.
- Calcium D-glucarate has the ability to bind to toxins. It may not work unless taken at the very beginning of symptoms.
- Probiotics might help. There may be bacterial vectors in ciguatera poisoning.
- Kombucha tea was found helpful by some people.
- Antihistamines can help with the histamine-type reactions. It might be worth a try to use quercetin instead, since it has a similar use.

Over the past few years, lab tests have improved and home test kits are now available. There has been some controversy about how accurate the home kits are. The FDA's seafood products research center has been working on a new lab test that may be ready soon. It gives the degree of toxicity for several toxins, including ciguatera and paralytic shellfish poisoning. Oceanit Test Systems has a test kit that they say provides quick, simple and reliable detection of ciguatera poison in fish. It is called Cigua-Check. You can contact them by phone (808) 539-2345 or fax (808) 531-3177, or visit their web site at www.cigua.com. Another company developing a similar product is Hawaii Chemtect at (626) 568-8606.

Scombroid poisoning (also called histamine poisoning) is thought to be another of the most common forms of fish poisoning in the United States. It results from eating foods containing high levels of histamine.

These histamines are formed by the growth of certain bacteria, found in improperly handled or stored fish, especially in warm climates. If fish are not quickly chilled after capture, bacteria on the surface will convert the amino acid histidine to histamine, resulting in an allergic response. Since reporting this particular type of food poisoning is not required and medical personnel may not suspect it because the symptoms resemble other illnesses, I suspect that it is underreported.

The severity of symptoms, which usually last between eight and twelve hours, can range from mild to moderate and can appear between a few minutes and four hours after consuming toxic fish. The face and upper body often become flushed, resembling sunburn. There can also be tingling and burning in the mouth and/or throat. The mouth will often feel dry, and the victim may have difficulty swallowing. Other symptoms include: fever, sweating, severe throbbing headaches, heart palpitations, a rash or hives, itching, dizziness, stomach pain, nausea, vomiting, diarrhea, respiratory problems, as well as muscular pain and weakness. The symptoms can be severe for the elderly and for those taking medications, such as isoniazid.

The fish most affected are primarily mahi mahi, tuna, marlin and bluefish. Less often it affects amberjack, anchovies, herring, jack, mackerel and sardines; however, any food that contains the appropriate amino acids and is subjected to this type of bacterial contamination may cause scombroid poisoning, even Swiss cheese.

Distribution of the toxin within an individual fish can vary, with some sections of the fish causing illnesses and others not. Neither cooking, canning nor freezing reduces the toxic effect. Fish may not even have a foul odor to warn you of danger. The only warning you may have about the presence of histamine in a particular food item may be a particular metallic or peppery taste.

Diagnosis of this type of food poisoning is usually based on a person's symptoms, time of onset, and the effect of treatment with antihistamine medication. The suspected food must be analyzed within a few hours for elevated levels of histamine to confirm a diagnosis. Chemical testing is the only reliable test.

Proper handling is the only way to prevent scombroid poisoning. Shipments of unfrozen fish packed in refrigerated containers have posed a significant problem because of inadequate temperature control. The FDA monitors the histamine levels in canned tuna and fresh/frozen fish, which is why you should only buy fish from a reputable dealer and immediately refrigerate your seafood after purchase (between 32–38°F).

Another seafood poisoning you should be aware of is amnesic shellfish poisoning. In 1987, four people died after consuming toxic mussels from Prince Edward Island, Canada. Since that time, Canadian authorities have monitored the water for the presence of the suspected toxin. Shellfish beds, especially mussels, are closed to harvesting when the toxic concentration reaches a certain level. Fish and crab viscera can also be contaminated, so the risk to human consumers and animals in the marine food chain, is more significant than previously believed.

Eating these contaminated shellfish can be a life-threatening syndrome. It is characterized by both gastrointestinal and neurological disorders. Gastroenteritis usually develops within twenty-four hours with symptoms including nausea, vomiting, abdominal cramps and diarrhea. In severe cases, neurological symptoms also appear, usually within forty-eight hours. These symptoms include dizziness, headache, seizures, disorientation, short-term memory loss, respiratory difficulty and possibly coma.

Diarrhetic shellfish poisoning has only been discovered in the last decade. It was first reported in Japan due to a toxin coming from dinoflagellates. The shellfish most likely to be contaminated are mussels, oysters and scallops. It causes gastrointestinal symptoms similar to ciguatera poisoning, usually beginning within thirty minutes to a few hours after eating toxic shellfish. The illness, which is not usually fatal, is characterized by incapacitating diarrhea, nausea, vomiting, abdominal cramps and chills. Recovery occurs within three days, with or without medical treatment.

This type of poisoning is not the only danger from eating shellfish like oysters. People who love to eat raw oysters have known for years that these delicacies can be hazardous. Even cooking them to the consistency of rubber bands may not keep you from getting sick. If raw oysters are contaminated with bacteria, cooking them usually eliminates the danger. If the contaminant is a virus, however, even cooked oysters can put you in harm's way. Current screening methods do not work well for this virus, which is a common cause of shellfish-related illnesses in the United States. This virus is spread through human waste, such as the waste dumped overboard by boaters, which is absorbed by the oysters. The symptoms are unpleasant with vomiting and diarrhea, but they are not usually serious and only last a few days. Until better testing becomes available, the only way to avoid the problem entirely is to stay away from oysters. If you just cannot resist them and you do become ill, you should report it to your state or local public health department so that officials can better track outbreaks.

Shellfish poisoning can also be caused by fungi. In one case, a forty-year-old man, who had suffered with nausea, vomiting and diarrhea for five days, went to the Veterans Affairs Medical Center for treatment. He told the doctors that he began having symptoms about two hours after eating a variety of seafood from the Gulf of Mexico. What concerned him was that he had a fever, was vomiting bile and was having intense stomach pains. His diarrhea was green in color and contained mucus, but he did not see any blood. He also suffered with severe halitosis and tenderness in the area around the stomach. His pulse rate and breathing were also faster than normal.

Doctors knew that he was generally in good health prior to the event and had an unremarkable medical history. He also had not traveled anywhere lately or been on antibiotics. After running the usual lab tests, however, they could not find anything. Then another type of test was done (methylene blue stain and iodine wet mount) showing a large amount of a particular fungus. The culprit was *Psorospermium haeckelii*, also known as "beaver body." It is a thick-walled, one-cell organism that is commonly found in the muscle, gills, connective tissue and liver/pancreas of many species of crawfish. It had been considered an algae, though it is now speculated that it might be a fungus. Once the diagnosis was made and an appropriate treatment was prescribed, the man quickly recovered. I include this case to make a point about lab tests. They may not initially reveal the correct organism. It is important to run other tests even if the initial ones come back negative.

In the southeastern United States, crawfish harvesting is an important industry. The local population and tourists eat this seafood in increasing quantities. Although the presence of algae or fungi is usually not reported in areas of crawfish harvest and consumption, they are commonly seen on human stool examination during crawfish season. While the finding of these organisms in stool specimens may not pose a big problem, it certainly may challenge lab personnel when visitors return home from crawfish-consuming areas and consult with their health care providers because of digestive upset.

Another danger, neurotoxic shellfish poisoning, produces an intoxication syndrome nearly identical to that of ciguatera. Gastrointestinal and neurological symptoms predominate. In addition, there can be asthma-like symptoms. No deaths have been reported, and the syndrome is less severe than ciguatera, but is, nevertheless, debilitating. Unlike ciguatera, recovery is generally complete in a few days. Monitoring programs based on *Gymnodinium breve* cell counts generally work for preventing human poisoning, except when officials are caught off-guard in previously unaffected areas. Neurotoxic shellfish poisoning is usually found along the Florida coast and the Gulf of Mexico.

Of all of the food poisonings, however, the most serious appears to be paralytic shellfish poisoning because of its extreme potency and unusually high death rate. This is a life-threatening syndrome caused by multiple species of the dinoflagellate, *Gonyaulax*, along the New England and Pacific coasts. Most prevalent in summer, it is often caused by algae blooms creating red (black, blue or brown) tides. The toxin is concentrated in filter-feeding mollusks: mussels, clams, oysters and scallops.

Standard cooking or steaming does not destroy the toxin, and there is no antidote. The best way to prevent paralytic shellfish poisoning is not to eat shellfish caught along the coast in warmer months. California mandates a May through October quarantine on local mussels, clams and oysters.

Symptoms are purely neurological and their onset is rapid, but they usually last only a few days. Poisoning begins with nausea and vomiting, often within thirty minutes after ingesting shellfish. Symptoms may also include tingling, numbness, giddiness, drowsiness, fever, rash and staggering, along with a floating sensation, headaches and muscle paralysis. The most severe cases result in respiratory arrest within twenty-four hours after eating the toxic shellfish. If the patient is not breathing or if a pulse is not detected, CPR may be needed. Poisoning with this toxin kills about 8 percent of its victims; however, it is often prevented when monitoring programs assessing toxin levels in mussels, oysters, scallops and clams find a problem and stop harvesting in suspected or confirmed toxic areas.

Probably one of the most notorious and violent seafood poisonings of marine world comes from the pufferfish. It is also found in some crustacean and certain species of salamanders, newts, ocean sunfish, porcupine fish and in the blue spotted octopus. This toxin has also been isolated from parrotfish, frogs of the genus *Atelopus*, starfish, xanthid crabs and angelfish. Recent studies suggest the actual origin may be bacteria, probably from the *Vibrio, Pseudomonas* and *Photobacterium* family. These are fairly common marine bacteria that are often associated with marine animals.

The flesh of the pufferfish may not be that toxic, but the poison is especially concentrated in the gonads, liver, intestines and skin. There is often sufficient poison to produce rapid and violent death. About 150 to 200 people a year are poisoned, and more than half die. Poisoning is a major public health concern in Japan where "fugu" is a traditional delicacy. It is prepared and sold in special restaurants where trained and licensed individuals carefully remove the viscera to reduce the danger of poisoning.

Importing pufferfish into the United States is not generally permitted, although special exceptions may be granted. Only a few cases have been reported in the United States, and outbreaks in countries outside the Indo-Pacific area are rare. Most of these poisoning episodes occur from home preparation and consumption and not from commercial sources. Deaths in other parts of the world are rare. Still, there have been several reported cases of poisonings from the Atlantic Ocean, Gulf of

Mexico and the Gulf of California. The diagnosis of pufferfish poisoning is based on the observed symptoms and recent dietary history.

The first symptoms usually begin with a slight numbness of the lips and tongue, appearing about twenty minutes to three hours after eating the fish. Then there is an increased feeling of paralysis in the extremities often followed by sensations of lightness or floating. Headache, stomach pain, nausea, diarrhea and/or vomiting may occur. Occasionally, there may be some difficulty in walking.

In the next stage of poisoning, paralysis increases. Many people are unable to sit and experience increasing respiratory distress. Speech is affected and their blood pressure often drops, leading to symptoms such as convulsions, mental impairment and cardiac arrhythmia. The victim, although completely paralyzed with fixed and dilated pupils, may be conscious and in some cases completely lucid until shortly before death. Death usually occurs within four to six hours after consumption.

After hearing about all of the potential dangers of eating seafood, you may ask yourself, should I eat sushi? In response to this question, let me tell you about one of my patients, Peggy. She came to see me after spending a few days in the hospital. It had all started with several days of vomiting and diarrhea. By the time she was admitted into the hospital she was dehydrated and had lost more weight than her slight frame could stand. When I first saw her she looked pale, thin and unhealthy. The hospital had run $37,000 worth of tests, even a mammogram, and concluded that she was under too much stress. They gave her a prescription for the antidepressant Prozac. She was also referred to a gastroenterologist who diagnosed her with gastric reflux and prescribed antacids. He had not taken into account why she had been throwing up for several days. Not once was she asked about her diet or what or where she had eaten, and no one had suspected food poisoning. However, one of Peggy's favorite places to eat serves sushi. She ate there so often that they had even named a dish after her. Eventually, I traced Peggy's symptoms back to this diner.

Most restaurants that prepare sushi and sashimi buy high-end, flash-frozen and well-preserved fish. They often have a chef that is specially trained in the preparation of raw fish. If you decide to eat sushi, there are precautions you should take. My advice about sushi diners is to inspect the place. Does the fish smell fresh? Are the fingernails of the person cutting the sushi short and clean? Check the restrooms since you probably can't see what the kitchen looks like. Is it clean? Do not eat raw fish unless it has been flash-frozen. Some people say that it does not taste as good if it has been frozen, but the taste may not be worth the risk. If you have to eat raw fish, only do it occasionally. The more often you eat these types of foods, the more likely you could become sick.

Sciatica

According to the medical journal *Lancet* (June 2001) there may be an association between sciatica and the bacterium *Propionibacterium acnes*. Investigators in England wanted to explain the systemic inflammation and laboratory markers seen in people with sciatica that could not be explained. After performing several studies, they found this bacterium and others in disk fragments. The studies are limited but suggest that these organisms may be causing the problem. Additionally, about half of the people who had these bacteria also had previous epidural injections.

Sinusitis

Sinus infections are one of the most common reasons people see a doctor and receive antibiotics. However, a study in the *Lancet* suggests that taking antibiotics may not resolve the ailment any faster, since sinus infections are usually triggered by colds and allergies.

For many people with unresolved sinusitis (up to 300,000 a year), sinus surgery is performed to enlarge the sinuses and improve drainage. However, between six months to a year following the surgery, many people experience a relapse. The cycle of sinus infections returns, as do the antibiotics and even more surgeries. This is because the underlying cause of the sinus infection is still there despite these treatments.

Normally, the microscopic hair-like projections that line the nose and sinuses move mucus and bacteria down to the throat, where they are removed by swallowing. The swelling and congestion of a cold or allergy prevent that process, allowing bacteria to become trapped in the sinuses. There they multiply, creating an infection from bacteria or possibly fungi. If fungi are primarily involved, antibiotics will only work temporarily. Soon after the antibiotics are discontinued, symptoms will usually return. People treated with antifungal agents often get better results.

Sinusitis sufferers may also harbor L-forms of bacteria (those without cell walls), which are more difficult to detect and treat. Many sufferers do not experience permanent relief because the offending pathogen is untouched by traditional treatments, due to a resistance to a particular drug or because the drug is not effective against it. Sometimes there is a need to prescribe antibiotics for both acute and chronic sinusitis, but there should always be a comprehensive program that addresses the underlying cause.

Strep Throat

In recent years, scientists have noticed an alarming increase in the antimicrobial resistance of the bacterium *Streptococcus pneumoniae*. Between the years 1994 and 1995, a survey conducted at thirty U.S. medical centers found 23.6 percent of the bacteria resistant to penicillin and 9.1 percent resistant to multiple agents. In a subsequent 1997–1998 survey conducted at some of the same medical centers, researchers found the overall rate of penicillin-resistance to have increased to 29.5 percent and the multi agent-resistance jumped to 16 percent. This rate is expected to continue to increase (*Antimicrob Agents Chemtherap* 2001).

What has caused this resistance? Inappropriate use of antibiotics for upper respiratory tract infections continues to be the single most important factor. Another factor is the use of less effective antibiotics. Often, managed care organization only want to pay for the cheapest antibiotic, not necessarily the most effective drug to treat these infections.

Some experts believe that if you must use an antibiotic for strep throat, then amoxicillin is usually effective if given for a shorter period at a higher dose. It is also cheaper than some of the newer and more potent antibiotics. It appears to minimize the impact of antibiotic use on the spread of drug-resistant *Streptococcus pneumoniae* as well (*Journal of the American Medical Association* 2001). There are herbal and homeopathic alternatives to antibiotics that may be helpful. If you must take an antibiotic, it is important to also supplement with a probiotic following this treatment to replenish the intestinal tract with beneficial bacteria.

Tuberculosis (TB)

Two decades ago, the United States Surgeon General announced that tuberculosis was a disease of the past, but he spoke too soon. The disease has since resurfaced in a potent new form that, once again, has turned TB into a public health hazard. Worldwide it is estimated that over fifty million people are infected with drug-resistant strains, making it truly a global problem. This new form, called "multi-drug-resistant TB" (MDR-TB), is caused by strains of the bacterium, *Mycobacterium tuberculosis*. Through mutation, this organism has developed the ability to resist two or more antibiotic drugs.

Moreover, this bacterium is not restricted to third-world countries. Areas of London and New York City have a higher incidence of TB than many developing countries. In fact, over the last few years, New York City has had a major outbreak of drug-resistant TB, and one of the worst outbreaks occurred in Britain. Most of those infected were Britain-born professionals around the age of twenty-eight. This TB has been described as a "clubbers" strain because it is rumored that crowded bars and nightclubs could be breeding grounds for the disease. Other places that are dealing with strains resistant to anti-TB drugs are India, Africa, China and the former Soviet Union.

TB is transmitted through the air and is no respecter of persons, so anyone who has been in a crowded, confined area (like a bus, subway or movie theater) is at risk. Airline flights could also be bringing in resistant strains from other countries. However, the majority of cases are actually associated with family and office contact, though there is also a link with intravenous drug abuse. Health care workers who are in frequent close contact with TB patients housed in poorly ventilated rooms are also at high risk for this disease.

In one recent outbreak in Kansas, a cluster of tuberculosis cases from 1994 to 2000 were found among women with a history of working as dancers in adult entertainment clubs and people who were in close contact with exotic dancers. Many of the dancers were also drug users, making them more at risk for infectious diseases.

Once infected, many individuals have a strong enough immune system to keep the bacteria in check. They will not feel sick and will not spread the illness to anyone else. In fact, without preventive therapy, *Mycobacteria* can survive in tissues for years in a latent state waiting for an opportunity to surface. A depressed immune system, weakened by illness, age, poor diet, drug use or a generally poor lifestyle, is one way this bacterium can become active and multiply.

A TB skin test is the only way to find out if you have an infection. There are several reasons to get tested: if you have lived or worked in close quarters with individuals who may have the active disease such as homeless shelter, migrant farm camp, hospital, prison, jail or nursing home; if you come from a country where TB is very common; or if you inject illegal drugs. It may also be wise to get tested if you spend time in bars and nightclubs.

At first, the only symptom is a mild cough, or there may not be any symptoms at all. Then there is usually weakness or fatigue, appetite loss, weight loss, a cough with occasional bloody sputum, a slight fever, night sweats and chills. There is also pain in the chest, back or kidneys, or perhaps all three. Since dormant infections can eventually become active, even people without symptoms should receive medical treatment.

Ulcers

It was not that long ago that people diagnosed with stomach ulcers were advised to watch their diet and reduce stress. Now, it is well established that most of these ulcers are caused by the bacterium *Helicobacter pylori* (*H. pylori*). *H. pylori* is a gram-negative bacterium that affects more than 50 percent of the population worldwide. It is believed that many people acquire the bacterium in childhood. Despite its prevalence, most people are unaware that nine out of every ten peptic ulcers are caused by this bacterium. If it is not properly treated, *H. pylori* persists chronically, causing chronic gastritis, peptic ulcer disease, and in some individuals, gastric cancer and gastric lymphoma (tumor).

One long-term consequence of *H. pylori* infection is the development of stomach cancer. This type of cancer is the second most common cancer worldwide. It is especially common in countries such as Colombia and China where *H. pylori* infects over half the population in early childhood. The cases of stomach cancer are less in the U.S. because infections with this bacterium are less common here, but it still occurs too often. Anyone who suspects they have these ulcers needs to seek medical help. Complications such as blood loss or ulceration can lead to perforation and obstruction. Even mild symptoms should be treated before things get worse.

Though ulcers may be aggravated by stress and diet, the best way to treat stomach ulcers is to start a protocol that will kill this bacterium, if present. It used to be thought that too much stomach acid, especially if brought on by nervous stress, caused ulcers. Now, it is known that stomach lesions can be cause even when there is normal or low stomach acid. Conventional treatments have been aimed at neutralizing or halting acid production, even though the role of too much stomach acid as the primary cause of stomach ulcers is losing ground rapidly.

In cases of stomach ulcers, attention should also be paid to factors such as immunity, oral hygiene, bile reflux, adequate mucus protection in the stomach, diet, stomach and digestive function, and response to stress. Although symptoms of an ulcer may be absent or quite vague, most symptoms are associated with some type of digestive discomfort. If you have had persistent or recurrent upper abdominal symptoms for more than four weeks, consider being tested for an overgrowth of *H. pylori*. Some of the most common complaints are indigestion, stomach pain, a sensation of fullness when eating, feeling full right after eating, nausea, an increase in acid belching, heartburn, loss of appetite and bloating in the upper part of the abdomen. There may also be stomach pain forty-five to sixty minutes after meals or during the night. The pain is described as gnawing, burning, cramp-like, aching or heartburn-like. Eating or taking antacids usually gives great relief. Symptoms are worsened by stress, alcohol, caffeinated beverages, tobacco and soft drinks. Some people will pass blackened, tarry or bloody stools. Other symptoms include fatigue, exhaustion, disturbed sleep, hot flashes, bladder irritation and increased symptoms after periods of stress.

Currently, the Food and Drug Administration approves several treatment regimens. Most of them use some combination of antibiotics and antacids. Although these regimens may provide some relief initially, these drugs can be expensive and potentially toxic, as well as interfering with the digestive process. There are some people who cannot tolerate the use of these drugs and will have some type of reaction to them. Because the underlying causes for bacterial overgrowth are not addressed, the ulcer often develops again after the drugs are discontinued. Moreover, H. pylori is developing a resistance to the various drugs being used in treatment. In fact, sometimes these drugs actually slow down healing if the ulcers are linked to the chronic use of nonsteroidal anti-inflammatory drugs (NSAIDs). See Section 4 for ways to treat this bacterium.

Also, keep in mind that in people that complete treatment for H. pylori infection, it is not unusual to find a 10 to 20 percent failure rate. Because of this and the risks of recurrent ulcers, chronic gastritis and possibly cancer, it is important to retest for the bacterium after finishing treatment. If treatment has failed to eradicate the infection, it is necessary to repeat therapy. Because treatment failures are primarily the result of antibiotic resistance, repeat treatment should utilize a different antibiotic regimen. It is also important to realize that there are alternatives to antibiotics when treating infection.

Urinary Tract Infection (UTI)

About one-third of the antibiotics prescribed in most nursing homes are for urinary tract infections. Women suffering from this condition account for approximately 5.2 million visits to healthcare professionals yearly. In fact, about half of all women get at least one bladder infection at some time in their lives. (Men rarely suffer from UTIs.) This type of infection is not usually dangerous unless the infection moves into the kidneys, and a one-time infection is generally not a cause for concern. Chronic, recurrent or frequent UTIs are a concern, however. Some of the most common symptoms are pain with urination, urinary frequency and sudden urgency to empty the bladder. Severe symptoms include a high fever, pain and blood in the urine.

Urinary tract infections are also common during pregnancy and can be very serious. UTIs in pregnant women are usually the result of not completely emptying the bladder due to pressure from the fetus, leaving potentially dangerous bacteria in the urinary tract. Women who experience an untreated urinary tract infection during their third trimester of pregnancy are at greater risk (40 percent greater) of delivering a child who suffers from mental retardation or developmental delay. In fact, fetal death was twice as high among women with UTIs in the third trimester. However, if the woman is treated within the first few days of a UTI, this risk is avoided. If you are pregnant and begin to show signs of a urinary tract infection, do not delay! Get it diagnosed and treated promptly.

Many affected women also have some type of gastrointestinal disturbance. The digestive tract is a major breeding ground for infectious microorganisms that infect the urinary tract. It is fairly easy for bacteria to spread from the anus to the urinary tract, and the most frequent cause is the transfer of bacteria after having loose stools or diarrhea. It is also very easy to contaminate the fingers when wiping with toilet paper. If the contaminated fingers or the toilet paper comes close to the opening of the urethra, then infection is possible. The most prevalent bacteria offenders are E. coli, Staphylococcus, Klebsiella and Proteus.

The urinary tract can also become colonized with pathogenic yeast as well as harmful molds, creating an environment that is predisposed to repeated infections. When accompanied by other harmful pathogens, infectious bacteria have an easier time upsetting the balance of the urinary tract. To achieve long-term wellness, all offending pathogens must be eliminated. In fact, the initial infecting strain of bacteria can persist in the fecal flora even after it has been eliminated from the urinary tract, causing repeated urinary infections for years.

Furthermore, at the 101st meeting of the American Society for Microbiology 2001, it was reported that bacteria have been found to survive in the urine even after antibiotic treatment. In as many as 30 percent of women thought to be cured by antibiotics, E. coli returned. According to conventional laboratory testing, it appeared that all the E. coli had been killed, but these bacteria may be reverting to a viable but inactive state to avoid detection. After further investigation, even after a month of antibiotic exposure, ten million of the original one billion E. coli remained. Now, investigators believe that antibiotic treatment may encourage many of the bacteria to change to a different form. The ability of bacteria to survive hostile circumstances and change may be what causes repeated UTIs.

After removal of the antibiotics, they repeated their testing using a "nutrient broth" (similar to the procedure that is needed to find gram-positive bacteria in cases of interstitial cystitis). When the researchers repeated the antibiotic, the bacteria again changed and could not be cultured, but a polymerase chain reaction (PCR) test confirmed their findings. If you suffer from chronic cystitis and routine urine cultures fail to identify the pathogen, you probably have the L-form or cell wall-deficient bacteria. Blood in the urine of unknown cause is almost always caused by L-forms and sometimes by the L-forms of two species acting together. L-forms need special laboratory testing to detect them. If you are prone to repeated UTIs, it is important that you bring research on L-form bacteria and testing procedures to your doctor's attention and that you receive follow-up testing two weeks and two months after antibiotic treatment to be sure the bacteria are gone.

Another theory about recurring UTIs hypothesizes that pathogenic bacteria may establish an intracellular reservoir in bladder tissue, making them inaccessible to antibiotics. Usually bladder cells only turnover about every six months. However, when there is an acute infection, the cell turnover occurs much quicker, to aid in elimination of the infection. Unfortunately, this protective mechanism may actually allow the bacteria to enter the bladder cells, where they can replicate safely out of the reach of antibiotics.

It is important that even minor bladder infections are properly diagnosed and treated, especially recurrent ones. You may think that an antibiotic is sufficient, but there is a growing concern among physicians that antibiotic therapy actually promotes recurrent bladder infections by disturbing the "good" bacterial flora of the vagina. It may also lead to antibiotic-resistant strains of bacteria.

Various strains of *Lactobacillus* are critical for maintaining a healthy ecosystem in the vagina. They have the ability to block infectious microorganisms that can cause urinary tract infections. They have been known to block the growth of these pathogens as much as 74 percent. These protective bacteria are most effective against *Pseudomonas aeruginosa* and *Klebsiella pneumoniae*. Pathogens can only cause trouble when they are able to fasten themselves to tissues and when the defense system is defective. The defense strategy of *Lactobacillus* seems to be one of adapting to the body's immediate needs.

One woman had a four-year history of recurrent bladder infections, some of which cultured positive for the yeast *Candida albicans* and the bacteria *Enterococcus faecalis*. She received a single vaginal suppository containing 0.5 grams of *Lactobacillus casei var rhamnosus* and became symptom free within two days. During the next six months, she received two more suppository treatments and has remained symptoms free. Vaginal application of probiotics has a long folk history as a treatment for recurring bladder infections and vaginitis.

Moreover, in a recent study from the *British Medical Journal* (2001), a mixture of cranberry and lingonberry juice taken daily for six months resulted in a 20 percent reduction in UTI risk (compared with women drinking a probiotic drink). Cranberry juice, capsules or tablets can be very effective in preventing bladder infections caused by *E. coli*. Bacteria must adhere to the surface of the urinary tract in order to cause infections. Cranberries contain a compound, mannose, which prevents this from happening. They also possess antibacterial properties. Unfortunately, most cranberry juices are loaded with sugar and contain very little pure juice. It may be better to take one-fourth teaspoon of mannose daily to prevent UTIs or cranberry in non-sugared capsules or tablets.

Vaginal Infections

It is common for chronic vaginal infections to be caused by a history of oral antibiotic use. Antibiotics can reduce the number of friendly bacteria, including *Lactobacillus acidophilus* in the vagina and create a pH of greater than 4.5. The result is a *Streptococcus* infection, also known as bacterial vaginosis. Loss of normal vaginal microflora predispose women to the overgrowth of bacteria, fungus or yeast, and even parasites. This condition is one of the most important causes of premature births (prior to thirty-two weeks of gestation).

There also appears to be a subset of women who do not have any symptoms but still carry a bacterial infection. Researchers reported in an issue of the *American Journal of Obstetrics and Gynecology* that these asymptomatic women did not benefit that much from common treatment for bacterial vaginosis using the drug metronidazole. Instead, many of them continued to have an infection after using the drug. Women like this may be better off seeking an alternative to antibiotics.

Of course, the predominant reason for recurrent vaginal infections is linked to sexually transmitted infections such as gonorrhea and *Chlamydia trachomatis*. Anyone with recurring vaginal infections that are not easily treated should also be tested for HIV, if there is any chance they could be infected. The greatest risk was among women who had more than one partner in the past three months along with having a sexually transmitted disease. However, there are several cases of women with this condition who do not have any STDs. These cases are probably caused by an imbalance in the vaginal ecosystem caused by antibiotics, diet, poor hygiene, tight-fitting or nylon clothing or a weakened immune system. Practices such as vaginal douching may also encourage overgrowth of pathogens by destroying healthy populations of protective microbes. Anyone prone to yeast infections should limit their intake of yeasty foods like bread, beer, sugar, alcohol and caffeine.

One defense to this problem is to replenish the "good" bacteria in the vagina. It may take extremely large amounts of *Lactobacillus acidophilus* (taken orally) to re-establish balance in the vagina, however. For chronic yeast infections, I have found that women respond best when treatment includes a daily douche with yogurt cultured with *Lactobacillus acidophilus* (or probiotic suppositories) plus daily consumption of a pint of unsweetened yogurt with active cultures and ten to twenty capsules of freeze-dried, *L. acidophilus* capsules. Most women will respond to this treatment.

The worst thing to do is ignore recurring vaginal infections. Bacterial vaginosis is linked to serious health risks in women, including increased rates of pre-term births, infertility and urinary problems. Before beginning any self-treatment, see your healthcare provider to rule out STDs and other serious conditions.

Wound Infections

Patients who are warmed (using a heated blanket or localized warming dressings) prior to a clean operative procedure are less likely to develop a wound infection than patients who are not warmed, according to a report published in an issue of the *Lancet*. The wound infection rate of non-warmed patients was 14 percent, while that of warmed patients was only 5 percent. Postoperative antibiotics were also prescribed more often in the non-warmed group.

CHAPTER 12

Invisible Killers: The Need to Know About Bioterrorism

IN PREVIOUS CHAPTERS, we have discussed ways in which common and sometimes benign bacteria can turn toxic and cause disease, but these bacterial invaders may seem somewhat inconsequential compared to the deadlier threats that are possible with bioterrorism. As discussed previously, *Mycoplasma* may have been used in biological weapons and could be a possible cause of Gulf War syndrome. The following are more examples of why protecting your internal terrain may be a matter of life or death.

Although it may seem like the increasing risks of terrorism and biological threats may be the result of September 11, 2001, possible security risks were surfacing long before the World Trade Center tragedy and subsequent anthrax mail contamination. In 1995, the deadly nerve gas sarin was released by the cult Aum Shinrikyo in a crowded Tokyo subway. Two years earlier the same Japanese religious cult ordered anthrax to be released from the top of a Tokyo building; however, the test failed. Unfortunately, these groups still pose a real threat and are believed to have an arsenal of biological weapons, including anthrax and botulinum toxin. In fact, it has even been rumored that Aum Shinrikyo members have traveled to Zaire in an effort to obtain the Ebola virus.

The threats are not just overseas. Intelligence agencies were stunned in 1993, when a Soviet defector involved in a bioweapons program revealed that the Soviet Union had made tons of smallpox virus for missile delivery, in violation of the 1972 Biological Weapons Convention. Another nasty shock came in 1995, when Saddam Hussein's son-in-law defected with news of Iraq's unexpectedly sophisticated bioweapons program. Now there's evidence that Iraq, Iran, Libya, China, North

Korea, Russia, Israel, Pakistan and Taiwan have all built biological arsenals, and the group is growing. Although only one or two of these nations is presumed to possess the most dangerous of the scourges, smallpox, verifying that information is difficult. Plus, countries and extremist groups without stockpiles of bioweapons themselves may easily buy them from Iraq or the former Soviet Union, legitimately or on the black market.

Of course, bioterrorist incidents do not have to involve anthrax or small pox to cause damage. Consider the incident that occurred in The Dalles, Oregon, some years ago. *Salmonella typhimurium* was used by the Rajneeshee religious cult to contaminate restaurant salad bars and a city water-supply tank. About 751 people were poisoned during a one-month period. Even bioterror hoaxes, such as the one that occurred in Washington, D.C. when a petri dish labeled anthrax was delivered to the mailroom of the B'nai Brith, are costly and destructive, even if only to our peace of mind.

Is it likely that we will experience a biological attack in the future? It is not so much a question of if it will happen, but when. Germ warfare is certainly not a pleasant subject to think about, but can we afford to bury our heads in the sand? Our lives may depend on being informed. Anyone who doubts the reality of this risk may want to remember a Presidential Executive Order declaring a national emergency in 1994 (extended in 1997). The order was released because of a belief that terrorist teams already in this country (or making plans to be here) were planning strikes with biological agents in hand.

Our city, state and national governments aren't taking bioterrorism lightly. In response to a 1999 anthrax scare in Spokane, Washington, the pharmacy department at Deaconess Medical Center developed an anthrax policy that incorporated the CDC's recommendations for the administration of vaccines and oral antimicrobials. After reviewing the recommendations, an interdisciplinary team requested that the pharmacy department develop a plan for bioterrorism preparedness. They formed a citywide disaster committee, comprised of representatives from local emergency departments and emergency medical services, to more aggressively address the issue of overall domestic preparedness, including readiness for nuclear, chemical and biological attacks. One aspect of their plan was to develop a correct antidote for multiple biological agents—and to make sure there would be enough available in case of an attack.

Moreover, in May 2000, dozens of emergency and medical personnel attended a day-long program on domestic preparedness against bioterrorism. The program was developed to help them learn about their community's response potential and how to improve it. The citywide network adopted recommendations from the medical management for each specific biological organism or toxin. Participants concluded that communities needed to be able to self-sufficient for at least twenty-four hours after an attack, since getting outside assistance could be difficult. If financially feasible, some local stockpiling of certain antidotes, like antimicrobials, may be necessary as well.

Of course, the gap between what should be done to prepare and what can be done often is wide, especially in hospitals. Financial pressures in the U.S. medical system have left hospitals and other healthcare providers ill-prepared to handle a health crisis stemming from a biological attack or a large epidemic. Dr. Robert F. Knouss, director of the Department of Health and Human Services Office of Emergency Preparedness, said a mock bioterrorist attack held in Denver in May, 2001, showed that the U.S. health system would not be capable of handling a large-scale disaster. Plus, healthcare facilities in local communities are already overwhelmed.

In June 2001, a mock smallpox attack showed that the U.S. government was still unprepared for bioterrorism. The exercise dubbed "Dark Winter" was based on a realistic scenario. In the simulation, fifteen thousand cases of smallpox with one thousand deaths occurred less than two weeks after twenty-four people first showed signs of an undiagnosed illness at an Oklahoma hospital. Experts told Congress that the failure of this exercise showed those government officials at the federal and local levels, as well as the medical community, were very unprepared for a bioterrorism attack. Involved experts determined that supplies of the smallpox vaccine were far less than needed, and it would take weeks to make enough to deal with an emergency of this magnitude. In the exercise, there was rioting and looting when the vaccine supplies ran out.

Managed care, healthcare funding, staffing issues and regulatory burdens have all conspired to prevent hospitals from preparing for a large epidemic. These burdens prevent them from planning for possible future crises and inhibit their ability to care for large volumes of people sickened from a biological attack. Furthermore, hospitals and healthcare providers often are not reimbursed when dealing with epidemics. For instance, hospitals responding to a meningitis outbreak in Mantako, Minnesota, 1995, took a heavy financial hit since they were not reimbursed.

Despite these inadequacies, probably the first place people would go in the event of a bioterror attack would be to their local hospital emergency room. However, the very healthcare professionals that are needed the most to detect bioterror agents—hospital pathologists and laboratory personnel—are the least funded and trained. According to Dr. Greg Evans at St. Louis University School of Public Health, about 80 percent of this country's public health workers lack adequate education and training and would not be prepared to respond to an attack.

Although physicians are most likely aware of bioterroism, few of them have been part of any local plans of preparedness, according to the chief of infectious diseases for Johns Hopkins Hospital and School of Medicine, Dr. John Bartlett. Physicians are already overwhelmed by the hectic demands managed care has placed on them and cannot properly prepare for such a crisis. In the end, the people you would depend on most in your community will most likely be unprepared for a bioterrorist strike of any scale.

Bioterrorism presents unique challenges because it differs dramatically from other forms of terrorism and national emergencies. While explosions or chemical attacks cause immediate and visible casualties, an intentional release of a biological weapon may spread over the course of days or weeks before it is identified, possibly causing a major epidemic and definitely causing widespread panic. Biological agents that are most likely to be threats are anthrax, smallpox, botulism and the plague. Let's look at the potential dangers of some of these agents in more detail.

Anthrax

Bacillus anthracis was studied by the Japanese starting in the 1930s and by the United States and Britain in the 1940s, as a means of germ warfare. *Scientific American* once showed drawings of U.S. cluster bombs designed for anthrax during World War II. In fact, there was a plan to use anthrax against six German cities if the war in Europe had persisted. However, the first large-scale use of anthrax that we know about was in Rhodesia, where it appears to have been used to kill cattle owned by black farmers to prevent them from harboring guerrillas. However, the farmers ate meat from the dead animals resulting in nearly two hundred human deaths and ten thousand human cases of skin-infected anthrax.

Anthrax is a naturally occurring bacterium found in domesticated animals. It is not spread from person to person but can still be deadly, as we saw in the months following September 11. Even though it is not contagious, anthrax is considered one of the most likely biological warfare agents because of the stability of its spores compared with other agents used in biological warfare. Moreover, it is easily inhaled and the mortality rate for inhaled anthrax is high. Anthrax can be produced as dry spores. If it were released by airplane, the aerosol cloud would be colorless, odorless and invisible. Anthrax spores are also very small, making those indoors just as vulnerable as those outside.

Anthrax is a very stable gram-positive, spore-forming organism that is today's most serious biological threat. It can be lethal when inhaled or ingested, and a lethal dose of anthrax spores can be as little as one-billionth of a gram. If there was just a little wind, a single container even with 2 pounds of powdered anthrax dropped from a plane could sicken many people if dropped over a highly populated area. For instance, if 100 pounds of anthrax were disbursed in a populated area, 95,000 people would be dead, and another 125,000 people incapacitated in just a few days—and these are conservative figures.

Inhaled anthrax has an incubation period of one to six days. The nonspecific symptoms could begin as soon as two days after inhalation, or as long as eight weeks after. Initial symptoms resemble the flu and can include fever, nerve pain, headache, cough and chest pain, followed by a period of improvement for a couple of days. Then there is rapid deterioration, and the disease progresses to the lungs leading to respiratory failure, fever, shock and tissue hemorrhaging. About half of the people who get this form of anthrax develop hemorrhagic meningitis. About 50 to 80 percent of those infected die, most within one to three days after the onset of acute symptoms. Antibiotics can significantly reduce the risk of death, but they must be taken with forty-eight hours after exposure. One of the reasons the anthrax mortality rate is so high is because the disease is usually not suspected until the course is irreversible.

The cutaneous (skin) anthrax is less dangerous because the infection is in the skin, not the lungs. It starts with the development of a painless bump at the site of contact that rapidly progresses to an ulcer-surrounded vesicle and then to necrotic tissue. There is usually massive edema and other systemic signs. The death rate with cutaneous anthrax is about 20 percent.

Until recently, the vaccine against anthrax had been studied mostly for its effectiveness in protecting veterinarians and mill and livestock handlers against skin infections from touching goats, sheep or cattle. However, the military hoped to inoculate all 2.4 million troops as protection against biological warfare. They began giving shots to personnel on active duty, and then to reserve troops if they were likely to encounter biological warfare overseas.

There have been complaints of side effects from the vaccine, such as fevers, muscle pain and dizziness. Some pilots testified that they would resign to protect their health and flying careers, while other soldiers have faced court martial, jail time or discharge from the service because of refusal to take the vaccine. Although there has been an attempt to develop a new and less invasive vaccine for anthrax, it is wise to avoid this vaccine unless absolutely necessary because of its potential immune-impairing actions. The anthrax vaccine should be considered experimental and its effectiveness against biological warfare is still uncertain.

The Centers for Disease Control and Prevention (CDC) in Atlanta has issued guidelines for the use of anthrax vaccine if anthrax were released in the civilian population as a bioterrorism agent. Concerns about a shortage of the vaccine in the case of a bioterrorist attack have peaked recently, in part because of the findings of U.S. Food and Drug Administration (FDA) inspections at the vaccine's manufacturer, BioPort Corporation in Lansing, Michigan. The FDA approved the use of the vaccine based only on the manufacturer's test data without subjecting the vaccine to outside testing.

When the FDA finally did their own inspection of the vaccine, they quarantined eleven formerly approved lots and forced the manufacturer to shut down and rebuild their facility. Their inspection identified several infractions related to product sterility and monitoring at the facility. This is one reason that critics have been saying that anthrax is inappropriate for mass inoculation. In fact, the reaction rate appears to be higher than for any other licensed vaccine, and the protection it offers is questionable. BioPort is hoping to be back in operation for the U.S. military by the year 2002. The firm recently completed a top-to-bottom, multimillion-dollar renovation of its manufacturing plant. Under government regulations, the overhauled facility must be inspected and cleared by the FDA before lots produced there can be released for use. For more information on the anthrax vaccine, refer to www.anthraxvaccine.org.

If American civilians ever do suffer a major anthrax attack, the federal government says the antibiotic ciprofloxacin should be the first line of defense and could be an antidote to anthrax. This is the first medication to be specifically designated for use in the case of bioterrorism. Federal officials say that ciprofloxacin could save people's lives if the first dose is taken within hours after exposure to anthrax. Unfortunately, taking Ciprofloxacin may result in many adverse symptoms. Ciprofloxacin had not previously been approved for use in children because of long-term safety concerns. The FDA based its recommendation on studies of monkeys. Once exposed to anthrax, only one of the nine monkeys died after being treated with ciprofloxacin. This antibiotic may save your life if taken in time, but once the symptoms of fever, chills, rash and respiratory problems begin, ciprofloxacin is of little use. Another antibiotic thought to be effective is doxycycline, but it has not received the approval of the FDA. Ciprofloxacin is thought to be more reliable, however, if the anthrax organism is altered in any way.

In several parts of southern India, human anthrax has reappeared.

Most of the people who develop the cutaneous (on the skin) form will recover if treated with antibiotics. There have been several small outbreaks of anthrax among cattle, sheep, and goats, in one area of India. Despite treatment with high doses of penicillin, twenty-seven out of twenty-nine people treated this way have died.

Indian experts are concerned that many strains of *Bacillus anthracis* are now resistant to penicillin. India is considered an endemic region for animal and human anthrax because of a large unprotected and uncontrolled livestock population. Conditions are favorable there for animal to soil to animal transmission. It seems like India would be a good place to test the effectiveness of the antibiotic ciprofloxacin.

Dr. Meryl Nass, an internist, played a major role in opposing the Pentagon's anthrax vaccine immunization program. She described the lack of information on the safety of the anthrax vaccine and pointed out that it has not yet been ruled out as a contributor to Gulf War syndrome (*Lancet*). She goes on to state that anthrax may have been used by the Germans against pack animals in World War I. She believes that the vaccine is better than nothing, but doubts it will be of much use when specially selected or genetically engineered strains of anthrax are used as biological weapons. Such highly virulent strains are very likely to override vaccine-induced immunity.

Mycoplasma: A Disease Agent Weaponized

According to Donald W. Scott, M.A., M.Sc., and President of The Common Cause Medical Research Foundation in Ontario, Canada, several strains of *Mycoplasma* have been "engineered" to become more dangerous. Most of the two hundred species of *Mycoplasma* are innocuous and do not harm us; only four or five cause disease.

Many doctors do not know about *Mycoplasma* as a disease agent because it was developed by the U.S. military in biological warfare experimentation and was not made public. The United States military and Dr. Shyh-Ching Lo patented this pathogen. Donald Scott says that he has a copy of the documented patent from the U.S. Patent Office.

Mycoplasma fermentans (*incognitus* strain) probably comes from the nucleus of the *Brucella* bacterium. This disease agent is not a bacterium and not a virus, but a mutated form of the *Brucella* bacterium. It was derived from biological warfare research starting in 1942 and resulted in the creation of more deadly and infectious forms of *Mycoplasma*.

Military scientists "weaponized" it, which means they made it more contagious and more effective. Then they began testing it on an unsuspecting public in North America. Dr. Maurice Hilleman, chief virologist for the pharmaceutical company Merck Sharp & Dohme, stated that everyone in North America now carries this disease agent and possibly most people throughout the world, and it continues to spread.

Since World War II, there has been an increase in all the neurosystemic degenerative diseases. In about 1970, we saw the arrival of previously unheard of diseases such as chronic fatigue syndrome and AIDS. This disease agent may be a contributing cause of many illnesses including AIDS, cancer, chronic fatigue syndrome, Crohn's colitis, Type I diabetes, multiple sclerosis, Parkinson's disease, rheumatoid arthritis and Alzheimer's.

Dr. Charles Engel, who is with the U.S. National Institutes of Health, Bethesda, Maryland, stated the following at an NIH meeting on February 7, 2000: "I am now of the view that the probable cause of chronic fatigue syndrome and fibromyalgia is the *Mycoplasma*."

The organism acts by entering into the individual cells of the body, depending upon your genetic predisposition. You may develop neurological diseases if the pathogen destroys certain cells in your brain. You may develop Crohn's colitis if the pathogen invades and destroys cells in the lower bowel. Once the organism gets into the cell, it can lie dormant for many years. If a trauma occurs or your immune system becomes compromised, then *Mycoplasma* can be triggered.

George Merck, of the pharmaceutical company Merck Sharp & Dohme, reported in 1946 to the U.S. Secretary of War that his researchers had managed to produce a crystalline bacterial toxin extracted from the *Brucella* bacterium. The bacterial toxin could be removed in crystalline form and stored, transported and deployed without deteriorating. Other vectors such as insects, aerosol, or the food chain could deliver it. The factor that is working is the *Mycoplasma*. Most of us have never heard of the disease brucellosis because it largely disappeared when milk was pasteurized. *Brucella* is a disease agent that doesn't kill people; it disables them. Because the crystalline disease agent goes into solution in the blood, ordinary blood and tissue tests will not reveal its presence.

In documents, the government of the United States revealed evidence of the cause of multiple sclerosis, but they didn't make it known to the public. In a 1949 report, it was suggested that the possibility that multiple sclerosis might be a central nervous system manifestation of chronic brucellosis. A 1948 *New England Journal of Medicine* report titled "Acute Brucellosis Among Laboratory Workers" revealed that many of them became ill with brucellosis because it is so infectious, even though these workers had been vaccinated, wore rubberized suits and masks, and worked through holes in the compartment. They were all military personnel engaged in making the disease agent *Brucella* into a more effective biological weapon.

The government knew that crystalline *Brucella* would cause disease in humans. Now they needed to determine how it would spread and the best way to disperse it. They first tested dispersal methods in Utah, in June and September 1952. Documented evidence proves that the biological weapons they were developing were tested on the public in various communities without their knowledge or consent.

A report from the *New England Journal of Medicine* reveals that one of the first outbreaks of chronic fatigue syndrome was in Florida in 1957. A week before people came down with illness, there was a huge influx of mosquitoes. It is suspected that the mosquitoes were bred and released on purpose. The cases kept occurring until finally 450 people were ill with the disease. The mosquitoes were released in other areas as well. For more information on this subject read *Nexus Magazine* Vol. 8, No. 5 September/October 2001.

Gulf War Germs

It is estimated that somewhere between fifty thousand and one hundred thousand Gulf War veterans and their close family members became ill since that war ended. There is also a high incident of unusual deaths among that population. Many of these men were healthy enough to pass their military physical exams, but died of congestive heart failure at unusually early ages. The suspected organism is *Mycoplasma fermentans* (incognitus) and *Mycoplasma penetrans*. It seems that the *incognitus* strain was being used as an agent of biological warfare. This brings to mind many questions. Where did the *Mycoplasma* come from? Was it released by our government or by Iraq? If it was released by Iraq, did our government give it to them back when they were our friends?

This airborne infection can stay inactive for long periods, has a slow onset, and is transmissible to immediate family members after prolonged contact with sick veterans. It has been found in the nucleus of white blood cells of 55 percent of sick Gulf War veterans and their ill family members. This organism may not be the only thing that made these veterans sick. Some may have been exposed to parasites, toxic chemicals, or from other causes that are not contagious. The main clue seems to be whether or not their immediate family members are ill with the same symptoms.

M. fermentans (*incognitus*) can be successfully treated with multiple courses of certain antibiotics such as doxycycline, azithromycin, ciprofloxacin or minocycline. Nearly all *Mycoplasma*-positive people in the study recovered after being given cycles of antibiotics. However, many people can not take the antibiotics because of severe reactions to them. It is important to treat the immune system and this can be done with less invasive methods.

Smallpox

A hypothetical situation: The place is a small town in Texas where a terrorist group has released a lethal virus into the air. The wind spreads the germs into the windows of the houses and finds even those people who are inside. The virus is an ancient enemy that now has been genetically engineered in a form far more deadly than ever before. It is smallpox. Within three days, hundreds flock to emergency rooms. There are not enough antibiotics and vaccines are not available. Those initially contaminated will spread it to many more. Now, the doctors and nurses are getting sick. Most will die. Thank goodness this is only one of many exercises that is being played out in this country to see how prepared we are to combat a possible new plague.

Smallpox is probably the ultimate weapon since people would continue to be infectious for months or years and transmit it to others. Smallpox is considered one of the highest-risk potential agents for bioterrorism. It kills 30 percent of those it infects. Before the World Trade Center attacks, 15.4 million doses of twenty-year-old smallpox vaccine were stockpiled. The CDC will publish explicit guidelines for use of this vaccine in those exposed to an initial release, their contacts, as well as healthcare workers and laboratory workers associated with their care. Because of the implied risk of smallpox to produce epidemic or pandemic disease, government, university, and private authorities need to be prepared to combat the threat.

New vaccine production is under way by a British company, Acambis, through a licensing agreement with the U.S. Food and Drug Administration. They announced in September 2001 that they expected to begin clinical trails on the drug by early 2002. The first of forty million doses is expected by 2004, with sustained production to 2020. Because of recent terrorist activities, the process will be speeded up. Smallpox has become a major threat again more than twenty years after the last reported case. There is some comfort in knowing that progress is being made to combat this organism.

Scientists say smallpox and anthrax pose the biggest germ-warfare threats, but only the smallpox virus has pandemic potential. The disease was eradicated in 1979 after a vaccination program, but military strategists are concerned that virus lots retained by the Soviet Union during the Cold War could fall into the hands of militant groups or rogue states. However, the old vaccine hardly meets modern safety requirements. The Acambis vaccine should have a shelf-life of five years.

Smallpox has an incubation period ranged from five to seventeen days. The virus enters and replicates in the respiratory tract without causing symptoms or contagion. Then the virus infects macrophages (white blood cells), which enter the lymphatic system and carry the virus to the lymph nodes causing the infection to spread to all the organs, followed by the characteristic skin rash. Then there is the development of additional lesions throughout the body followed by either death or recovery.

Where Will These Germs Come From?

The British experimented with anthrax during W.W.II because of its high kill rate, but never used it during the war. They ended their program during the 1950s, but the U.S. did not stop. In 1969 the U.S. operated extensive tests one thousand miles southwest of Hawaii involved the spraying of biological agents in powdered form over caged monkeys. Jets sprayed these biological agents over hundred of barges containing hundreds of monkeys. One half of the animals died—showing how effective this weapon was.

Even thought we had developed the technology, we had no need for it since we also had nuclear deterrent weapons. To prevent anyone else from developing these biological agents, the government renounced them. In 1972, the U.S., the Soviet Union, and the United Kingdom pushed for an international treaty to ban any research of these agents. In time 140 other countries also signed the treaty.

Decades later, information was released that the Soviet Union had violated this treaty and continued to research and develop biological agents such as smallpox in spite of the treaty. Today, we know this because of Soviet defectors. Their work was conducted with high intensity and new weapons were developed. This took place in secret locations in western Siberia. The work was conducted on some of the most dangerous viruses and bacteria known to mankind: smallpox, plague, anthrax, etc. They were not being developed primarily for the battlefield, but as agents of mass destruction against civilians in New York, Los Angeles, and Chicago. The plan was to put them in cluster bombs and in the warheads of missiles.

You might ask, why use smallpox? During the 1970s, the United Nations conducted a decade of vaccine programs and by 1980 had eradicated small pox worldwide. The Soviets realized that no one in the future would have any immunity to smallpox because there was not any need to be vaccinated. Smallpox is one of the deadliest of all plagues. Once the smallpox virus takes hold, it produces a high fever with distinctive and very painful pustules. Then the body's tissues break down and the immune system is overwhelmed. The person can die a horrible death.

By the 1970s there was suspicion by the U.S. that the Soviets were very involved in biological agents. We accused them, but they denied it. In March of 1979 the Soviets had an anthrax outbreak next door to a facility that had been suspected of developing it. One hundred people died who were downwind from this facility. It was claimed that the deaths were due to eating tainted meat. Some cases showed up as long as six weeks later. Symptoms caused by anthrax should have occurred within a few days, so it began to look like the tainted meat story might be true. It would be years before the Soviet government would admit that the anthrax had been released accidentally from a military lab. We had given them the benefit of the doubt and they continued to develop and research their program of biological weapons unheeded.

One of the stories that a defector related was of a lab accident more than ten years ago that exposed one of their scientists to an even more deadly virus than its cousin, the Ebola virus. It took him two weeks to die a horrible death. Then the virus was taken from his body and made into a more virulent biological weapon. In 1985, with the election of Gorbachev came the death of the old guard, or at least we thought. From 1986 to 1990 it now appears that there was new secret work being conducted on biological agents. The Soviets denied that they had any such organisms. To quote Gorbachev, "Don't you trust us?"

A top scientist of the biological weapons program defected to the United Kingdom and revealed many of the Soviet's secrets to the British. He said that the Soviets had a secret, sophisticated and extensive program throughout the entire Soviet Union that had been going on uninterrupted. When the first inspections were launched by an U.S. and British team, it confirmed that the Russian deception was extensive. They used false accounts and misleading information that was well planned in advanced. The main purpose was to hide what was really going on: plague, anthrax and legionnaires' disease development. Our government completely underestimated just how massive their program was.

The Russian program continued into the 1990s. By this time the old Soviet Union had crumbled and Yeltsin had taken charge. He admitted that they had been breaking the biological weapons treaty and was going to do away with this program. There are still doubts that this is entirely true, with suspicion that the military is still working on their offensive capabilities.

When Yeltsin visited Britain he was quoted as saying, "They had undertaken the research into the influence of various substances on human genes." It is believed that he was talking about genetic weapons. There were rumors that they are attempting to combine genetically deadly bacteria with viruses, such as the smallpox bacteria and Ebola virus. That would bring the kill rate up to 100 percent. This would be the ultimate and perfect doomsday weapon, since no one infected would survive. Of course, these allegations are totally being denied.

The biggest concern today is that with the Soviet Union in shambles will their ex-scientists sell their expertise to terrorists? Many of these experts in biological weapons are unemployed because of the financial problems Russia now faces. At Russia's State Research Center of Virology and Biotechnology, also known as VECTOR, laboratories held quantities of smallpox, Ebola, and Marburg viruses and other viruses associated with hemorrhagic fever. With the lapse of security at VECTOR and with key research scientists gone, those who remain are poorly paid. Could these materials of doom been distributed to other parts of the world?

Tracking these scientists is hard without the Russian government's help, but they have not seem interested in helping us, at least so far. There is the belief that the former Soviet biological warfare program remains largely intact. Another point to consider is that at least eleven other nations are suspected of having some type of biological agent, as well as several terrorist groups. Many more seek these "poor man's" nukes.

In the last few years, hundreds of millions of dollars are being spent by our government to set up more training, military inoculation, vaccine stockpiles, early warming equipment, emergency team training, etc. But are we working hard, fast, and smart enough to get policy makers to see that all the money being thrown into bioterrorist does not impact these events without including state and local health departments and local emergency management? If we do not develop a better program for dispensing vaccines and antibiotics, we will remain largely unprepared for bioterrorism.

With the advancements in biotechnology today, additional unknown threats may be waiting to be discovered. To date, except for the Rajneeshee attack with *Salmonella*, there have not been any major acts of bioterrorism in the United States. Now, after what has happened to the U.S. on September 11, 2001, the Bush administration has concern that there will be an attack in our near future. Our government needs to be prepared for such an event.

Some antidotes and vaccines can be obtained only from the Centers for Disease Control and Prevention (CDC). Treatment for exposure to some infectious agents, such as anthrax, can be accomplished with antibiotics that most pharmacies currently have on their shelves. The challenge is to ensure that there are sufficient quantities of these crucial drugs.

Failed Safety Measures

Recently, London's Imperial College was fined after pleading guilty to failing to ensure the safety of a research project that involved the construction of a genetically modified virus. This major medical research institution had failed in their safety measures before starting this potentially hazardous project. They were working on using genetic modification techniques to construct a new virus by combining genes from the hepatitis C virus and the dengue fever virus.

The research lab did not have means to fumigate the area in event of an accidental spillage and did not have the correct instruments to inactivate waste. They also were found using the wrong safety cabinet for some of their experiments. That's not all. Rules covering the procedures to be used in the lab were inadequate. It is not believed that anyone was hurt or that any of the genetically modified viruses were released from their lab, but if this lack of care can happen at Imperial College, what could happen at other places that don't even pretend to use good laboratory technique?

The Germans used *Burkholderia mallei* as a biological agent during World War I. Now, in July 2001, a microbiologist working at the U.S. Army Medical Research Institute for Infectious Disease, Fort Detrick, Maryland, became the first reported human case of *Burkholderia mallei* infection in this country in fifty years. The person worked with this organism without wearing latex gloves and the pathogen was probably transmitted through the skin (*New England Journal of Medicine* 2001). Again, we see the lax protocols of major research laboratories when dealing with potentially hazardous organisms that could be released onto an unsuspecting public.

Are Chemtrails Delivering Danger?

Would our own government test its chemical and biological weapons on an unsuspecting public? There is suspicion by some people that discolored skies are being polluted by jets spraying chemical aerosols. Could bizarre and unpredictable weather be conjured up by our military? What is being suspected is that people are becoming increasingly ill and their immune system is being compromised from such ecological tampering. Just how many laboratories across this country are developing new technologies and strategies for killing human beings in the name of national security?

Congressional hearings in 1975, 1977 and 1994 revealed that our Department of Defense has used the American population as guinea pigs since WWII without their knowledge or consent. Rutgers professor Dr. Leonard Cole collected lists from the U.S. military records of biological and chemical agents tested on American and Canadian civilian populations. In 1999, Jonathan Moreno confirmed in his book, *Undue Risk*, decades of military-intelligence experimentation on civilians.

Before a Senate committee in 1994, Dr. Cole testified that he feared the military might develop new and genetically engineered pathogens. He did not know then that our government had been working on such pathogens since the 1960s, when it initiated a special virus cancer program in order to create contagious cancers for biowarfare. The Rockefeller Committee also issued a report confirming fifty years of secret government testing on both civilians and military personnel.

During the summer of 1994, a gel substance was dropped on the tiny town of Oakville, Washington, near the pacific coast. People in town came down with flu and pneumonia-like symptoms. Some people were hospitalized and remained ill for months. Pets and barnyard animals died. The gel material was tested to find a modified version of *Pseudomonas fluorescens* along with human blood cells. This bacterium is cited in many military papers as an experimental biowarfare agent. The television program, *Unsolved Mysteries*, aired the story on national television in May 1997. In 1999, a CBS affiliate covered the story again.

In 1996, Dr. Leonard Horowitz confirmed in his book *Emerging Viruses* that both AIDS and the Marburg-Ebola complex were manmade in America's biowarfare labs. He says that the military continues with open-air testing in populated areas across the United States, using dangerous live microbes to test biowarfare detection gadgets.

In Caldwell, Idaho, 1999, eyewitness reported seeing a dark fibrous material that looked like feces falling on homes, cars, and lawns shortly before seven people were found dead in their sleep after their lungs collapsed. Medical journalist Ermina Cassani has investigated nationwide reports of such biological waste being dropped on neighborhoods from low-flying planes. Cassani investigated over thirty different drops during the years 1998 and 1999. One sample looked like dried blood and contained the bacteria *Pseudomonas fluorescens*. It is thought that the reason that this particular bacterium is being used is because of its glowing properties, allowing the military to track its path.

Some samples also contained the bacteria *Staphylococcus* and several fungi, which can cause lung disease. Cassani also reported twenty-nine biological cases in the state of Utah. Utah is home to Dugway Proving Grounds, a chemical-biological test center where hundreds of former workers have contracted Gulf War-like symptoms, according to a 1997 testimony before a government committee.

After several chemtrail spray (the "trails" visible behind flying planes) episodes on the small town of Sallisaw, Oklahoma, a web-like material was found to contain a mutant of *E. coli*, *Salmonella* and anthrax. A Sallisaw resident reported on the internet that the entire town was made extremely ill by the spraying and that the town now has epidemic rates of both lupus and cancer. When this web-like filament was examined, it appeared to be man-made fibers of the type developed by both industrial companies and the military. People in South Africa also reported web-like filaments falling from aircraft that formed a blanket-like appearance across vegetation, telephone poles and fences. When the cattle ate it they developed large bumps on their hides, became listless and went blind.

Chemtrail researcher Clifford Carnicom and his associates have documented many atmospheric samples containing biological components. There is evidence that gels, webs, fecal matter, powders and blood cells may be used to harbor viruses, *Mycoplasma*, and/or other bioengineered toxins until they can reach their intended hosts. For more information on the biological aspects of the ongoing chemtrail project see www.carnicom.com/contrails.htm.

A Wakeup Call

In the wake of the terrorist attacks on New York City and the Pentagon, Secretary of Health and Human Services Tommy Thompson reported that the dispatch of vaccine and other drugs represents the first time the government has mobilized the country's emergency pharmaceutical stockpile, a cache of medicines and supplies stored at eight secret sites around the nation. Several hundred medical personnel and thousands of medical supply items were sent to the attack sites to assist state and local authorities with the rescue of injured victims and the recovery of the dead. Hopefully, we will no longer be unprepared for a national disaster no matter where it comes from.

It may be prudent to have disaster-type contingency preparations including food, water, and planning for no electricity would seem wise insurance measures. If bioterrorism attacks do occur they will most certainly happen in densely populated urban areas. They are not likely to be disbursing these biological weapons in sparsely populated areas. These agents will likely be dispersed by the wind.

The interesting thing about bioterrorism is that, unlike the World Trade Center attack, there will be virtually no warning or explosions. This first thing I thought I might need was some type of gas mask, but I later found out that they probably would not be effective except in cases of chemical agents. For biological agents I would need a much better filter and that could cost me as much as $500.

All that is required is a relatively tight seal against your face around your mouth and a good filter. Surgical masks fit the bill. There are high-quality masks designed to filter out particles larger than 0.1 micron, which is smaller than all of the agents that would be used for germ warfare, including the most deadly anthrax spores. There are several models of masks to choose from and if you are going to use them, you want to make sure that you don't purchase surgical masks that only filter out 3 or 5 micron sized particles. These masks are not expensive.

You can increase the effectiveness of these surgical masks by using tape to seal the edges of the mask against your face and then you will have biological warfare protection for you and your whole family. Here is all the information you need to order the face masks. They are Isolation Face Masks, product number 28-370C. You can reach MD Depot at their web site www.mddepot.com. They will sell to consumers.

The good news is that the U.S. has begun to face this potential horror. Even back in 1999, the Clinton Administration launched a bioterrorism initiative. This effort had already begun to step up the ability to quickly identify suspected biological agents and created a national stockpile of antibiotics and drugs that can be rushed to fight an epidemic.

Meanwhile, states have set up offices to handle the complex coordination among hospitals, rescue teams, law enforcement, and others needed to fight a terrorist bioweapons attack. "We have a ways to go, but we're better prepared now than we've been before," says Dr. Julie A. Casani, medical coordinator for emergency preparedness and response for the state of Maryland. Not only will such plans lessen the toll from bioterrorist attacks, their existence will discourage the use of the organisms in the first place.

For more information on the use of and prevention/treatment options for bioterror agents, see my publication *Natural Defenses Against Bioterrorism*.

Section 4

Prevention and Treatment Options for Bacterial Overgrowth

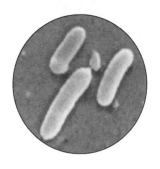

Introduction

WHEN IT COMES to bacterial overgrowth and resulting disease, prevention is just as important as treatment of existing conditions. The chapters in this section will discuss the various approaches (through lifestyle factors and other therapies) that can help one prevent and treat bacterial infection and overgrowth.

Keep in mind that many of these approaches involve improving the body's immune function and the state of its internal "terrain." As previous chapters have explained, a malfunctioning immune system and unhealthy tissues, blood and cells are principal players in allowing bacteria to intrude and take over.

Freedom of Choice in Healthcare Options

If you are currently experiencing a problem with bacterial overgrowth or a chronic condition that you feel requires help beyond your own, a competent health provider is certainly an excellent option. However, it is usually quite difficult to find doctors who will treat you for medical conditions such as the overgrowth of bacteria, parasites, yeast, multiple chemical sensitivities and chronic fatigue syndrome. You might not know that your very own doctor is unwilling to prescribe medication for any of these conditions until you ask. Sometimes, you can find a doctor in your state by looking on the internet. If that does not work, try calling a few medical offices to see if any of these doctors recognize the connection between your condition and infectious agents.

One reason that most medical doctors prefer not to deal with chronic illnesses is that time is money, and most doctors simply do not want to waste precious office and staff time dealing with these hard-to-diagnose, hard-to-treat conditions. Another unfortunate truth is that many doctors simply do not have the knowledge of how to treat the overgrowth of fungus, parasites, or bacteria, and they seem unwilling to learn more.

Sometimes doctors do not order the correct lab tests to determine what is really going on with their patients. A recent example concerned a local doctor who did not know the best test for diagnosing *H. pylori* infection. He ordered a less reliable test that often does not reveal this organism. The patient had previously had this test done with negative results so the doctor refused to treat her for *H. pylori* infection. When the correct test was finally done, the results were positive that she did have *H. pylori*, and she could finally receive treatment.

Lawmakers recently passed healthcare legislation that interferes with the doctor-patient relationship by making it illegal for Medicare recipients to contract privately with doctors or to pay with private funds for their own preferred medical treatment. This law discriminates and denies freedom of choice in healthcare. It is also becoming much more difficult for doctors in any state to accept Medicare patients, especially if those doctors wish to practice medicine freely and according to their conscience.

"Freedom of access" is imperative to quality healthcare in this nation. Nine states have already passed legislation designed to protect complementary and preventive healthcare professionals. These states are Alaska, Colorado, Georgia, New York, North Carolina, Oklahoma, Oregon, South Dakota and Washington. For more information, contact Citizens for Health, PO Box 2260, Boulder, CO 80306 or (303) 417-0772 or www.citizens.org. Another web site for information is www.healthlobby.com.

Health Management Organizations (HMO)

HMOs are "for-profit" organizations and must answer to their stockholders or their board of directors. They only want to hold down cost with policies directing doctors not to acknowledge many conditions and treatments that will cost them money. They will not allow doctors to diagnose or treat certain conditions or to prescribe certain medications. There are always other patients waiting in the wings that are easier and cheaper to treat.

Naturopathic Physicians

There is certainly a need for change, but until changes occur you can reach out for other types of non-MD doctors, called naturopathic physicians. These are physicians that practice a more holistic type of medicine. Hopefully, there is a licensed professional in your area that can guide you to better health, but you may not get insurance coverage to pay. For more information about naturopathic medicine read my book, *Allergies and Holistic Healing* or go online to www.naturopathic.org.

CHAPTER 13

Detoxification: Cleaning from the Inside Out

YOU SHOULD KNOW by now that the nutrients taken into your body are important factors in determining your health. But what about the elimination of waste and toxins from your body? This is an area often not discussed when it comes to health maintenance. While it is certainly important that you put good things into your body, it may be even more important that you get the harmful things out. Unfortunately, neglect of this practice is common.

The Basics of Detoxification

Detoxification is the process of simply ridding the body of toxins. This process requires patience and understanding. An overload of toxins destroys the body's balance and leads to a number of health problems. Alternative health practitioners such as naturopathic physicians, view the body as an integrated whole, not as separate components. A health condition is not an isolated problem; it is a manifestation of the entire body. Whether we succumb to the adverse effects of toxicity depends on our knowledge of the subject and the choices we make. It takes many years to get into a state of chronic toxicity, and it takes time to come out of it.

Three things have to be addressed: chronic dehydration, chronic toxicity and chronic nutritional deficiencies. They all affect the integrity of the cell membranes and establish a state of general acid waste. With the number of bacteria in the colon being estimated at ten billion per gram of fecal material, there are greater numbers of bacteria in the body than there are numbers of human cells. All these bacteria release by-products, some of which have healthful effects, while others can become toxic to the body. The accumulation of unnecessary wastes that cannot be eliminated properly is the primary cause of chronic disease.

Detoxification is the removal of toxic debris traveling through the lymphatic system and bloodstream for elimination by the liver, kidney, bowel, lungs, skin, etc. This will not happen properly if you are dehydrated or if any of these avenues of elimination are clogged up. Often, the health of these elimination organs is not considered before detoxification begins. This means that the toxins will again circulate and have the potential to create a temporary resurgence of old symptoms or a feeling of un-wellness. There are lab tests available today that can evaluate the ability of your body to successfully detoxify. This is especially important for those of you who find yourself getting sicker every time you try to detoxify your body.

Signs of a toxic body include a bad taste in the mouth, coated tongue, constipation, dizziness, foul-smelling flatulence, fatigue, headaches, lowered immunity, offensive breath, personality changes, poor circulation, acne, allergies, boils, colitis, eczema, gastritis, hemorrhoids, or skin conditions such as itching or psoriasis.

Understanding the Process

It is important to understand the cleansing process. Eating too much grain, meat or sugar makes your intestinal fluid too acidic. Then your digestive tract cannot properly digest foods, nutrients are not absorbed, toxins are stored rather than eliminated, and disease-causing pathogens are busy increasing their numbers. As the digestive tract becomes more imbalanced, healthy bacteria can manufacture less of their beneficial products. Now digestion is no longer optimal and abnormal fecal substance lines your intestinal tract and accumulates.

When considering a general detoxification plan, the role of the gastrointestinal system and liver becomes the main focus. If healing is to be complete and lasting, the toxic load on the liver must be dealt with. It often comes from the underlying gut dysbiosis, be it bacterial, fungal, viral, or parasitic. Your diet, emotions and stress levels are also part of the detoxification process. There are several self-tests you can do to see how your body is functioning: the saliva test, the lemon test and the urine test (see pages 273–274). You will know that you have been successful when you have an increase in energy, a sense of well being and improved digestion. A healthier body should also produce a stronger immune system.

Supporting The Cleansing Process

In the past, a water or juice fast was thought to be the best way to detoxify. The body was thought to clear stored toxins and heal itself faster when the stress of digestion and the further accumulation of toxins were eliminated. Now, we know this is not true. The body's detoxification mechanism is a heavily nutrient-supported process. A more modern approach is to nourish the body thoroughly, fueling its natural detoxification mechanism with the nutrients needed to achieve optimal detoxification activity. There is a need to provide high-quality proteins, complex carbohydrates, and essential fats. The following are actions that support your body's ability to detoxify:

- Cut back on high-fat foods, dairy products, meat, processed and fiber-depleted foods. When you eat foods that are hard to digest, you use energy not available for detoxification. Meat should be free of antibiotics and hormones.
- Eat more raw fruits and vegetables. They are easier to digest, especially if slightly steamed. Raw vegetables and fruits also contain live enzymes and valuable nutrients to aid detoxification. The fruits and vegetables should be organically grown, if at all possible. See Chapter 14 for more information on diet recommendations.
- Avoid caffeine, which is found in tea, coffee, chocolate and some soft drinks. Also avoid alcohol and processed sugar.
- Drink water. You need to drink at least eight glasses of pure water each day for proper lubrication. Water is needed to carry toxins out of the system. It is best to drink between meals. Filtered water is best; distilled water can leach minerals from the body.
- Do all you can to clean up your work and home environments. Avoid or eliminate the source of any toxic materials or household offenders or cleaning agents. Use an effective air purification system. Wear protective clothing and a breathing mask when using toxic materials. The last thing you want to do is to continue exposing yourself to harmful substances when you are trying to rid them from the body.
- Avoid antibiotics and anti-inflammatory drugs, especially during this time, because they destroy the beneficial bacteria of the body.
- Exercise to a sweat so the open pores allow toxins to escape.
- Find time to relax and relieve stress.

The Liver's Role in Detoxification

After the bowel becomes toxic from a lack of adequate elimination, the blood stream is forced to pick up these bowel toxins and deliver them to the liver. As your liver becomes more congested with these toxins, it cannot function as well as it once could. Gradually, every organ in the body is affected. A body cannot be healthy when all the parts are affected, and all its parts affect the whole.

The liver plays a vital role in the detoxification of the human body. Sometimes liver function is below optimum, although no medically observable liver disease or liver damage is present. A poorly functioning liver can have widespread impact on your health, with symptoms including sluggish digestion, fat intolerance, nausea, chronic constipation and the intolerance of chemicals, foods or drugs. A poorly functioning liver may also contribute to a number of disease states such as psoriasis, autoimmune disease, irritable bowel syndrome, allergies and cancer.

Endotoxins are cell wall constituents of bacteria that are absorbed from the gut. Normally, the liver plays a vital role by filtering these toxins before they reach the general circulation. If the amount of endotoxins absorbed is excessive, or if the liver is not functioning adequately, it can become overwhelmed and endotoxins will spill into the bloodstream. If endotoxins are allowed to circulate, they can be responsible for much of the inflammation and cell damage that occurs in many diseases, including gout, arthritis and psoriasis.

There are herbs that boost liver function and are particularly beneficial if digestive symptoms are also present. They include *Berberis vulgaris* (barberry), *Chelidonium* (great celandine) and other bitter herbs. However, you should avoid them if you have a history of liver damage. If you need to improve the health of your liver, then take the following natural supplements: *Silybum marianum* (St. Mary's thistle), *Cynara scolymus* (glove artichoke), and *Taraxacum officinale* (dandelion root). *Schisandra chinensis* is useful since it also enhances the detoxifying capacity of the liver. Other herbs helpful for liver detoxification are *Arctium lappa* (burdock) and *Rumex crispus* (yellow dock).

The Intestines

In a healthy body the intestines promote the elimination of toxins through regular bowel movements. The intestines also provide a strong and intact barrier to prevent the leaking of toxic materials into the bloodstream.

The intestines eliminate roughage, water, salts and dead cells. If the small intestines build up excessive mucus from foods, absorption will be reduced, slowing down all nutrient utilization. The cleaner the intestines, the faster any course of action will show results. It is also important to have one or two bowel movements daily before attempting any detoxification program.

The Skin & Lymph System

The skin is an important organ of elimination. Toxins can be released more efficiently if the skin is in proper working condition. To aid this process, try a detoxification bath (explained below). Another way is to use a body brush to stimulate lymph and blood flow by dry-brushing the skin from the ends of the limbs toward the heart, including the abdomen. Repeat this process daily, especially during your detoxification process to keep the lymphatic system in good condition. The lymphatic system also benefits from a lymphatic drainage massage from a massage therapist trained in this procedure. This should be preceded and followed by an adequate intake of pure water. A dehydrated and congested lymphatic system will poison your body. Another aid to lymphatic drainage is the addition of heat.

Detoxification Baths

Having a fever is your body's way of attempting to liquefy toxic fats. It also kills pathogens in order to discharge them. You can create your own fever with a hot bath. Keep the bath water hot and soak for about an hour. The body temperature should be kept at about 102°F and the head kept cool.

Both alternating hot and cold showers and foot soaks are excellent circulatory stimulants. The bath water should not contain chlorine or fluoride. Pet shops sell water purifiers (liquid drops for instant detoxification of chlorine and heavy metals) usually used for fish tanks. There are also water-purifying systems for filtering your water or shower units. You really do not want to soak in and breathe in chlorine and fluoride.

If you are a person with a history of toxic chemical or pesticide exposures, you may do well with sauna therapy. This is because the toxins are stored in the fat cells and must be eliminated through the sweat. The heat of a sauna can be harmful to some people. Heat may cause disease progression in MS patients and in some people with an unknown infectious component to their illness.

The Healing Crisis: It "Hurts" So Good

A cleanse can be demanding on your body. For this reason, your body might suffer what is called a "healing crisis." This might include symptoms such as digestive upsets, diarrhea, headaches, fatigue or dizziness. If any of these occur, it is important to remember that it is not only natural, but it is a good sign that your detoxification program is working. However, if it becomes too uncomfortable, you may need to reduce what you are doing until your symptoms decrease. Wait until your body has adjusted to the cleansing process before moving ahead. Once you feel better for at least three days, then you can go back to the program and begin to increase the dosage. Nearly every discomfort associated with a healing crisis should disappear within a few days to a week, depending on your toxic "status." And the best part? Afterward, you'll feel better than you have in a very long time.

It is important to remember that detoxification needs to proceed at a rate that the body can handle. The lymphatic system and the liver, kidneys, etc., may become overloaded unless handled correctly. Some toxins take a while to clear out. As the tissues become less toxic, they work more efficiently. Most people push the envelope and want detoxification to happen quickly. They cannot just relax and let their body detoxify at a comfortable rate. A healing crisis can be brought on if you proceed too rapidly. Others have a frantic fear of symptoms and refuse to believe that unless these symptoms disappear instantly, they will never go away at all. The point to remember is that whatever caused your illness is the enemy, not the symptoms. Symptoms are the warnings that indicate there is a problem and direct us to its detection and resolution. Disease and symptoms are not the same thing. For instance, joint pain is a symptom, but dehydration may be the enemy. When you treat the dehydration, the joint pain goes away. Unfortunately, many doctors who practice conventional medicine sees the joint pain as the enemy and use drugs to suppress the pain so it cannot be felt.

Cleansing the Colon

Since the earliest times, the large intestine has been known to play a major role in a wide range of diseases. Colon irrigation (also known as a colonic, high enema or colon cleanse) is a treatment that flushes out the colon and is of great value in treating many diseases, especially those that have resisted other forms of treatment. The first thought of a holistic physician should be to aid intestinal elimination and restore balance. Plans should include changing the intestinal microflora,

Detoxify with Exercise

Excess fat provides a ready storage site for fat-loving toxins entering the body. Once deposited there, it is very difficult to remove them, and they may continue to be a source of toxicity. Exercise aids in the elimination of these stored toxins. Many people begin an exercise program with the best of intentions, only to find that it is either too difficult or requires too much time. Find an exercise program that is fun, and not so ambitious that it is impossible to continue. After you find one that works for you, gradually increase your level of exercise.

Toxins can be eliminated through the sweat glands. One of the best ways to do this is to walk fast. Your walking distance and pace can be upgraded as time allows. Walking twenty to thirty minutes three to five times a week will help to prevent toxins from overloading the body and being reabsorbed, further allowing the body to eliminate more toxins. Any exercise is better than none at all.

increasing peristaltic activity, and overcoming stasis without resorting to toxic measures. This can be done with diet, exercise, herbal and homeopathic medications, colon irrigation, and other natural and non-invasive methods.

It was once said that having a good reliable set of bowels is worth more than any quantity of brains. You may not realize how true this is until your bowels do not function properly. All body cells take in nutrients to nourish themselves. Then they need to get rid of the waste material generated. You have approximately one hundred trillion cells all needing to do this. If you are going to maintain optimal health, it becomes necessary that the body eliminate this waste efficiently. Otherwise, you become overloaded with toxins, with the end results being illness and disease.

Bowel Movements: What Is Your Transit Time?

The colon eliminates the bulk of the most toxic and putrid waste in the body, usually within twenty-four to thirty-six hours after eating. You can check how fast your feces move through your intestinal tract by ingesting activated charcoal, beets, corn kernels, or anything else that can mark your stools. Write down when you first swallowed the substance and again when you first see it appear in the stool. This is called your "transit time."

The typical American diet is a prescription for disaster. There are too much fried and over-cooked foods, sugar, salt, white flour, starches, and dairy, along with artificial chemicals. They are all hard to digest and contain few nutrients, causing the colon to move slowly, and producing too much toxic waste. If you eat too much fat, it will slow down your transit time. Eating too much meat can do the same thing, if there is not enough hydrochloric acid in the stomach. When you have a stagnant colon filled with toxic and putrid feces, the result is a poisoned blood stream, as well as toxins accumulating in the cells and organs of the body. It also feeds critters in your intestinal tract.

I am amazed that many people do not have a bowel movement every day. Some do not even have one every other day. One woman who had a bowel movement approximately once every ten days thought this was normal. What is even more amazing is that these people do not think that there is something wrong. I explained to her that this may be average for her, but it certainly was not normal for anyone.

In addition to sluggish bowels, they often have other colon-related problems such as diverticulosis, hemorrhoids, irritable bowel syndrome, spastic colon and inflammatory bowel disease. All these health problems can be the result of a slow-moving, hard, dry stool. A diet high in fiber and water, and low in fat, produces soft and moist stool that can be easily eliminated along with the toxins it carries. Also, it is estimated that the average colon contains five pounds of putrid meat particles and another five to ten packed pounds of toxic fecal matter. To minimize toxins being absorbed into the blood stream from the colon, mucus is created as a barrier. There is also mucus buildup from people who eat too many mucus-producing foods every day. In fact, you could have built-up layers of mucus or encrusted fecal matter for years. Inside those layers, pockets can form that harbor pathogens. This is a great place for bacteria, fungus, and parasites to live.

Just because you are having daily bowel movement does not rule out colon dysfunction. Bowels full of waste material often show up on x-ray despite laxative and enema treatments. When defecation is unduly delayed, a person may experience mental depression and restlessness. The odor of the breath is in part due to gases produced in the colon. Foul odors coming from the body are a good indication for treatment of the colon and diet changes.

The Saliva Test

The saliva test is an important first step to any cleansing program. With saliva from your mouth, wet a small strip of pH paper. Read the pH. Record the results and the date.

Interpreting Test Results

• 6.0 or below: You are seriously acidic. Before starting any cleansing program, it is important to replenish your alkaline reserves. This means more vegetables. For now, it is best to avoid strenuous exercise or fasting.

• 6.2 to 6.3: You are still too acidic. Continue to increase your alkaline foods.

• 6.4 to 6.8: Now you know what a proper pH should look like. This is much better.

• 7.1 or above: This is too high. Wait about one hour and retest. If you continue to stay at this pH or higher, you are probably eating a diet that is too alkaline, experiencing psychological stress, or have an overgrowth of microbes.

The Lemon Test

Fast for at least two hours before doing this test. Cut and squeeze the juice of half a lemon into 2 ounces of distilled drinking water, without using any sweeteners. Before you swallow the juice, swish it around in your mouth. After swallowing, wait one minute before checking your saliva using the pH paper. Wait another minute and recheck the pH. Continue to record your results every minute for a total of six times.

Interpreting Test Results

• 7.5 or higher: This is a healthy indicator. Your liver has adequate alkaline reserves available.

• 7.0 to 7.4: You have some alkaline reserves, but it is still not high enough to be healthy. Increase your alkaline foods.

• 6.9 or lower: Your alkaline reserves are still too low. This could indicate a possible problem and could be affecting your liver and digestion.

The Urine Test

For an entire day eat only vegetables and vegetable juices. The next morning wet a strip of pH paper in a midstream of urine. Record your results.

Interpreting Test Results

• 7.0 or above: Your body has a good supply of alkaline reserves. The excess is being eliminated in the urine.

• 6.5 to 6.9: Your alkaline reserves are somewhat depleted. Before starting a cleansing program, it is important to replenish your alkaline reserves.

• 5.6 to 6.4: Your pH is too low. Before starting a cleanse, you need to focus on replenishing your reserves by eating a diet rich in alkaline-forming foods.

• 5.6 or below: Your body is very depleted and you do not have adequate alkaline reserves. Do not start a cleansing program until your alkaline reserves have returned to normal.

Once you begin a cleanse, your kidneys will remove stored acids resulting in a lower than normal urine pH. You will not be able to detect the correct pH in the urine at this time. The saliva and lemon tests should continue to give you reliable readings while continuing the cleansing program.

*For a list of alkaline foods, refer to my book *Allergies and Holistic Healing*.

Colonics

Since it appears possible for viruses to live inside bacteria, then it may be of use to have a colonic to decrease the viral load as well as the overload of other harmful organisms. Never let a colon therapist use ozone as part of the treatment. The colon is an anaerobic chamber (without oxygen). This means that your beneficial bacteria will be exposed to oxygen from the ozone, which will destroy them.

Colonics are most effective if they are done at least once a week for four to six weeks, along with an intestinal cleanse. Some of the bacterial overgrowths are up in the small intestines where the colon irrigation cannot reach them, but a healthy immune system will usually deal with them. If not, you can take supplements that will.

The book *Achieve Maximum Health* by colon hydrotherapist David Webster is highly recommended for anyone who wants to try an enema for improving colon health. He recommends using a "whey wash" because it is slightly acidic. Plain water is too alkaline. Whey may be a problem for those of you who are sensitive to dairy products. There are also other ways to use enemas such as the coffee enemas discussed in the book, *Wellness Against All Odds*, by Sherry Rogers, M.D. Enemas are an excellent way to easily and safely rid your body of toxic waste and thereby ease the symptoms of a cleansing reaction. Another book helpful in creating a healthy digestive tract is Brenda Watson's *Renew Your Life: Healthy Digestion and Detoxification*.

A lack of awareness among physicians about colon irrigation is a sad consequence of the fact that few hospitals and medical schools are equipped with modern, easily operated equipment. Fewer have knowledgeable staff. Colon therapy works best in conjunction with other natural therapies and while supervised by a knowledgeable technician.

Why Have a Colon Cleanse?

One of the main objectives of a bowel cleanse is to remove the build-up, or plaque, from the intestines. This plaque can be somewhat shiny and often looks like pieces of leather or rubber. Some of it may appear stringy or rope-like. When a large piece of plaque come from the upper part of the small intestines, it may show definite striations. Plaque from the lower part of the small intestines is smooth, usually shiny, with no bumps, striations or curvy shapes. Plaque from the large intestine (colon) has bumpy shapes and overlaps.

The plaque can be up to a quarter-inch thick, but occasionally may be even thicker. Sometimes it is hard and stiff, but usually it feels soft and flexible. At other times, it can be gooey and mucus-like. The color ranges from light brown to black, and often is a blackish-green. The average length is 6 to 18 inches, but pieces commonly come out more than 2 to 4 feet long. Some people have mistaken this plaque for the presence of worms.

People who consume too much table salt have trouble removing this plaque. It seems that salt causes the plaque to harden to the point that it resists removal. Also, simply drinking more water, juice fasting, or having colonics, will not remove this hardened mucoid plaque. There are various cleansing programs that do remove it from the colon, but for best results, it is necessary to cleanse the stomach and the small intestines, as well as the colon. A cleanse should last for about four weeks, depending on the amount of toxic buildup. It involves changes in diet and a regiment that demands a significant level of commitment to improving your health.

How to Make A Cleansing Shake

Ingredients:
1 tablespoon liquid bentonite clay
2 teaspoons psyllium husk powder (or flaxseed powder)
8–12 ounces filtered water

Bentonite clay has highly absorptive properties that will draw out heavy metals, drugs, and toxins for release from the body. This clay can assist the removal of the excessive mucus layers and other debris. Psyllium husk powder is a fibrous bulking agent that gels and thickens when mixed with water. It works with the bentonite clay to help detoxify the digestive tract and loosen the plaque. The psyllium helps to push these toxins and waste materials out of the digestive tract.

Mix the bentonite clay with water in a 16-ounce shaker bottle with the lid tightly closed. Add the psyllium and shake again. Drink immediately before the shake begins to thicken. If you mix the ingredients in a blender, it will have a smoother texture. During the cleanse, drink three to five shakes a day, but between meals. It is best not to take supplements near the time you take this shake, because it will take much of the nutrients out of the body.

When you first start any new cleansing program, it is important to begin with low doses and slowly work up to the desired amount. This will prevent you from detoxifying too quickly.

CHAPTER 14

The Role of Diet in Conquering
Bacterial Overgrowth

THE ROLE OF diet is crucial in strengthening the immune system, enhancing the body's internal terrain, and supplying the body with the tools necessary for fighting bacteria. I believe that the one factor that can affect a person's health more than any other is diet. This chapter will discuss some important points related to both overcoming bacterial overgrowth and promoting overall optimal health.

The Healthy Diet

What is the point of eating healthful (and hopefully organic) foods if you cannot properly digest, absorb and assimilate these foods you so carefully choose? When we think of a healthy diet, the first thing that comes to mind is not usually the state of our intestinal tract. However, digestion is the very basic foundation for good nutrition. When our digestive tract does not function properly it becomes the underlying problem of so many health issues. The gastrointestinal tract is not just a long tube filled with waste material, but a complex system with its own unique ecology. An estimated 58 percent of the U.S. population suffers from some form of digestive problem.

When there is balance in the bowel microflora and normal motility of stool, the results are usually normal intestinal immune levels and a strong overall immune system. As this healthy cycle continues, it prevents toxins from developing from bacterial overgrowth in the intestines. Then the liver is not under excessive stress and does not have to be exposed to more toxins than it can handle at one time. In this state, a person can be exposed to a great number of toxins or organisms before an illness or disease develops.

There is no single diet that fits everyone. Over the last few years, I have seen a lot of success with the blood type diet for many people who have tried it. But it did not work for some. A few simple dietary changes may be all it takes to put you back on the road to better health. Even if your diet needs to be more individualized, there is still some information that is common to almost all of us.

Adequate chewing reduces food to a mash. The stomach acids break down large molecules preparing the food to pass into your intestines. The pancreas releases digestive enzymes through the bile duct into your small intestines where trillions of friendly bacteria help process the food. Then the intestinal wall absorbs nutrients into the blood stream. The leftovers go on to your large intestine where liquid is absorbed before the waste material passes out of your body. When all goes well, the body stays healthy.

Along this route, there are many factors that can contribute to poor digestion. If you are under stress, blood rushes to your limbs or brain to help you with the "fight or flight" response. If you eat when you feel this way, your digestive tract will not be able to properly digest your food. Stress and aging impairs the body's ability to produce adequate stomach acid and other digestive enzymes. Digestion has been compromised and the body gets less nourishment. If this continues, you are faced with a downward spiral.

A good diet and plenty of rest contribute to an adequate enzyme supply, and therefore, normal digestion. A diet heavy in meat and cooked foods, but low in raw vegetables, impairs enzymatic performance. Many fruits are picked green and therefore do not contain the proper enzymes that help to digest them.

Eating meals on the run or at irregular hours can weaken the body's natural ability to digest. It would be much better to eat slowly in a tranquil setting listening to relaxing music. Wait two or three hours before eating again so your stomach can recuperate after a digestive challenge. On the average, people who skip breakfast struggle with lower energy levels later in the day and more weight problems than people who take the time to eat breakfast. This is because those who skip breakfast in order to cut calories often end up snacking more and overeating at evening meals.

What you eat and how much you eat for lunch sets the tone for the rest of the day. Eating about 500 calories will refuel energy without leading to drowsiness, whereas fatty meals trigger feelings of fatigue. Low-fat lunches result in a "get things done" afternoon. An all-carbohydrate lunch, such as pasta with marinara sauce, raises levels of a brain chemical called serotonin. This is almost guaranteed to make you drowsy.

Protein, on the other hand, triggers the release of norepinephrine, which boosts energy and mood. A mix of low fat, reduced carbs and protein may be better. Then you can maximize the fuel needed from carbohydrates while getting the energy lift from protein.

Frequent stops to refuel throughout the day can be a great way to sustain energy, if you choose your snacks right. Sugary treats may provide a quick fix to lagging energy levels, but you will be setting yourself up for a big crash later on, resulting in fatigue. Too much sugar also depresses your immune system. Frequent small meals and snacks rather than two or three big meals are your body's best bet for maintaining adequate blood sugar levels and avoiding fatigue.

Coffee, tea, cola drinks and other caffeine-containing beverages are quick "pick-me-ups" with the promise of instant energy, but they will put you into a nose-dive later. At a moderate intake, coffee helps some people think faster, concentrate better, stay alert and work more efficiently; however, this means maybe one to two cups a day, not a coffeepot full. In addition, many of these beverages will dehydrate your body; not having enough water in the body puts you at a greater risk for disease.

Pick Your Proteins with Care

Meat can be an important part of a healthy diet, contrary to what many people would like you to believe. However, a vast majority of the meat available today is from unhealthy animals. They are almost never fed their natural diets and are filled with antibiotics and growth hormones and fed grain that contains pesticides.

Proteins provide the building blocks for the synthesis of enzymes, hormones and nucleoproteins. Certain proteins transport oxygen while others facilitate muscle constriction. Many vitamins and minerals are bound to specific protein carriers that facilitate their absorption. Proteins play a vital role in virtually every structural metabolic and physiological process necessary for overall health and well-being.

Dietary protein is broken down into its component parts, amino acids, before being absorbed and used by the body. The body manufactures all but nine or ten of the amino acids, so these "essential" ones must be obtained from the diet or supplements. Protein does not have to come from just animal products, but it still has to contain all of the essential amino acids each and every day. The number-one problem that I see with many vegetarian diets is the lack of complete and usable proteins. Many vegetarians do not even know about complementary proteins and their necessity for good health.

Why Don't You Have Energy?

Americans spend billions of dollars every year on stimulants such as caffeine, nicotine and other such products, yet one out of every three people suffers from fatigue. How do stimulants like caffeine and nicotine affect energy? The calorie is the unit of energy, but how many calories are in a cup of black coffee? The answer is zero. If there are no calories, then there is no energy. Since most coffee drinkers experience a boost of energy from their morning cup of java, where does the energy come from? It comes from your body's reaction to caffeine. This is energy that would otherwise be used for healing and repair.

Increase Your Water Intake

Most people fall short of drinking the recommended eight 8-ounce glasses a day (or 64 ounces). Although nearly three quarters of Americans are aware of the fact that they should drink more water, only 34 percent actually drink adequate amounts, while 10 percent said they do not drink water at all. However, Americans drink an average of nearly six servings a day of caffeinated beverages such as coffee and soda. These drinks can actually cause the body to lose water, making proper hydration even more difficult to attain. A book that is worth reading is *Your Body's Many Cries for Water*, by Dr. Batmanghelidj.

Drinking adequate amounts of water is one of the most important health habits you need to establish. Water is essential and if you do not get enough clean water you will suffer health problems. Your body is 55 percent water and it must be replenished daily. Be good to your millions of tiny cells, and they will continue to supply you with abundant and reliable energy. You may need to invest in a water filter system for your drinking water. You will also need a filter for your shower. Most of us will absorb far more toxins from bathing or showering than we will from drinking tap water.

If you exercise regularly, you will need to consume more water than the average person does. During the summer months, even more water may be necessary. If you sweat a lot, then it is important to drink plenty of water. It is better to sip water throughout the day then to gulp it in a few drinks so that you don't put too much stress on your kidneys.

It would be best to drink water that has been left at room temperature. Ice-cold water can be a trauma to the delicate lining of the stomach, unless you are overheated. If you buy bottled water, try not to purchase the one-gallon cloudy plastic (PVC) containers from your grocery store as they transfer far too many chemicals into the water. The five-gallon containers and the clear bottles (polyethylene) are a much better plastic and will not give the water that awful plastic taste. Do not drink chlorinated or fluorinated tap water. These are toxic chemicals and should not be consumed in large quantities.

Do not use distilled water as your main source of water. Although it is free of contaminants, it also acts like a vacuum and will suck out many of the beneficial trace minerals you need to stay healthy. Obtaining good mineral balance is hard enough. You do not want to put a metabolic drain in your system by drinking distilled water. I will quote Dr. Zoltan Rona when he said, "Distillation is the process in which water is boiled, evaporated and the vapor condensed. Distilled water is free of dissolved minerals and, because of this, has the special property of being able to actively absorb toxic substances from the body and eliminate them. Studies validate the benefits of drinking distilled water when wanting to cleanse or detoxify the system for a short period. Fasting using distilled water can be dangerous because of the rapid loss of electrolytes (sodium, potassium and chloride) and trace minerals such as magnesium. Cooking foods in distilled water pulls the minerals out of them and lowers their nutrient value."

Many other health advocates have found that drinking only distilled water is not such a good idea either. This water is dead and so foreign to the body that it is actually possible to get a temporary high white blood cell count in response to drinking it. Dr. Rona also says, "The longer one drinks distilled water, the more likely he is to develop mineral deficiencies and an acid state. I have done well over three thousand mineral evaluations using a combination of blood, urine and hair tests in my practice. Almost without exception, people who consume distilled water exclusively will eventually develop multiple mineral deficiencies."

The body maintains the best health when it maintains a body chemistry (pH) that leans slightly to the alkaline side rather than the acidic side. Distilled water quickly turns acidic, about 5.8 in an open air container. Does it still make sense for you to drink eight glasses a day of distilled water? But tap water has all those chemicals and pollutants and other unknown factors contained in it.

I hope you will give your source of water more thought. Do consider investing in a good water filter system. For more information about what to look for in a water filter system refer to my book *The Parasite Menace*. If you cannot afford a reverse osmosis filter system, the Culligan filter is a better choice than the Brita filter. They are easy to install and can usually be found locally.

It Could Be Wheat Gluten

Intolerance to wheat gluten often goes undiagnosed or is misdiagnosed as irritable bowel syndrome or lactose intolerance. Many people who have chronic health complaints benefit when they stop eating all forms of wheat. One of the most common symptoms I see is hard-to-treat skin rashes that disappear within days once wheat is eliminated. If you have a chronic health complaint, try avoiding gluten for at least two weeks and see if you improve. You may need to avoid all gluten-containing grains, not just wheat.

Does Milk Really Do A Body Good?

Pasteurized and homogenized cow's milk has been promoted as the perfect food for humans, especially for our children. Most people believe that the healthy growth of their children's bones depends on drinking milk. The milk industry certainly wants us to think that this is so. Countless articles on the subject show that processed cow's milk is not healthy for humans and has been linked to a wide range of illnesses. The list of health problems includes allergies, sinusitis, skin rashes, arthritis, diabetes, ear infections, osteoporosis, asthma, autoimmune diseases, diarrhea, colic, cramps and gastrointestinal bleeding.

Even as far back as 1939 the book *Back to Eden* stated that cow's milk is unfit for human consumption and causes the symptoms of intestinal auto-intoxication. What must it be doing now with the addition of bovine growth hormone, antibiotics and pesticide-laden feed given to the cows?

The average person in this country consumes 375 pounds of dairy products a year. One out of every seven dollars spent on groceries goes to buy dairy products. We have been told to drink plenty of milk in order to build strong teeth and bones. The U.S. has the highest consumption of dairy products in the world, yet it also has the highest incidence of bone fractures and osteoporosis in the world.

The major cause of chronic ear infections in children and frequent trips to the doctor's office is due to the consumption of dairy products. Many cases of over-mucus conditions such as sinus problems are often eliminated when dairy products are avoided. One germ, group A beta-hemolytic streptococcus, will not usually establish an infection in a child who is not consuming dairy products or drinking milk. What can you drink instead? Try drinking some clean water, organic herbal teas, and fresh extracted vegetable juices. If you have a newborn infant, then the obvious choice is breast milk.

Healthy Choices for Today's Teen

Teenagers nowadays consume fewer calories, especially from necessary and healthy fat. They also eat less fresh fruit and vegetables and are more likely to load up on junk food. There are significant increases in soft drinks as well as harmful foods such as French fries, pizza, and macaroni and cheese. They do not eat enough high fiber foods such as beans and salads.

The average teen diet is compromising nutrition and health and may contribute to important increases in chronic diseases. The fact that teenager's total calories have dipped, but their junk food consumption has gone up, makes things even worse. This means that the percent of total calories obtained from empty carbohydrates has increased. With girls, the intake of foods with adequate iron, folate and calcium, continues to be below the recommended amount.

School Lunches Need Improvement

This is one area that certainly needs a makeover. Many families that are trying to have healthier meals at home still send their children off to school allowing them to eat very unhealthy lunches and snacks. Thanks to a program that is designed to improve the nutritional quality of school meals called the School Meals Initiative for Healthy Children, some schools lunches have already improved. They include less fat, cholesterol and salt in these lunches, as well as an increased number of fruits and vegetables.

At Berkeley High School in Berkeley, California, students are offered foods such as hormone-free chicken and chow mein made with fresh vegetables from the local farmer's market. In another school near Santa Cruz, California, students cook breakfast and lunch in the food lab using ingredients grown in the school's organic garden. There are more salads being served. Changes are desperately needed in more schools and on college campuses. It takes parents' involvement as well as concern from the school and other organizations to make sure these students have healthy food available to them. Do you as a parent even know what your child is served for lunch?

In many cases schools contract out food services. Do you know who has that contract? It would be worth your time to check out what kinds of meals are being served. Because many school lunch programs compete with fast-food establishments, they need to make lunches appealing, yet still nutritional and healthy. It is hard to sell these healthy alternatives when next to them are foods from such chains as Pizza Hut, Taco Bell, and Arby's.

Part of any school education should also be an education in better food choices. It is important to let children known why healthy food is so important before many of them will choose to eat it. Also, if children are not taught to eat healthy at home, how can we expect them to choose these foods at school?

Schools should have a responsibility to offer good nutrition to children instead of serving fast food, soda, and snack foods. Since many schools are strapped for cash, they market unhealthy choices of foods and drinks to their student body. In the end, schools that do not change are contributing to unhealthy children and putting them at a higher risk for a compromised immune system that will allow the presence of pathogen organisms.

Dangerous Low-Fat Diets

Low-fat diets are not recommended for very young children because adequate and healthy fat is essential for proper growth. A new study looked at forty-five children that were twelve to eighteen months old. They found that many of these toddlers were eating diets too low in healthy fat. Current pediatric nutrition recommendations call for children up to the age of two to get at least 30 percent of their calories from fat. Intake of zinc, vitamin E and iron was also below recommended levels. The period between the first and second year of life is an important transitional phase as regular food starts replacing breast milk and/or formula.

Why Eat Organic Foods?

Eating organic foods was once dismissed as the pastime of crackpots and idealists, but today the organic food business has grown to well over $15 billion a year worldwide and growing. The number of organic farms has soared in the last few years because consumers have grown to distrust chemical-dependent farming and the biotech industry. This country is seriously trailing the Europeans, who have taken a massive interest in organic farming. Since World War II the world of agriculture and horticulture has been significantly altered by the general use of synthetic fertilizers, pesticides, and drugs. On the other hand, the organic farmer uses crop rotation, beneficial insects, and plant biodiversity. This is the best defense against an imbalanced ecosystem and the best protection for our environment and for us.

The Agriculture Department received a record number of comments from the public that included environmentalists, farmers, celebrities, and the entire Vermont legislature. The vast majority of the responses opposed allowing the organic label on foods that are grown using biotechnology, irradiation, and sewage sludge. This massive, unprecedented consumer interest shook up the USDA and forced them to back off on plans to degrade organic standards and allow biotech and corporate agribusiness to take over the rapidly growing organic food market.

The USDA bureaucrats bowed to these grass root pressures. They agreed that any product bearing the label "USDA Certified Organic" would have to be produced without toxic pesticides or toxic inert ingredients. No synthetics or chemicals will be allowed in organic production without the approval of the National Organic Standards Board. Factory farm-style intensive confinement of farm animals will not be allowed either. It just goes to show you that many people standing together on an issue can change the outcome.

In March 2000, this public demand won out to ban biotechnology and irradiation procedures on foods labeled and sold as "organic." The U.S. Department of Agriculture (USDA) now provides us with a standard for food and clothing marketed as "organic." This label previously fell under a hodgepodge of state, regional, and privately certified standards, giving rise to confusion about its meaning. These new standards make it easier for consumers to determine which products are genuinely organic and which are not. Having a single national organic standard, backed by consistent and accurate labeling, will greatly aid the organic industry.

The new rules ban foods from the organic category if they contain any ingredients that are genetically engineered, fertilized with industrial sewage sludge, or irradiated to kill bacteria. Meat and poultry must be fed 100 percent organic feed in order for such products to be labeled organic. This means that they cannot be treated with antibiotics or growth hormones.

Products containing at least 95 percent organic products will be labeled USDA certified organic. Food and clothing with between 50 and 94 percent organic inputs will be able to claim that they were made with organic ingredients. Any products made with some, but less than 50 percent of organic materials, can only make organic claims on the side label. These products may have the following characteristics: genetically engineered, irradiated, derived from sewage sludge, or produced with pesticides, growth hormones, or antibiotics.

HERE'S THE BAD PART

Big business very much wants to muscle into the organic sector and dilute the standards of organic farming. Manure from factory farms can be used as a fertilizer on organic farms. Although the proposed regulations on organic animal husbandry requires access to the outdoors, there is no clear definition of what actually constitutes pasture, nor does the USDA delineate exact space or spacing requirements for humane housing and outdoor access for poultry, pigs, cattle, and other animals. Another problem is the genetic contamination of organic crops by "drift" coming from farms growing genetically engineered crops. This is one of the most serious environmental threats to organic agriculture and to all nongenetically altered plants on Earth.

SO WHAT ARE ORGANIC FOODS?

The use of organic techniques in growing plants and raising animals has been around since humans first tilled the Earth and cared for animals. The main guidelines for organic production are the use of materials and practices that enhance the ecological balance of natural systems. Organic foods are grown or raised without materials known to be harmful or disruptive to people and other aspects of our environment. Such foods enrich rather than deplete, balance rather than disrupt, contribute to health rather than pollute. Not all "natural" foods are organic. There are fertilizers, pesticides, hormones, drugs, and other harmful substances that may be called "natural." So natural foods are not necessarily organic, but organic foods are always natural.

Organic farmers use natural insect predators or other alternative substances that are broken down and harmless to the environment and to the consumer. Rather than killing or suppressing every ill that affects crops and livestock with an arsenal of poisons and drugs, organic agriculture views pests and other infestations as symptoms of underlying problems. They look at the need for nutrients to make the plants stronger or ecological imbalances that need to be addressed. Insects, weeds, and disease are not necessarily the real problem, but rather the results of an imbalance that needs to be corrected for optimal plant health.

More Reasons To Buy Organic

Synthetic fertilizers provide nothing to benefit the soil and leave residues and contamination. These fertilizers repel and kill beneficial soil microorganisms and earthworms. They are harsh and interfere with the natural chemical, physical and biological systems in the soil. The nitrates found in these fertilizers end up in our lakes, streams and aquifers. Pesticides can destroy the microorganisms of the soil as well, virtually sterilizing it. Each year, U.S. farmers use more than 200 million pounds of insecticides, 450 million pounds of herbicides, and 40 million tons of chemical fertilizers on croplands. Manufacturers produce new and stronger pesticides every year, which are finding their way into our food chain. There is not any adequate toxicity evaluation on these substances or the way they are being combined. Dependence on these toxins is so pervasive it is affecting the very center of our ecological web of life.

Government testing records from 1992 to 1993 revealed sixty-six different illegal pesticides were detected in forty-two fruits and vegetables. Americans eat an estimated two billion pounds of produce containing illegal pesticides each year. More than 80 percent of apples, peaches, and celery samples contain unsafe levels of pesticide residues even after washing and peeling. Generally, 77 percent of conventionally grown fruits and vegetables contain unsafe pesticide residues. Produce is contaminated with insecticides, fungicides, herbicides, and growth regulators. With the inclusion of grains, milk, and processed foods, over 70 percent of non-organic foods have unsafe residues. Many people with food sensitivities find that they are actually sensitive to the toxic pesticides or herbicides, and not to the food itself.

About 95 percent of the toxic chemicals found in U.S. food comes from meat, fish, dairy products, and eggs. Huge amounts of toxic chemicals are applied to crops used for livestock feed and accumulate in the tissues of the animals eating these crops. Beef contains the highest concentration of herbicides than any other food and ranks third in insecticide contamination. Farm animals receive an average of thirty times more antibiotics than people do. The drugs are used not only to treat disease, but also to make the animals grow faster. Almost half the antibiotics produced in this country are given to livestock. Up to eighty-two drugs are used on dairy cows, but the FDA tests only a few of them. Non-organic milk may contain traces of many antibiotics without disclosing that information on the label. European countries have banned most beef, poultry, and dairy products coming from the U.S. because of detectable levels of these drugs.

Organ meats tend to accumulate pesticides, drugs, and hormone residues in even higher concentrations. Some poisons accumulate in the fat, so fatty meats and some fish, and dairy products, especially cheese and butter, have higher residue levels. Fish harvested close to shore or from inland water suffer the most from pollution. Farmed fish are raised similar to farmed animals, complete with toxic drugs and pesticide residues. On the other hand, organically raised animals and fish are fed organic feed (no pesticides or other foreign substances), graze in unsprayed areas, and are not given growth stimulants, antibiotics, or hormones.

Each day, our children consume foods with pesticides on them. The worst fruits and vegetables are spinach, peaches, pears, winter squash, green beans, grapes, apples and celery. Commercial baby food poses the greatest risk to infants. Many pesticides are known or suspected endocrine disrupters. These are substances that mimic or interfere with hormones. They raise the risk of cancers and weaken and compromise the immune system, besides posing other health issues.

Biotechnology is big business. Gene-altered potatoes may be spliced with chicken genes, tomatoes spliced with fish genes, corn spliced with virus genes, pigs spliced with human genes. Bacteria, insect, animal and various plant combinations are being produced. Manufacturers can sell bio-engineered foods without adequate safety testing or disclosure, whereas organic methods do not employ genetic engineering at all.

COMPARE THE NUTRITIONAL VALUE

There are usually higher amounts of trace elements and other nutrients in organically grown foods. Several years ago *Science News* related the outcome of a study comparing the nutritional value of organic and nonorganic vegetables. Guess which foods scored higher? The organic ones, of course. Other studies have confirmed the same results. In fact, trace elements may be totally absent in some of the commercial foods, since they are grown on virtually sterile soils except for what has been added to the fertilizer. These nutrients are usually in the form of synthetic vitamins and inorganic minerals.

Trace minerals are key elements in the structures of enzymes that govern all biological and metabolic processes in life systems. The mineral and enzyme components built into the food crop not only give it nutritional value, but also improve plant resistance to insects and disease. When you have healthy soil, you have healthy plants, and that leads to healthy consumers. A Rutgers University study comparing organically grown vegetables to supermarket produce revealed substantial differences. Organically grown tomatoes were over 500 percent higher in calcium, and much higher in magnesium and iron compared to nonorganic samples. This type of increase was found in other produce as well.

The biotech industry claims that some of their foods will have higher nutritional value. What are they comparing it to? It is highly doubtful that they compared their findings to organically produced foods. And what is the ultimate cost to us and our environment by this manip-

Digestive Tips for Optimizing Your Health

- First you have to recognize the cause of your health problem or have a diagnosis.
- Remove the cause. These are the harmful bacteria, yeast, fungus, and parasites. You may need to take specific herbs and supplements to accomplish this. Remove any known food allergens from the diet. The most common ones are dairy and wheat. Remove from the diet any other foods that cause problems.
- Replace digestive enzymes. The pancreas burns out working overtime to make enzymes for food that has not been properly broken down, often leading to blood sugar problems. Supplementing with digestive enzymes can help restore balance to the gut. You will need to take them for at least four to six months. There are many different enzymes. You may need some help from a trained health professional to find out which ones you need.
- Reinoculate the friendly bacteria. If helpful bacteria have been wiped out by antibiotics or became overpowered by aggressive bacteria, they can be replenished by taking probiotics. Many commercial yogurts and supplements do not contain reliable stains of these bacteria. Some species pass through the intestines and do not colonize. You want ones that will stay and do their job.
- Repair the intestinal lining. Pathogens damage the intestinal wall causing a condition known as "leaky gut." You may need to begin a specific nutritional program to help repair your intestine.
- Now it's time to restore normal function to the digestive tract and the body through a better lifestyle and dietary changes, adequate chewing, fiber, and decreasing the toxic load on the body by avoiding substances such as NSAIDs, etc. You will need to be on a digestion revitalization program for a minimum of six to eight weeks. This will need to include a restrictive organic diet and supplements to detoxify the liver.

ulation of nature? Will we just see more genetically engineered foods, pesticides, herbicides, and the like? The biggest complaint I hear concerning organic foods is that they cost more. The higher nutritional value and the better taste should be worth it, as well as the freedom from all those toxins. It is difficult to be healthy when you continue to consume poisoned and non-nutritious foods.

WHAT ABOUT THE TASTE?

If I have not convinced you to eat certified organic food by now, I have one more reason to tempt you. There is the taste difference. The soils used to grow organic foods are well balanced and yield strong, healthy plants, which taste better. The color, aroma, and taste of fresh organic foods reflect their nutritional value. The succulent taste of an organically raised fruit is incomparable to its commercial counterpart.

IN THE SUPPLEMENTS?

Why would you buy a multiple vitamin/mineral supplement to provide health-giving nutrients, but not make sure that the ingredients are from healthy sources? That goes for any supplement that you put into your body. Many people eat organic food and filter their water, but their supplements are from questionable sources.

Commercial Food Toxins

Not only can toxins create adverse effects, they also deplete nutrients and energy as the body attempts to get rid of these toxins. They interfere with digestion, transportation, and the incorporation and utilization of nutrients. Data as far back as 1987 from the National Academy of Science indicates that pesticides in our food supply add up to more than one million additional cancer cases in the U.S. over our lifetime. I'm sure that it is much higher today with all the additional toxins being applied to foods.

The Danger of Pesticides

Many of today's pesticides are systemic. That means that the pesticides do not just stay on the outside of the plant, but actually become a part of the plant and cannot be washed off or removed by peeling. Pesticides also frequently remain in the environment for a long time. One pesticide, toxaphene, has a half-life of fifteen years in the soil. This means that half of the pesticide still remains active in the soil fifteen years after it is applied. Pesticides accumulate in the soil over time and often lead to contaminated lakes, streams, and ground water.

Since pests have the remarkable ability to rapidly adapt to toxic chemicals in their environment, more and more pesticides have to be used to produce the same degree of crop protection. Modern agriculture

Holistic Treatments For H. pylori

If you are diagnosed with the *H.pylori* bacteria, holistic treatments should be considered first. Continue treatment for a minimum of two months. Repeat the lab test before discontinuing your treatment plan to see if the bacteria are still there. The following are suggestions for promoting good health in general, but people who are recovering from stomach ulcers should pay special attention to them.

- Maintain an acid environment in the stomach.
- The stomach needs adequate levels of vitamins C and E.
- Eliminate sugar and refined carbohydrates from your diet.
- Increase whole grains, legumes, and vegetables.
- Get a juicer and drink 16 to 24 ounces of vegetable juice per day; make sure to consistently include fresh cabbage juice.
- Include a high-potency vitamin-mineral formula with meals.
- Drink twelve glasses of pure filtered (not distilled) water each day. Stop drinking alcohol, soda, fruit juice, milk, black tea, and coffee.
- Take a good probiotic such as *Lactobacillus acidophilus* and *L. bifidus* cultures to help create an environment that does not support the growth of *H. pylori*.
- Reduce or eliminate smoking and tobacco products.
- Eliminate analgesics such as aspirin, NSAIDS, and cortiosteroids.
- Employ stress reduction techniques such as exercise, hobbies, relaxation techniques, and meditation.
- Eat a high-fiber diet so that you will not be constipated.

uses increasing quantities of pesticides that continue to put poisons into the human food chain. It is more than interesting that pesticide use has increased some 3,300 percent since 1945, but crop loss due to insects has still increased some 20 percent over the same period. This should make it clear that the use of pesticides is not the answer. For additional information about the Food Quality Protection Act, see the website www.ecologic-ipm.com.

What About Our Safety?

Here's how the scenario goes. Synthetic fertilizers deplete the soil.

Pesticides incorporated into plants deplete nutrients. Other modern farming practices result in lower quality foods. There are fewer nutrient reserves in the individuals who eat these foods, which increases the chance for a weakened immune system. Now, the body is ripe for pathogenic bacteria to invade it.

Just because a pesticide is produced here in the U.S. doesn't mean it is safe, no matter what the government says. Pesticide residues were found in 48 percent of the most frequently consumed fruits and vegetables. Only 38 percent of the pesticides on the market have been tested for cancer-causing properties as required by law. Only 30 to 40 percent have been tested for birth defects, and fewer than 10 percent have been tested for their ability to cause genetic damage. And what about the safety of herbicides, genetically altered foods, and other toxic substances applied to crops and animals? Can we really trust the very companies that profit from these products to keep us safe?

We Are What We Eat

Our food choices have a high impact on the state of our health. The best health can only be achieved when we consume nutrient-dense whole foods free of harmful poisons. Nutrition and digestion are undeniably important. This belief must be fundamental to a person wanting to be healthy. We are what we eat, absorb, and assimilate. Excellent health is not possible otherwise.

A proper diet can have a near miraculous effect in most people who improve theirs. If you have done any gardening, you know that altering the conditions of the soil can optimize plant growth. Our intestines work in a similar way. If the terrain in the intestines is not optimized, the stage is set for the growth of bacteria that will promote illness. The most effective and least expensive approach involves using the diet to adjust the internal terrain. This will support the growth of the beneficial bacteria and suppress the growth of the harmful ones. I hope you will read my book, *Allergies and Holistic Healing*, for more information about healthful eating.

CHAPTER 15

Good Hygiene for Good Health

WITH SO MANY food scares in the news, it is understandable that people are concerned. Bacteria are impossible to avoid; they are nearly everywhere: in our food, every room in our house, everything we touch, the air we breathe. That doesn't mean we can't live with them. We just need to know where they are in the highest concentrations and how to protect ourselves from them. The highest levels of bacterial contamination are found in areas that remain damp, such as the kitchen sponge or dish-cloth, kitchen and bath sink drains, and the kitchen faucet handle. Bathroom countertops, bathroom floors, and toilet seats usually have the lowest bacterial levels.

Even a very clean house is teeming with bacteria, but the chances of contracting the really bad ones are actually pretty slim, if you take a few precautions. The best way to battle common germs is with regular hand washing, cleaning of surface areas, and safe food handling. Limit harmful bacterial by adopting a lifestyle of good habits and a constant awareness of how you interact with your environment.

When it comes to the food we eat, prevention should start on the farm, then in processing, distribution, and at the retail level. Unfortunately, most of the burden of making sure the food is handled and cooked properly is put on you, the consumer. Good hygiene needs to start at the source, but until that changes, there are a few strategies that will keep those nasty germs from making you sick.

Old-Time Cleansers

We now know that kitchen and bathroom surfaces in most homes show high levels of contamination that can lead to disease. Commercial household cleansers and soaps, now commonly spiked with antibacterial agents, do eliminate more germs than many of the natural products. They also increase our chances of breeding drug-resistant bacteria in our homes.

Ingredients in antibacterial soaps and cleansers intended to fight bacteria have the potential of creating "superbugs" that might otherwise be kept in check with little more than a vigorous scrub. Dousing everything with antibacterial agents and taking antibiotic medications at the first sign of a cold can upset the natural balance of microorganisms in and around us, leaving behind only the most powerful germs. Strong antibacterial cleaners are needed only when someone in a household is seriously ill or has low immunity.

The old time cleansers such as soap and hot water, alcohol, and hydrogen peroxide are sufficient for most purposes. Vinegar and baking soda still kills about 90 percent of the microbes. It is usually sufficient to use a dilute solution of bleach and water to wipe down counters and for soaking cutting boards. It may not sell products, but the above items can deal with most germs. Liquid soap is best because damp bars sit around and grow microbes. Do not use bathroom cleaners in the kitchen, because many contain chemicals that could be harmful if they get on your food.

What we do not know yet is whether disinfecting drains, handles and toilet seats would actually decrease infection rates among family members. It may be that more direct contact, such as touching, kissing, sneezing, and sharing food or eating utensils, plays a much bigger role in spreading infections.

How To Make A Food Wash & Disinfectant

As more foods are imported from underdeveloped countries, it is likely that bacteria contamination will find its way to your dinner table unless you take some precautions. It is important to wash your food prior to eating. Simply rinsing with water may not be enough. Adding a food-grade soap is not always available or effective, especially for sprouts and softer fruits and vegetables.

Soaking produce in a solution of grapefruit seed extract (GSE) and water will go a long way toward preventing foodborne illness. Depending on the strength of the grapefruit seed extract, add twenty to thirty drops of GSE to a quart size mister bottle filled with distilled water. You could also add drops of GSE to water in your sink. Follow the product's directions for a food wash. Soak your produce in the solution, then drain, rinse and dry. Using GSE extends the refrigerator life of many produce items.

GSE is ideal as a safe and simple way to disinfect drinking water when camping and backpacking. It is also practical in an emergency situation when safe drinking water is not obtainable and boiling is not possible. The available water should be filtered first. At the very least, let suspended particles settle to the bottom of the container. Retain the clear water and add twenty or more drops of GSE for each gallon of water. Shake well or stir vigorously and let sit for a few minutes. A slightly bitter taste may be noticed. This is the natural flavor of grapefruit seed extract. White vinegar can kill bacteria on vegetables intended for eating. Leave vegetables in a vinegar solution for fifteen minutes.

You can make your kitchen even a safer place without exposing yourself and your family to toxic chemicals that also damage the environment. You can use 3 percent hydrogen peroxide, the same strength available at the drug store for gargling or disinfecting wounds, and plain white or apple cider vinegar. You will also need a pair of clean sprayers. For cleaning produce, just spritz them with both the vinegar and the hydrogen peroxide, and then rinse them off under running water.

It doesn't make any difference which one you use first, but best results come from using one mist right after the other one. It is more effective to use both of these products than using either one by itself and more effective if you do not mix the vinegar and hydrogen peroxide in one sprayer. You should not get any lingering taste of vinegar or hydrogen peroxide, and neither is toxic to you if a small amount does remain on the produce. This protocol worked exceptionally well in sanitizing counters and other areas used to prepare foods, including wood cutting boards. They killed virtually all *Salmonella, Shigella,* or *E. coli* bacteria on heavily contaminated food and surfaces when used in this way (*Science News* 1998). There is additional information about washing food in my book, *The Parasite Menace.*

What About Those Sponges?

Do you wash your hands before handling the kitchen sponge, especially after going to the bathroom or changing the baby's diaper? Kitchen sponges can host many different bacteria. After an investigation of fifty sponges used for only three weeks, they were tested for coliform or fecal coliform bacteria (found in soil, water, or the intestinal tract).

All of these bacteria can cause illness in humans. At least 70 percent of the sponges had high levels of coliform bacteria and 38 percent showed high levels of fecal coliform bacteria. What the researchers discovered was that most of the bacteria found on the sponges came from food left on dirty dishes, especially raw foods such as meat or poultry, and even vegetables.

What can you do? Make sure your sponge is squeezed dry and free of food residue. It is also important to clean the sponge after using it to wash the dishes. Keep it away from the cutting board, especially where you cut up raw meats. Cutting boards are notorious for harboring bacteria. You may even think you are cleaning your cutting board when you are not. Instead, you are just moving the bacteria deeper into the board to grow and contaminate the next item put there. One way to clean your sponge is to put it in the dishwasher with the dishes. Hopefully, the hot water kills the bacteria. More effective ways are rinsing them in a 10 percent solution of chlorine bleach or putting them in the microwave at the high setting for five minutes. Replace the sponge about every ten days.

Toxic Laundry

J.P. Kilbourn, Ph.D., Director of Consulting Clinical and Microbiological Laboratory, Portland, Oregon, experimented with germs and washing. She washed contaminated towels in a washing machine either with cold water and detergent, or in hot water with detergent and bleach. Then she refrigerated the towels for a week. Bacteria were killed when using the hot water, detergent, and bleach method. After being washed in cold water and detergent, a few tiny bacterial colonies of Staphylococcus aureus were found, but not E. coli.

This experiment suggests that using cold water and detergent might be inhibiting the growth, but not killing some of the Staphylococcus aureus, while killing the E. coli. Take additional precautions when undergarments are mixed in the wash load. If you share a washing machine, wash the first load with bleach to kill any microbes left from previous washes. Household bleach does kill bacteria.

How Clean Are Those Restaurants?

The silverware and dinner plates in some restaurants are home to hazardous microbes. Investigators sometimes found the dinner plates more contaminated than the toilet seats and faucets. The microbes could harm immune compromised people and indicate poor hygiene practices among the staff. The best way to find a safe meal is to frequent facilities with clean floors, clean-appearing silverware, good lighting, and a tidy bathroom with soap in the dispenser and disposable paper towels. This at least indicates the appearance of good sanitation. Also, note the way the employees handle your eating utensils. Are they also the same people who handle money, which is known for harboring germs?

Improper Food Handling: Worth the Risk?

Do you ever sniff at a container of leftovers in the refrigerator to see if it is still safe to eat? What you see and smell may provide some clues to the food's safety, but how that food was handled and stored may be more important. Most people could use a class in food safety because they do not use caution when preparing and consuming their food. Taking just a little extra care with your food buying and preparation can greatly reduce your risks of getting ill.

A new government survey found that 25 percent of men and 14 percent of women did not wash their hands with soap after handling raw meat. Half of those surveyed said that they ate undercooked eggs during the previous year. This is a risk factor for *Salmonella enteritidis*. Despite recent publicity about *E. coli* contamination linked to undercooked hamburger meat, 20 percent of the people said they ate hamburgers without cooking them thoroughly. More men reported eating rare hamburgers compared to women. Men generally had riskier food safety behavior than women. Younger people took more risks than older folks did. People with higher incomes handled foods improperly more often than those with lower incomes. City residents were not as careful as rural residents were.

The first rule of the kitchen is to wash your hands before handling anything. This is to avoid contamination from the bacteria already present on your skin. The next most important rule for preventing food-borne contamination is to wash and scrub your fruit or vegetables carefully with a food wash, especially when eating them raw. Even without soap, a good rinse can rid food of most harmful organisms. It may not completely eliminate bacteria in the tiny crevices of berries, but it should decrease the risk if you have nothing else to use.

If the skin of the produce is broken that you plan to eat raw, toss it out or cook it. Microbes can crawl into the pulp beyond the reach of your scrubbing. After washing, refrigerate all cut or peeled fruits and vegetables, and do not mix them with other produce that remains unwashed. If you are unsure about a liquid preparation, briefly heat it and then rapidly cool it. This can kill most feces-associated bacteria and makes even contaminated drinks safe. If you buy raw cider at a roadside stand, you are really taking a chance if you drink it there. Take it home and boil it before drinking to insure its safety. When eating out at a party, or mass-prepared lunch, avoid any raw foods that do not look washed, been sitting out for more than two hours, or implicated in a current outbreak. Eating raw fruits and vegetables at home where you can wash and prepare them safely may be a better choice.

Cook meat until it is no longer pink in the middle and juices run clear. Use a meat thermometer to make sure that the middle of the meat has reached the correct temperature to kill bacteria. Use hot, soapy water to wash and scrub all cooking utensils, cutting boards, pots and pans, and countertops that have come in contact with raw meat and their juices. Wash and scrub your hands after handling raw meat to avoid contaminating other foods, products, countertops, and appliances, etc.

Do not forget to scrub under the fingernails. Personally, I just wear disposable gloves whenever I handle raw meat. The last thing to do before leaving the kitchen is to wash your hands again just in case you did get some microbes on them. This will keep you from transferring them to other objects in your house.

Taking Care With Fruits and Vegetables

It is recommended that we eat more fresh fruit and vegetables, and consumers have listened to the call. So it is not surprising that the number of outbreaks of foodborne disease related to fresh produce has nearly tripled since the 1970s. Foods as diverse as alfalfa sprouts, mangoes, orange juice, strawberries, and raspberries have been linked to outbreaks of bacterial and parasitic infections. So has the addition of convenience foods such as shredded lettuce. Just as we are learning about the benefits of fruits and vegetables, your gastrointestinal health may suffer severely for your efforts.

The list of disease-causing organisms in fruits and vegetables is almost as varied as our supply of fresh produce. Here are several ways to protect yourself and your family from *Salmonella* on the cantaloupe, *Shigella* in the parsley, and other pathogens. Before cutting open melons, rinse them in a food wash, and scrub their skins with a good food brush. Their rough skin can cause the transfer of pathogens from the rind to the flesh when you cut them open. Wash berries, lettuce (even if they have already been pre-washed), and other hard-to-scrub fruits and vegetables with fast-running water. You can also soak them in a grapefruit seed extract wash or other good food wash. Wash fruit even if you plan to peel it. If there are microbes on the peel, it can contaminate the rest of the fruit.

When In Doubt, Throw It Out

How long has that food been in the refrigerator? One of the worse things you can do is to leave food out at room temperature for any extended period before heating it up. Some people do this several times before eating all of the leftover food. This is a sure way to put yourself and your family at high risk of bacteria contamination and food poisoning. Here are some additional things you can do to insure your safety:

- Do not just wipe clean cooking utensils, pots, and pans, allowing bacteria remaining from contaminated food to contaminate the next food you place in them.
- Keep hot foods hot and cold foods cold.
- Heat leftovers thoroughly and refrigerate them promptly.
- Throw out any leftovers that have been sitting at room temperature more than two hours.
- Eat leftovers within two days or freeze it.
- Thaw frozen meats in the refrigerator, not at room temperature.

Do you still have some Thanksgiving turkey in your freezer? Pay attention to the age of leftover meat and fish to reduce the risk of food poisoning. Even frozen foods go bad eventually, just more slowly than the refrigerated edibles. Nonanimal foodstuffs can also make you sick. The life span of different foods vary so much that there is no fixed rule of thumb other than to toss out perishables that sit at room temperature for more than two hours. The Food Marketing Institute in Washington, D.C., publishes a booklet listing how long many foods will keep.

Even mayonnaise, if handled correctly, can weather a fairly long stint in the refrigerator. Mayonnaise is actually a very stable food and its high acid content actually deters the growth of bacteria. One of the biggest safety concerns is not refrigerator shelf life, but cross-contamination. This is when bacteria are transferred from one item to another. How often have you double-dipped a knife from your mayonnaise or favorite condiment to something else? To avoid cross-contamination use a clean utensil each time you dip. Do not put a utensil back into the same container, or even a different one, after using it to spread something on the luncheon meat, cheese, etc. You could also put a small amount in a bowl for use and not return it to the original bottle.

Here are some tips to consider:

- Know the differences between "sell by" and "use by" dates. The sell by date is determined by the manufacturer and tells the store how long to keep a product on the shelf. The "use by" date indicates when the manufacturer believes that the product is no longer at peak quality. To be on the safe side, do not use foods after the "use by" date.
- To guard against the pathogen *Listeria,* the U.S. Agriculture Department recommends that unopened luncheon meats sit in your refrigerator no longer than two weeks. Anyone with a compromised immune system would be wise to recook the meat before eating it.
- Mold develops an intricate root structure long before it appears at the surface of your food. If your mozzarella is turning green or your salsa is a little fuzzy, throw it out. You can cut away mold on hard cheeses such as cheddar and Parmesan, because they are too dense for the mold to penetrate far. Just be sure to make your cut at least one inch away from where the mold is.
- Set your refrigerator to 40°F. Refrigerate groceries promptly and remember these six simple words: When in doubt, throw it out.

Packaging Leftovers

Your holiday feast may leave you with leftover turkey and dressing, cranberry sauce, and pumpkin pie. Since many people have leftovers for days after holiday eating, it is good to know the right way to package the food. Put the leftovers in several small containers rather than one or two large ones. They will cool down quickly this way and reduce the risk of bacteria growth.

More Ways To Reduce Foodborne Illness

To minimize the risk of foodborne illnesses, start before the food reaches your kitchen. First, buy foods only from reliable sources. Once potentially harmful bacteria are present, dirty surfaces can promote their growth. Cutting boards that are used for raw foods, especially meat, can spread their germs to cooked foods or salads. To avoid this, use separate chopping boards for raw plant foods and cooked foods, and another one for raw meats. Clean boards thoroughly with hot soapy water and allow them to dry between uses. Periodically soak sponges and cutting boards in a bleach solution. Sponges and cutting boards made of plastic, glass, or solid wood, can be disinfected in chlorine bleach or put them in the dishwasher where the high temperatures kill most harmful bugs; put sponges in the microwave. Better yet, throw out sponges frequently.

A recent study discovered that even at chill temperatures typical of food storage, ten percent of the pathogen bacteria *E. coli* were still alive on stainless steel tiles after thirty-four days, whereas bacteria were completely eradicated on brass tiles within twelve days, and on copper tiles in just fourteen hours. It was found, for example, that in acidic environments representative of fruit juice processing, *E. coli* survived for as little as forty-five minutes on copper, versus two days on stainless steel.

In environments containing animal feces loaded with *E. coli,* copper and brass tiles were found to exhibit superior bactericidal effects when compared to stainless steel tiles. It may be possible to achieve important public health benefits just by changing the surface material commonly used in food processing. Stainless steel is the most widely used surface in food preparation, but this material appears to be a repository of microbial food contamination for very long periods. Plans are under consideration to investigate the antibacterial effect of copper and selected alloys on other toxic bacteria.

What About Swimming?

Here are some things you can do to reduce your chances of bacterial contamination when swimming in a lake. If you use goggles when you swim, do not fill them with lake water. This can increase your chance of eye infections. You do not have to drink the water for it to make you sick. A fast-flowing river can carry infectious organisms. In 1996, five Americans became ill with *Leptospirosis* after they whitewater rafted in Costa Rica.

If you begin to feel flu-like symptoms after swimming in a natural waterway, consult your doctor. You may have a waterborne disease. It is important to do your part. Do not go to the bathroom in or near the water, and always wash your hands with soap and water after using the toilet. Recently, in Oregon and Washington, there were a couple of outbreaks of *E. coli* at campgrounds. One occurred after people swam in a contaminated lake and the other one happened because of contaminated drinking water.

The Facial Wash

Your nasal passage is teeming with good bacteria that compete and help protect you from the more dangerous ones. Rubbing the eyes with unwashed hands introduces germs that travel down the tear duct and grow in the nasal passageway. A facial wash cleans and warms the nasal passageways, eyes, and the rest of your face. It should be done each morning using a safe water supply. Perform the facial wash in very warm water at approximately 100°F, using five to eight quarts of water.

During the facial wash open your eyes several times to cleanse the lens. Wash any debris from the eyes and eyelids and clean out the tear ducts. Always use a clean water basin and rinse with hot water first. In cases of infections, you may want to do the wash longer. About half the time, add one teaspoon of salt to the water. Wait about thirty seconds for the salt to dissolve before using.

Washing Your Hands Can Keep You Healthy

As discussed elsewhere, contaminated fingertips and fingernails transfer germs easily. This area accumulates dirt, makeup, oils, and microscopic pieces of skin, hair, mucus, saliva, sexual fluids, feces, and other body tissues. All this material combined with an enormous concentration of germs is self-inoculated constantly into the nose, eyes, mouth, ears, and skin. Fingernails also damage the tissues and reduce the number of germs required to cause an infection. This can stress and overload the strongest immune system in the healthiest person. Since the fingertips and nails are used extensively in sexual contact, make sure you and your partner both have clean hands and clean fingernails.

The fingernail region has the least natural disinfecting power of the skin. It is also the most difficult to clean and the most neglected. To wash your hands effectively, wet your hands and apply about a dime to a quarter-sized drop of liquid soap. Rub your hands together vigorously and lather for at least fifteen seconds. Be sure to scrub between your fingers and around the tops and palms of your hands. Do not forget the thumb. Use a nailbrush to scrub under the fingernails. Rinse under warm, running water. Wash this way at least four times each day.

Dry the hands with a clean, disposable, or single-use towel, being careful to avoid touching the faucet handles or towel holder with your clean hands. Turn off the faucet using the towel so your skin does not touch the faucet handle. Avoid touching door handles after your hands are clean. Use a paper towel to open the door, especially if you are in someone else's bathroom.

If you use hand lotion, use the kind you can squirt out of the bottle or tube, and do not touch the spout with your hand. This might inject bacteria onto that surface that will later grow and contaminate your clean hands. Teach your children to do the same. Regular hand washing is one of the best defenses against the spread of colds and gastrointestinal infections. Even though antibacterial agents have been added to many hand soaps and lotions, ordinary soap works just fine for everyday use. Do not forget to wash off your toothbrush, and occasionally disinfect it with bleach. It is best to keep your toothbrush covered. When you shower, lather all over the body, and then rinse. Use a clean cloth each time you shower or bathe.

Barbecuing? Start With A Clean Grill

Millions of Americans take out their grills in the summer to enjoy outdoor cooking. It is always best to scrub and wash the BBQ grill with hot soapy water before using it. Some people feel that this is not necessary. They believe the food particles just burn off, not causing any health hazards, but this is not true.

Be sure to use clean dishcloths and clean kitchen utensils, since bacteria are known to hang out on those items. Use disposable towelettes and paper towels for cleaning surfaces and hands. The sponge is one of the best ways to transfer bacteria to another surface. Grillers should carefully wash their hands before and after handling any food.

It is important to separate raw meats from other foods. Use separate cutting boards for raw meats, raw vegetables, and cooked foods, to prevent cross-contamination. Check the food with a meat thermometer to make sure that all meats, poultry, and fish are sufficiently cooked. The recommended cooking temperatures are between 145°F and 160°F for large cuts of meat, and 160°F for hamburgers. Cook skinless, boneless poultry breasts to an internal temperature of 160°F; bone-in breasts to 170°F; and drumsticks, thighs and legs to 180°F.

When people marinade food before throwing it on the grill, they increase the risk of bacterial contamination when they double dip. For example, you brush raw meat with the marinade, then dip the brush that touched the raw meat back into the bottle before marinating again. Pathogens such as *Salmonella*, *Listeria*, and *E. coli*, are often on the surface of meats. It would be better to just pour out the amount of marinade needed for that meal into a separate container and never pour what is left back into the original bottle. If you are in doubt as to whether the marinade has been contaminated or not, you can boil it first.

Summer Food Safety

If summer and picnic season have arrived, there are a few rules that will insure that foodborne bacteria don't leave you with a nasty case of food poisoning. Here are some safety tips:

- Wash your hands and work areas; be sure all utensils are clean before preparing your food.
- Make sure to wash your hands before eating. Use disposable moist towelettes in resealable bags.
- Keep perishable food cold, below 40°F. Make sure your ice chest or insulated cooler can stay this cold for the duration of your trip. Ice in blocks will keep longer than ice cubes. Some of the newer packs that are put in the freezer before using work very well.
- Foods cooked ahead of time need to be cooled thoroughly in the refrigerator before being packed in the cooler.
- Pack your food directly from the refrigerator to the cooler. Do not leave them out of refrigeration for any length of time.
- Pack foods in the reverse order of how you will eat them so you do not have to unpack your cooler each time you go looking for an item.
- Pack a full cooler. A full cooler stays cold longer than one that is only partially filled. If there is space in the cooler, fill it with more ice or nonperishable foods.
- Do not put the cooler in the trunk where it can heat up. Keep it inside the air-conditioned car.
- It would be better not to leave perishable foods out for over an hour, especially if the temperature is over 90°F.
- Leftover grilled foods and other perishable foods should be placed back in the cooler as soon as possible. Do not leave them outside for more than one hour, even in the shade.
- If there is ice left in the cooler when you get home and the food did not stay out for over an hour, the food is probably safe to put back into your refrigerator. It is a good idea to invest in a thermometer that you can put inside the cooler so that you actually know how cold your food is being kept.

If you are at the beach, plan to take some foods that don't require refrigeration. It is better to keep your perishables in a separate cooler from the drinks, since the drink cooler is opened more often. Put the cooler under your beach umbrella and out of the sun. You could cover it with a blanket for more insulation. Spray sun tan lotion or insect spray away from the food.

When you are hiking on the trail choose foods that do not require refrigeration, unless you are going only a short distance. They now make insulated coolers that look like daypacks. Always assume that water in lakes, ponds, and streams is not safe to drink. Bring purification tablets or filtering equipment that you can purchase from camping supply stores and learn how to use them effectively. Bring along bottled water if you can. Bring soap or disposable wipes to clean your hands and dishes. Wash dishes immediately after eating so bacteria do not have a chance to grow on them. Pack carefully so that you use your fresh foods first.

Keep Your Kids Healthy This School Year

Lax hygiene and parents who permit their children to attend school when they are sick are the main reasons that thousands of cases of colds and flu leapfrog from child to child each school year. Millions of school attendance days and adult workdays are lost each year when schoolchildren get ill. In addition, schoolchildren can get and give a host of other illnesses including bacterial infections such as strep throat, conjunctivitis (pinkeye), and impetigo. Sick children should stay home; a single child can easily infect ten others. One proven way to reduce this problem is basic hygiene. In one daycare study, kids caught fewer colds after they washed their hands regularly and the toys were disinfected three times a week.

Those who track infection among children say that the best way to give infectious organisms an express path into the body is by nose picking, eye rubbing, wedging fingers into the mouth, and putting objects into their mouth. Children are not careful about handling their secretions. Some germs that cause upper respiratory tract infections spread in the air when a child sneezes, releasing germ-laden droplets that can remain in the air for up to forty-five minutes. It is important to teach children to cover their mouth and nose with a tissue while coughing or sneezing and then to discard the tissue and wash their hands.

There are other ways to pick up germs: touching objects contaminated by other classmates, bringing germs home from school and giving them to other family members, and using public restrooms. The majority of the time bacteria and viruses are transferred from hand to hand, then hand to mouth, hand to eye, or hand to nose. It stands to reason that this is something to avoid.

With all the things that are important to learn in school, one of the most important is good hygiene, which certainly includes washing hands before eating and after using the restroom. Schools do not always provide enough paper towels or adequate soap for proper hand washing. Since regular hand washing is one of the best defenses against the spread of colds and gastrointestinal infections, your child may need to carry his or her own hand wipes or convenient size soap and disposable towelettes.

Avoid any raw food that does not look washed or any item that has been implicated in a current outbreak of food poisoning. Eating raw fruits and vegetables at home, where you can be certain they are washed, may be a better choice. If you are unsure about the drinks served, have your child carry their own water. Any meat that is eaten should be checked to see if it is cooked all the way through until it is no longer pink in the middle and juices run clear.

The best way to fight back against these germs is to enhance your child's immune system, the first line of defense against infection. It should be no secret that proper nutrition builds good immunity and plays a key role in fighting infections. Adequate nutrients are the backbone of health. Even marginal deficiencies of a single nutrient can profoundly impair the immune system. The least you should do is give your child a good quality multiple vitamin and mineral supplement every day.

Food is one of the biggest challenges facing the immune system. Eating too much sugar in the form of glucose, fructose, sucrose, or honey, significantly reduces the body's ability to have an effective immune system. These negative effects start within thirty minutes and last for several hours. The white blood cells will not have the ability to gobble up those nasty bacteria the way they usually do.

More than 50 percent of the immune system takes its signals from the digestive tract. It represents one of the largest immune organs of the body in order to defend against the barrage of toxins and extraneous materials ingested daily. Intestinal microflora also impact human health. "Friendly" bacteria living in us compete with the "not so friendly" germs and help us stay healthy. When there is complete digestion, healthy bowel microflora, a healthy constitution, and minimal exposure to toxic foods and a toxic environment, all goes well.

The new U.S. Food Pyramid suggests we consume five servings of fresh vegetables daily and three to four servings of fresh fruits daily. Sounds easy enough, doesn't it? Yet, only 20 percent of the population do this. It is also important to get adequate protein and fat in the diet. How much quality water is your child drinking each day? Dehydration may be a big factor in whether they stay healthy or not. Are your children eating food and drinking beverages that contain pesticides, preservatives, and other chemicals that depress the immune system? Then it should be no surprise if they often get sick. If you make some changes in your child's diet and lifestyle, you might be amazed at how few illnesses they get this school year.

CHAPTER 16

Probiotics: Using Friendly Bacteria To Beat Chronic Infections

ALMOST ONE HUNDRED years ago, Nobel Prize Winner Elie Metchnikoff wrote *The New Hygiene*, speculating about the importance of the intestine as an entrance for infection and the role of bacterial balance in human health. After all this time, health-minded people are finally incorporating this idea of fighting bacteria with bacteria. Increasingly, probiotic therapies are becoming an alternative to antibiotics. They are one strategy for combating the increase in resistant strains of bacteria. Hopefully, this will become standard medical practice.

Antibiotics tend to kill both the good and bad bacteria indiscriminately. The word *antibiotic* means "anti-life." Often Western medicine's emphasis is on destroying the harmful bacteria, not replenishing the beneficial ones. One of the best and least emphasized methods you can use to protect yourself is to promote the growth of beneficial bacteria in your intestinal tract. Taking these friendly bacteria can lower your dependence upon antibiotic use. They are as important as any other supplement used to improve health. In fact, they may be more important.

The relationship between humans and beneficial bacteria has a long history. Even at the turn of the century, yogurt was considered the elixir of life, because it contained beneficial bacteria that limited the growth of harmful bacteria in the intestines. Not having enough of these beneficial bacteria was believed to shorten life. For years these claims were considered unscientific and just folklore. We now know for a fact that *Lactobacilli* play a significant role in human health. These bacteria found in some fermented foods have been of great importance to the diets of people all around the world. Most cultures have some form of fermented food such as kefir, yogurt, or miso.

What is a Probiotic?

The word probiotic means "pro-life." Probiotics are beneficial, naturally occurring bacteria residing in the mouth, digestive, and vaginal tract, which positively influence human health. One of the most successful approaches to treating diseases of the intestinal tract is to use these beneficial living organisms for the treatment of various types of health problems. There should be a balance of about 85 percent beneficial bacteria to about 15 percent harmful organisms in the intestinal tract. Today, those numbers are more likely to be reversed. There are many illnesses due to harmful intestinal bacteria dispersing their toxins throughout the body.

Probiotics restore the healthy intestinal microflora normally depleted by the use of antibiotics and from years of poor eating habits and lifestyle. The proper kinds of intestinal bacteria are essential for a strong immune system. You need them to aid in the assimilation of vitamins, proteins, fats, and carbohydrates. They break down dietary fiber and mucus, yielding energy from the fermentation of these substances. Fermentation makes protein more available. It also produces a mixture of desirable enzymes not present in the original residue such as vitamins B12 and K.

Other Benefits of Probiotics

Your intestinal tract is teeming with life, some good, and some not so good. There is a constant battle for healthful bacteria to keep the harmful ones in check, creating a healthy balance that contributes to your overall well-being. Disruption of this balance is frequently the underlying cause of constipation, diarrhea, and other digestive disturbances.

Lactobacillus acidophilus and bifidobacteria occur naturally in the human intestine. It is important to have a sufficient amount of them present in the stool, as well as the presence of human *E. coli*. The first two are noted for their contributions to intestinal health by increasing the body's natural antibiotic production, detoxification of cancer-causing substances, as well as controlling intestinal pH.

In a healthy digestive tract, beneficial organisms make up a substantial portion of the more than four hundred species of bacteria found there. Bifidobacteria comprise up to one-fourth of the total bowel microflora in a healthy adult. Reduced numbers of these beneficial organisms leave the intestine susceptible to invasion by pathogens.

They also help in the synthesis of vitamins, and the production of enzymes, and to reduce cholesterol. They degrade toxins, prevent colonization of pathogens, and stimulate a normal immune response. Maintaining a healthy level of these friendly organisms is important for the well being of the digestive system, and the well being of the entire body. Think of them as your body's recycling machine. While human *E. coli* does not share some of these direct beneficial effects, it usually does no harm, and ample amounts of this organism are present in healthy intestines.

Lactobacillus acidophilus and bifidobacteria also help maintain the proper population balance between the different forms of microorganisms in the intestine. They do this by producing organic acids that reduce intestinal pH and inhibit the growth of acid-sensitive, undesirable bacteria. They have the capacity to secrete numerous substances, including a wide range of natural antibiotics that kill pathogenic bacteria, viruses, and yeast. The bacteria they inhibit include some species of *Bacillus, Salmonella,* or *Vibrio* as well as *Clostridium perfringens, Escherichia coli, Klebsiella pneumoniae, Proteus vulgaris, Pseudomonas aeruginosa, Shigella, Staphylococcus aureus* and *S. fecalis.*

In the intestinal tract and vagina the beneficial bacteria have the ability to use defense strategies against those bacteria that can harm us. Some release powerful chemicals that stunt the growth of potential pathogens. Others have strategic positions in the inner lining, preventing harmful microorganisms from gaining a foothold. Still others knock loose pathogens that have already fastened themselves to the surface of tissues.

Various strains of *Lactobacillus* are critical for maintaining a healthy ecosystem in the vagina. They also have the ability to block infectious microorganisms that can cause urinary tract infections. They have been known to block the growth of these pathogens by as much as 74 percent. These protective bacteria are most effective against *Pseudomonas aeruginosa* and *Klebsiella pneumoniae.* Pathogens can only cause trouble when they are able to attach themselves to the tissues and when our defense system is defective. The defense strategy of the helpful *Lactobacilli* seems to adapt to the body's immediate needs.

An article in the *Journal of Pediatric Gastroenterology and Nutrition* (1998) emphasizes the importance of balancing the diverse range of microbes in the gastrointestinal tract. In children with inflammatory bowel disorders. this will prove effective prevention and treatment of conditions such as diarrhea, irritable bowel syndrome, and inflammatory disorders. The article explains how these "good" bacteria can displace potential pathogens in the intestine such as *Helicobacter pylori*, the trigger for ulcers and gastritis. The article also confirms that beneficial microbes can secrete natural substances that deter the growth of harm-

How Many Bacteria Live In Us?

The stool and digestive tract of healthy human beings contains more bacteria than there are human cells in the body. Twenty species of bacteria comprise 75 percent of the total number of colonies. Anaerobes (bacteria that do not live in oxygen) predominate over aerobes (bacteria that need oxygen) by a ratio of 5,000 to 1. Organisms cultured from the surfaces of intestinal tissues are significantly different from those found in stool. They also vary in different parts of the gastrointestinal tract. There are fewer bacteria in the stomach and first part of the small intestine than in the colon.

ful bacteria, lower the pH in the colon, take away nutrients from pathogens, and stimulate immune antibodies against viruses.

New research suggests that giving near-term pregnant women and newborns doses of beneficial bacteria may prevent childhood allergies and asthma. There is now evidence that harmless bacteria can train an infant's immune system to resist allergic reactions. Researchers in Finland used a type of bacteria found naturally in the gut called *Lactobacillus rhamnosus*. This bacteria is safe to take at an early age and has been effective in the treatment of allergic inflammation and food allergies.

This hypothesis holds that the worldwide growth in allergic disease or asthma is in part due to our increasingly sterile surroundings. When babies are exposed to germs early in life, it is thought that their immune systems are guided to an infection-fighting mode and away from the tendency to overreact to normally benign substances. Support for this idea comes from studies showing that infants who have more colds and other infections have lower asthma rates later in life.

The measurement of beneficial bacteria levels is available from specialty laboratories and may indicate the need to supplement. To correct any bowel microflora deficiency, take a preparation containing strains of *Lactobacillus acidophilus* and bifidobacteria in a dose of at least five billion units per day. It is best to supplement with a strain that has the ability to colonize in humans. Many are dairy strains and will not colonize once the product is stopped.

What Special Property Do Beneficial Bacteria Have?

Beneficial colon bacteria have the ability to take soluble fibers and convert them to short chain fatty acids (SCFA). These fatty acids supply the majority of the energy needed for healthy colon cells and play an important part in establishing and maintaining a balanced ecosystem in the colon. SCFA may also prevent pathogens, such as *Salmonella* and *Shigella* species, from establishing themselves in the gut. When there are elevated levels of SCFA, it usually reflects colon malabsorption, bacterial overgrowth, and active colitis.

According to an issue of the journal *Science* (2001), colonization by some gut bacteria, such as *Bacteroides thetaiotaomicron,* can influence intestinal function by altering human gene expression. This and other commensal (nondisease-causing) bacteria can change the expression of genes involved in several important intestinal functions, including the absorption of nutrients, protecting tissues, postnatal intestinal maturation, and the metabolism of toxins.

They can also affect changes in the composition of indigenous microflora. By identifying which human genes are manipulated by microbes and how, we may gain new appreciation of their influence on our health. The wide scope of functions provided by microbes in the gut suggests the need to carefully examine the consequences of manipulating this flora, both in early postnatal development and during adulthood.

What Disrupts the Body's Intestinal Tract?

Now we know that the intestines are home to a wide range of life forms. They need to live in harmony with our body tissues and with each other. If conditions are unsuitable because of antibiotic treatment or poor diet, they get out of balance. Many antibiotics kill harmless and beneficial bacteria, as well as the pathogens they are meant to destroy. Consuming too much alcohol, caffeine, sugar, junk food, and many drugs (both legal and illegal) can have negative effects on your intestinal microflora.

Low levels of stomach acid create conditions favorable to the overgrowth of unhealthy organisms in the intestines. It can also occur as a result of a parasite or bacterial infection, yeast overgrowth, or maldigestion. The imbalance can be profound and lead to chronic illness and diseases, as well as gastrointestinal disturbances. Often, because doctors do not know what is really going on, they just call this condition "irritable bowel syndrome" and try to stop the symptoms with prescription drugs.

What Type of Diet Is Best for Friendly Bacteria?

When the diet is healthy and adequately supplied with unrefined carbohydrates and fiber, the stools flourish with about 85 percent of the microbes being beneficial ones. When the ecology of the gut reflects this balance, the production of toxins in the colon is almost completely eliminated. In experiments on animals changing the diet from pure protein to pure unrefined carbohydrate sources and back again to protein, created a tendency for the bowel microflora to become uniform, crowding out undesirable bacteria. Lengthy exposures to either pure protein or pure carbohydrates can cause problems. This type of diet is recommended in books on proper food combinations such as in *Fit for Life*.

Taking Probiotics After Antibiotics

It is difficult to prevent the destruction of healthful intestinal bacteria when it is necessary to take antibiotics. That is because antibiotics do not distinguish between the good and the bad microorganisms. This creates the ideal breeding ground for antibiotic-resistant pathogens to reproduce, since they are left alive and face little competition. Every antibiotic given by mouth causes alterations in the intestinal microflora. It seems reasonable that the first step during and after taking antibiotics is to reestablish the intestinal microflora balance with a probiotic as soon as possible.

Take probiotics for at least a month after any antibiotic treatment. Since there are also antibiotics and toxic chemicals present in most nonorganic foods and unfiltered drinking water, it is probably a good idea to take these beneficial bacteria every day. A probiotic supplement is very important. It is also critical to realize that a poor diet will neutralize the benefits of most probiotic supplements. Rid your diet of as many sweets and junk foods as possible. It is one of the single most important things you can do to stay healthy.

Vaginal Yeast Infections

Lactobacillus strains are normal constituents of the vaginal microflora, where they contribute to the maintenance of the acid pH, block the attachment of pathogens to the vaginal lining, and are able to excrete substances that inhibit the multiplication of pathogens. Broad-spectrum antibiotics suppress this ability and often lead to the overgrowth of yeast and other harmful microbes. Douching or using suppositories with *Lactobacilli* inhibits many yeast reinfections. Eating live culture yogurt has been a folk remedy for most forms of vaginitis. Other cultured dairy products show similar effects, probably due to the presence of lactose, which favors the growth of *Lactobacilli*. It is important to use products that contain minimal sugar, since many forms of sugar appear to increase the incidence of vaginal yeast infections and promote intestinal yeast.

The Link Between Probiotics and the Immune System

It has been known for a long time that the "good" bacteria can overtake the "bad" bacteria within the intestinal tract. These beneficial bacteria in the bowel enhance your immune system by increasing the production of immunoglobulin A (IgA), which functions as your body's natural defense. Since you are constantly going to be exposed to new and more virulent forms of pathogens, it makes sense to strengthen your immune system by enhancing the beneficial microflora in your intestinal tract.

Take Care When Choosing a Probiotic Product

One of the problems with probiotics is that they sometimes fail to live up to their expectations and promises. Some of them only create a temporary re-colonization, but cannot reproduce after being exposed to gastric acid when taken orally. Others may not have the ability to colonize once the product has been discontinued. A probiotic needs to be hardy enough to survive gastric acid and then to replicate so that they can repopulate the intestinal tract. Many of them are not able to do this.

In 1999, a disturbing and revealing article appeared in the medical literature. It said that none of the *Lactobacillus* species commercially available today are capable of creating permanent, self-sustaining colonies in the human gastrointestinal tract. They said that even if the strains tested were able to survive stomach acid exposure, none could be recovered from stool cultures just ten days after last taking the supplement. This is not good news. This means that taking probiotics may only benefit you while you are taking them. Once you stop, they are unable to sustain themselves and provide long-term benefits.

Many people think that they can just eat yogurt and that will supply the necessary beneficial bacteria. Raw or unpasteurized yogurt is loaded with bacteria, but most commercial yogurt is pasteurized, a process that kills bacteria. Though a few investigators have found promise in pasteurized yogurt with live bacteria added, most research has focused on capsules containing specific strains of bacteria. If a probiotic is not capable of colonizing the intestinal tract, it cannot influence human health once the product is stopped. This requirement disqualifies many of the strains currently used in fermented dairy products.

Having studied fifty-five probiotic products, Belgian biologists conclude that not every product that claims to be probiotic actually contains the bacteria associated with this claim. In many cases the researchers found bacteria other than those named on the label. The researchers studied the microflora of twenty-five dairy products and thirty powdered products that are used as nutritional supplements. More than a third of the powdered products contained no living bacteria. They found that only thirteen percent of the products contained all bacteria types included on the label. In one third of all the products the researchers found other bacteria not listed on the label. However, these could be classified as harmless. This research will be published in the *International Journal of Food Microbiology.*

Which Bacteria Should You Take?

Various *Lactobacillus* species are used commercially, but the most common ones are *Lactobacillus acidophilus* and *Lactobacillus bifidus*, sometimes called bifidobacteria. They are first introduced during the birth process to the sterile gut of the infant. Later, other bacteria become established in the gut through contact with the world. They include such beneficial strains as *Lactobacillus casea, L. fermentum, L. salivores,* and *L. brevis.*

The Probiotic "Die-Off"

Some people experience a "die-off" reaction from taking probiotics. This is often the result of killing off the more harmful organisms. Your symptoms appear to get worse for a few days. You may even feel that you are coming down with a cold or the flu. The more toxic you are, the more likely you will experience a die-off. Usually these symptoms are temporary and transient. If you are really uncomfortable, you will need to reduce the dosage or stop the probiotic. When you start taking the probiotic again, build back up slowly to the recommended therapeutic dose.

There are several things you can do to enhance the survival of beneficial bacteria in the intestinal tract:

- Select products that have been enteric coated or micro-encapsulated so that they are resistant to both gastric acid and bile in order to be released directly into the colon.
- If you have lower-than-normal levels of stomach acid, you may be able to dilute it even further by drinking several glasses of nonchlorinated and nonfluoridated filtered water at the same time you take the probiotic. This will allow the acid-sensitive bacteria to pass through unharmed. It is important to deliver bacteria safely past this acid barrier and directly into the small intestine. This will not be successful unless a special bile-tolerant strain of *Lactobacillus* is selected. Bile is the second defense after stomach acid designed by Mother Nature to protect us from foreign invading pathogens.
- Bypass the route through the digestive tract entirely and get the bacteria into the colon rectally as a retention implant.
- One strain of *Lactobacillus acidophilus* reproduces after exposure to bile and is now available. It is the NCFM strain, named for the University of North Carolina Food Microbiology Department, where it was developed. It has the unique capacity to adhere to the surface cells in the intestines. Adherence is the first necessary step towards reimplantation and eventual recolonization.

It is an advantage to obtain this formula when it has been grown on lactose (milk sugar), since lactose is the natural substrate for the NCFM strain. Traces of calcium in the substrate act as a glue to assist adherence. Unless the bacteria are able to adhere, the moving force of the fecal stream carries them away before they can multiply and become established. The NCFM strain is a human strain of probiotic and this is an important advantage. However, in the beginning you may need to take a dairy-free form, especially if you are intolerant to milk-based products. In time, the bacteria themselves can usually produce enough enzymes to digest lactose. Then you may be able to tolerate the NCFM strain that includes dairy.

If the label does not clearly state that it is a human strain, then assume it is a dairy strain instead. Many of the probiotic products on the market today are dairy strains because these strains are relatively cheap to produce. However, the dairy strains do not do well when exposed to gastric acid or to bile. Few survive, and those that do may not produce enough survivors to sustain colonies in the intestines. That means that within a short time after you quit taking these bacteria, they will not be present in your intestinal tract. The strains of lactobacilli derived from sourdough bread, or from other fermented grains, excel for their ability to grow after exposure to bile. Unfortunately, none of these strains are available on the U.S. market at the moment. Your best bet is the NCFM strain.

In a recent issue of *Journal of Infectious Diseases*, the authors described seven strains of probiotics as having "sufficiently substantial data published on their properties that are required of an antipathogen probiotic." They are *Lactobacillus reuteri, Lactobacillus rhamnosus GG, Lactobacillus acidophilus NCFM, Lactobacillus casei (Shirota), Lactobacillus casei CRL-431, Lactobacillus rhamnosus GR-1,* and *Lactobacillus fermentum RC-14.*

All strains of the *Lactobacillus* bacteria are destroyed at high temperatures, such as you might find inside delivery trucks during hot weather. Be sure that your source can assure you that it was shipped under refrigeration or at a low enough temperature that the bacteria survived. It is important to know how the product was handled up to the time it reached you. Otherwise, you are taking a chance of buying a product that will not do you much good.

When using multiple beneficial organisms in the same product, you run the risk that they inhibit each other more than they inhibit pathogens. It is important to find out if this product was developed with compatible organisms. Otherwise, it is best to take the fewest organisms possible.

Bulk powders are a good buy economically, but keep moisture out of the jar by using a clean dry spoon each time. The capsule form is more expensive, but it is easier to protect from moisture and convenient to carry with you for use away from home. Avoid probiotics that come in compressed tablets because the mechanical process of compression damages the fragile living bacteria. Ignore claims of a higher cell count on tablets because manufacturers count even fragments of bacteria that are no longer viable.

Always read the label of a probiotic carefully. It is best if the manufacturer guarantees potency until a given expiration date, not just at the time of manufacture. Probiotics sold as refrigerated products retain their original potency longer than those do that are not refrigerated. Usually, you can carry them for a short time without refrigeration as long as the temperature is less than 70°F. Do not leave probiotics in a hot automobile in the summertime, because temperature can rise above 100° F quickly. Put them in a container with an ice pack if you think the temperature will get too hot.

Before attempting to re-innoculate the bowel with a massive dose of any form of probiotic, take the extra precaution of testing yourself. Do this by gradually increasing the dosage over the period of a few days to weeks (depending on how sensitive you are). It is important to be sure that the probiotic will agree with you before proceeding to higher doses.

Tested Products

There are many probiotic products on the market in the United States, but only a few commercially available agents have actually been tested in placebo-controlled, double blind studies. These are *Lactobacillus rhamnosus GG, Saccharomyces boulardii, Lactobacillus acidophilus, Lactobacillus bulgaricus,* and *Lactobacillus reuteri.* This is not to say that other probiotic products might not be effective; there have simply been no well-controlled studies.

How Should You Take Probiotics?

Usually, you should take a probiotic on an empty stomach at least thirty minutes before or two to three hours after eating, so that the gastric acid secretions are at their lowest. Do not take probiotics with chlorinated water. Many people forget that chlorine was put into the drinking water to kill bacteria. Probiotics are still bacteria, even if they are good ones. For best results, follow the directions on the label of whatever brand you are using. Each manufacturer knows its product best. You cannot just rely on yogurt with added acidophilus for your "friendly bacteria" because it probably contains bovine growth hormone as well as residues of many antibiotics, unless you buy an organic brand. Also, *L. acidophilus* mainly grows in the small intestine and beneficial bacteria, such as *L. bifidus,* are also needed for the large intestine.

HOW MUCH AND HOW LONG?

There are not really any clear-cut answers. Some people require extremely large and persistent probiotics to establish enough organisms in the stools. In cases of acute food poisoning the best solution is large doses of good quality beneficial bacteria taken every hour until you feel better. This usually works within hours. If you are taking a human strain, it will usually maintain a self-producing colony after about three weeks. Ten standard capsules per day for one week seems to be the minimum required dose for initiating reimplantation. Not everyone can tolerate these high doses of beneficial bacteria without consequences (die-off). At first, you may need to work up to such a high dose of probiotic. Eventually, a reduced maintenance dose should work fine.

During this time, it is best to also clean up your diet by avoiding junk food, eating more fiber, and emphasizing unprocessed carbohydrates. If you eat out often, consider that most nonorganic meats contain antibiotics. Many foods also contain substances (preservatives, pesticides, genetically engineered, etc.) that will keep your bowel microflora imbalanced. If you eat out often, you would be wise to take a probiotic every day.

The dosage of a commercial probiotic supplement is based upon the number of live organisms it contains. The ingestion of one to ten billion viable organisms daily is a sufficient dosage for most people. Current data seems to indicate a range of ten to one hundred billion live organisms as being best for a variety of health conditions. Amounts exceeding this may produce mild gastrointestinal disturbances while smaller amounts may not be able to colonize the intestines.

We have learned that low-dose commonly used probiotics such as *Lactobacillus acidophilus* and *L. bifidus* can work just fine for a general maintenance program. A much higher dose of a different bacteria may be required to achieved success initially. It is becoming apparent that strains such as *Lactobacillus rhamnosus* or *Lactobacillus plantarum* can have dramatic effects. Multiple strains may be beneficial for a specific condition and play an important role.

If the clinical effect begins to change, it might be time to change the probiotic supplement for a period of time, followed by a repeat application. Sometimes it is best to withdraw all probiotics for a time, substitute with another product that contains different organisms, or to use higher doses. This probiotic rotation will be useful in a variety of situations.

It is important to follow up with stool cultures several months later after supplementation has stopped. This will show whether or not you have achieved self-sustaining colonies. You may need to consult with a health professional that has access to laboratories that specialize in detecting these beneficial bacteria in the intestinal tract.

Are Probiotics Safe?

Probiotics are very safe and effective for a wide variety of disturbances including antibiotic side effects, diarrhea/constipation, lactose malabsorption, and cholesterol reduction. Dosages ranging from one to almost five hundred billion organisms have been used without complications.

The available probiotic microorganisms are considered nonpathogenic, but even benign microorganisms can be infective when a patient is severely debilitated or their immune system is suppressed. To date, there have been only isolated reports linking probiotics with adverse effects. There is a theoretical risk of transfer of antimicrobial resistance from the probiotic to other microorganisms with which it might come in contact, but this has not yet been observed during therapy. The use of probiotics must be carefully considered when these "living drugs" are used therapeutically in people at high risk for opportunistic infections or when the gastrointestinal tract is badly damaged.

Probiotics are probably safe enough for most people. One of the problems with megadosing is that it can produce D-lactic acidosis, which is a condition of low acid pH in the bowels. A person with diarrhea is more at risk than someone with constipation, because diarrhea is often associated with low pH. Most physicians are not familiar with this condition, and may not realize that the probiotic is causing the acidosis. D-lactic acidosis must be measured by means of a special enzyme assay. Since it is an expensive test, few labs are equipped to perform it.

Another concern is the possibility of contamination by some unidentified species in the mixture, such as *Enterococcus faecium*. This hardy species may cause additional health problems for some people who already have a compromised immune system. Contaminants might not be listed on the label. Check with the manufacturer to see if each batch is assayed for all the common contaminants, especially if the probiotic seems to be causing adverse symptoms.

Occasionally, some people have an overgrowth of "good" bacteria. In most cases this only occurs to people taking megadoses of probiotics. Their thinking is that if the recommended dose is good for them, a whole lot more would be even better. They begin having what first appears to be a relapse with some of their old symptoms returning, but lab tests do not reveal any noted pathogens overgrowing in their intestinal tract. I usually give them calcium D-glucarate and quercetin. Calcium D-glucarate has the ability to bind up toxins coming from bacteria. Quercetin can aid in allergic type reactions, especially involving food and other bacterial toxins. Taking these products along with stopping the probiotic will reduce their symptoms quickly.

Probiotics Won't Solve Every Health Problem

There are some health conditions that cannot be fixed by any amount of probiotic therapy. It seems that about 80 percent of dead teeth harbor anaerobic bacteria that are a constant source of toxins to the body. The only solution is to remove the source of infection. Other chronic conditions that cannot be treated by probiotics alone are blood-borne infections caused by intracellular bacteria.

What is FOS?

FOS stands for fructo-oligo-saccharide and is included in many probiotic products. This sugar is not absorbed by the body and in most cases is thought to improve the microflora in the intestinal ecosystem. It not only feeds the "good bacteria," but it may also feed some "bad" bacteria, such as *Klebsiella*. People who harbor *Klebsiella* should avoid FOS. There are indications that the yeast *Candida* is also able to grow on FOS in some situations.

Why Have Follow-Up Tests?

Follow-up stool cultures are helpful to monitor progress. The goal is to achieve self-sustaining colonies of beneficial bacteria. This means that the probiotic you have been taking needs to reproduce on their own. You should not stop probiotics until these beneficial bacteria can be found at normal levels in at least two or more consecutive stool cultures. *Lactobacillus acidophilus* and *L. bifidus* should continue to show up in stool cultures long after you have stopped taking them. To be sure you could test the stool approximately six to eight weeks after probiotic replacement therapy has stopped and again at six months. Only certain labs will be able to perform these tests.

When Does The Need For Bacterial Balance Start?

For premature infants, it starts very early. Having enough beneficial bacteria in the intestines can make the difference between life and death in their encounter with dangerous gastrointestinal diseases. This may help explain why breast-fed infants do better in general than babies fed formula in a bottle. Unfortunately, premature infants are kept in the hospital, often for weeks or months, where they are not breastfed nor given any probiotics.

In other researchers, researchers found that bifidobacteria drastically reduced the number of toxins produced by harmful bacteria migrating across the intestinal barrier into the bloodstream. Probiotics also decreased inflammatory response linked to gastrointestinal distress. Taking these beneficial organisms play a central role in protecting gastrointestinal and systemic health.

Probiotic Use When Traveling

If you happen to be traveling here or in a foreign country, it is always wise to bring along a high quality probiotic and take it a few times a day to prevent any intestinal infections. If you do develop an infection overseas or even from eating at your local restaurant, taking the probiotic every thirty to sixty minutes usually resolves the problem in a few hours. Even though probiotics should be refrigerated if you want maximum potency, you can find some that can be kept at room temperature or even at higher temperatures for a few weeks. If you do have access to refrigeration, then use it.

Beneficial Probiotics

BACILLUS COAGULANS

This is a hardy species that helps to lower the pH of the fecal stream. The acidic pH that it creates helps the other resident bacteria to colonize better. *Bacillus coagulans* is a transient organism and does not colonize the intestinal tract.

BACILLUS LATEROSPORUS

This bacterium is considered nonpathogenic to humans and produces unique metabolites with antibiotic, antitumor, and immune enhancing activities. This organism is now available in the United States. It seems to be an effective addition for control of symptoms associated in some people with small bowel imbalances.

BIFIDOBACTERIA OR LACTOBACILLUS BIFIDUS

The presence of adequate bifidobacteria in the colon has been associated with health and longevity. Bifidobacteria, also called *Lactobacillus bifidus*, is found abundantly in the intestines, especially the large intestine. They are normally the first microflora to colonize the human intestinal tract, appearing as early as the second day of life. In the intestines of breastfed infants, these beneficial bacteria account for more than 95 percent of the microflora. This is why breast-fed babies usually do better than formula-fed infants.

Adolescents and adults have fewer numbers, but bifidobacteria still remains the single most common probiotic group in the intestines. As the body ages, or because of illness, bifidobacteria are depleted. This is why supplementing may be important to a healthy body.

Bifidobacteria prevent pathogenic bacteria and yeast from flourishing in the intestines. Researchers found that adequate amounts of bifidobacteria drastically reduced the number of toxins produced by harmful bacteria migrating across the intestinal barrier into the bloodstream. They also blocked inflammation linked to gastrointestinal distress. This bacterium, and other *Lactobacilli*, does not cause problems the way harmful bacteria can. The end result is a reduction in infection and overgrowth of pathogen bacteria and a healthier microflora environment.

Bifidobacteria produce lactic acid the same way that *Lactobacillus acidophilus* does, but they also produce acetic acid. Acetic acid, which is also found in vinegar, is important because it helps to break the adherence bonds of unfriendly microbes. If pathogens cannot adhere to the intestinal lining they cannot cause disease. This allows these friendly bacteria to attach themselves instead so that they can recolonize the gut. *Bifidus longum* is an adult strain; *Bifidus bifidum* is the strain given to infants and small children.

This organism helps us produce vitamins B and K. It assists our macrophages in digesting the toxic by-products of bacteria. They also help to control allergic reactions from undigested foods. Yeast infections are inhibited by the addition of bifidobacteria to the diet. They also have the capacity to produce some enzymes and take up iron from the intestines helping to buffer against iron overload. They have the ability to use attachment sites in the intestine that otherwise could be occupied by pathogens. Some of the undesirable organisms that bifidobacteria help to protect against are the yeast *Candida albicans* and pathogenic *E. coli, Salmonella, Shigella, Clostridium* and *Enterobacter spp.*

Too much of the wrong kinds of fat in your diet cause a series of reactions that end up inhibiting bifidobacteria. Their growth in the colon is also altered by factors in the diet such as indigestible carbohydrates. There are some substances that are likely to harm bifidobacteria more than other microflora residents. These include alcohol, caffeine, and drugs. Their numbers can be decreased by ill health and advancing age. Because a large part of the human population is sensitive to dairy products, it is best to start supplementing with a dairy-free product.

ENTEROCOCCUS FAECIUM

See *Streptococcus faecium* for more information.

HOMEOSTATIC SOIL ORGANISMS (HSO)

Humans used to eat food that came from soil rich in bacteria, mostly beneficial bacteria. After World War II, it became popular to kill disease-causing pathogens with chemicals and pesticides and to put chlorine in the drinking water systems. Not just harmful bacteria were killed, but many of the beneficial bacteria as well. Since we do not acquire the beneficial bacteria from the soil as we did in the past, it may be important to supplement them.

The use of HSO is intended to improve the intestinal terrain. They encourage the return of the slower growing, beneficial, resident organisms that have become depressed because of hardier and more aggressive pathogenic species. These soil-based organisms are a recent innovation among the probiotic supplements. These are not permanent resident organisms of the gastrointestinal tract, but temporary transients only.

When these soil organisms are ingested, they end up in the intestinal tract where they reproduce to form colonies that attach to the intestinal wall. After they establish themselves in the colon, HSOs multiply into larger colonies. They are very hardy and will grow where many of the beneficial organisms cannot. They can even grow where there are overgrowths of yeast, parasites, or harmful bacteria.

HSOs produce many chemicals to assist in fighting invading organisms and diseases. One of them is alpha-interferon, the key to fighting viruses such as herpes, hepatitis, and influenza. HSOs do not just eradicate harmful organisms. They change the environment by taking over receptor sites so harmful organisms cannot establish themselves again. This allows the immune system to save its strength for more urgent needs.

The putrefaction of food in the intestinal tract is the perfect place for parasites, yeast, and other germs to live and thrive. These HSOs can burrow behind the rubbery substance that has become attached to the intestinal walls and dislodge it. They can actually eat this putrefied substance off the walls and prevent its re-establishment. As the HSOs increase in number, they change the colon's pH. This begins the changes that lead to balancing the intestinal tract and the entire body.

The small intestine is where the absorption of nutrients takes place. This is where the villi fill the small intestine and make contact with enzymes, enabling the digestion and assimilation of food. When putrefaction occurs, it causes the villi to flatten. Flattened villi reduce the ability of digestive enzymes to break down food, leading to a reduction in digestion and absorption. The HSOs can remove this putrefaction from the villi. Some people have increased their ability to absorb nutrients by as much as 50 percent after taking a therapeutic trial of HSOs.

When people are anemic, especially the elderly, iron supplements are usually given. When excessive iron is in the body, it just feeds iron-loving parasites and harmful bacteria. It might be better to give HSOs instead. HSOs are able to enhance iron absorption by stimulating the body to produce lactoferrin. This allows the iron to be carried back into the small intestine for proper absorption by the digestive tract. Iron carried by lactoferrin is well assimilated and does not readily feed the harmful organisms.

When taking HSOs, proceed gradually. HSOs will begin to clean out toxins and pathogens quickly. If you take too many or too often, the cleansing will occur faster than the body can eliminate the accumulated toxins and may cause some discomfort or die-off symptoms. It is usually recommended to start with one capsule a day and work up to about ten each day for an average of three months. If you have been very ill, then proceed much slower. During the three month period, you will saturate the body with these beneficial bacteria. After three months you can gradually decrease back to the recommended maintenance dosage of five capsules per day.

Friendly bacteria, such as HSOs, must battle overwhelming odds to crowd out harmful bacteria. This does take time. You did not arrive at your current health situation overnight, and you cannot expect a miracle pill to make you well overnight either. So you will need to take HSOs for a minimum of ninety days. Either be committed to this program, or do not bother to even start.

LACTOBACILLUS ACIDOPHILUS

Often, the word "acidophilus" is used generally to mean any beneficial bowel microflora occupying the intestinal tract. It is important to realize that many other bacteria reside in the intestines besides *L. acidophilus*. The word "acidophilus" means acid-loving. Its name is derived from its ability to produce lactic acid, which helps to acidify the colon. That makes the intestinal environment inhospitable to unwanted pathogens. *Lactobacillus acidophilus* is probably the best known of all the various probiotic bacteria. They live mostly in the small intestine and are one of the most important beneficial bacteria found there.

LACTOBACILLUS BIFIDUS

See "Bifidobacteria" for more information.

LACTOBACILLUS BULGARICUS

Lactobacillus bulgaricus is commonly used as a yogurt culture, but is unable to proliferate in the human colon. That is because it is not a normal resident. They are only transient bacteria, rather than permanent residents. There is some concern that *Lactobacillus bulgaricus* does not increase the viability of other beneficial intestinal microflora and may reduce populations of *Lactobacillus acidophilus*. However, they are friendly bacteria and serve a useful purpose. They help to re-acidify the colon so that the intestinal terrain is favorable for the return of the acid-loving resident organisms. They also provide an environment that is not favorable to pathogens.

LACTOBACILLUS CASEI OR LACTOBACILLUS RHAMNOSUS

There is a strain of bacteria called *Lactobacillus casei,* subspecies *rhamnosus.* It is also known as *Lactobacillus GG* (GG stands for the initials taken from the names of its co-developers, Gorbach and Golding). People who tried this product often claimed that they notice an immediate improvement in their energy level and relief from deep fatigue. Its claim to fame is the unusually high potency, ranging from thirty-eight to forty-two billion colony-forming units (cfu) at the time of manufacture. It has a guaranteed potency of ten billion at the end of its one year expiration date when stored at room temperature. If refrigerated, it maintains its original full potency for much longer.

L. *casei* is able to colonize the human gastrointestinal tract, but only temporarily, and fails to create a self-sustaining, permanent re-colonization eighteen days after it is discontinued. It does seem to decrease many types of diarrhea, particularly the type that develops after a person has taken an antibiotic. *Lactobacillus GG* has the ability to readjust the acidity of the gastrointestinal tract long enough for other friendly strains of bowel microflora to become established. It is more resistant to bile salts, guards against gut permeability defects, provides the last chance for protein to be digested, and prevents several pathogens from attaching to the intestinal wall.

There is some speculation that the alarming increase in allergies and asthma may be due to an overactive immune system in the first months of life. One of the things thought to help is to provide beneficial bacteria to keep the immune system in check. A new Finnish study in the medical journal *Lancet* provides some evidence that it may be helpful to give beneficial bacteria to expectant mothers and their newborns that are predisposed to eczema, hay fever, and asthma. The researchers recruited near-term pregnant women who had a family history of allergic diseases and gave some of them *Lactobacillus GG*. The bacteria prevented the immune system from going into an alarm mode when it detected an otherwise harmless intruder such as dust, pollen, or a particular food. This same Finnish group has also published that infants taking probiotics have decreased milk allergies and fewer skin complications.

In one study (*Journal of Pediatrics* 1999) *Lactobacillus GG* was given to children taking antibiotics for a variety of bacterial illnesses, such as bladder infections. Many children who did not get the probiotic ended up with diarrhea. The diarrhea is often caused by the pathogenic bacteria *Clostridia spp*. Hospitalized infants are at high risk of acquiring intestinal microbes, which can cause diarrhea and possibly lead to infant death. In another study, 80 percent fewer children developed diarrhea when given *Lactobacillus GG* (*The Journal of Pediatrics* 2001).

LACTOBACILLUS REUTERI

Discovered in 1986 as a distinctive new strain, *Lactobacillus reuteri* is being studied as an alternative to pharmaceutical antibiotics in combating *Salmonella typhimurium* in flocks of poultry. *Lactobacillus reuteri* produces an antimicrobial substance that can inhibit the growth of gram-positive and gram-negative bacteria, yeasts, fungi, and protozoa. At even higher concentrations, it can kill lactic acid bacteria and lower the numbers of *Salmonella typhimurium* even further.

Lactobacillus reuteri has also been identified in the vagina. In a recent issue of the *Journal of Infectious Diseases,* it is one of seven strains described as having antipathogen properties. The handful of studies using *Lactobacillus reuteri* with humans has focused on shortening the duration of viral diarrhea in children. One study reported the safety and tolerance of *Lactobacillus reuteri* on people infected with HIV who also are likely to suffer gastrointestinal complaints. These bacteria colonize the human intestinal tract well, where it appears to inhibit the adherence of pathogens. It is available commercially as a probiotic in the United States and in several other countries.

LACTOBACILLUS SALIVARIUS

Highly prolific, *Lactobacillus salivarius* doubles its population every twenty minutes and helps crowd out the unfriendly microflora. Extensive research and testing has shown that this organism alone can assist in reestablishing normal intestinal ecology. These bacteria are transient organisms that flourish in the small intestine, but will not last for long once the supplement is stopped.

LACTOBACILLUS SPOROGENES

This is a particularly hardy organism closely related to *Lactobacillus acidophilus*, but more resistant to physical and chemical insults. *Lactobacillous sporogenes* has developed survival mechanisms that cause it to resist antibiotics and other toxic chemicals. Taken orally, they resist the stomach acids and begin reproducing rapidly within a few hours after they reach the small intestine. The spores also resist heat, radiation, drying, and freezing, and remain viable for long periods without refrigeration. Like their beneficial relative, *Lactobacillus sporogenes* helps to maintain the acidity of the intestine, crowding out unwanted bacteria and contributing to the intestinal probiotic barrier effect. They also help reduce the toxins produced by harmful bacteria.

SACCHAROMYCES BOULARDII

Saccharomyces boulardii is not a bacterium, but a yeast that was originally isolated from lychee fruit found in Indochina. This therapeutic yeast has been available in Europe for over fifty years and is currently sold in many countries worldwide. Now it is available in the United States. *Saccharomyces boulardii* helps with several types of diarrhea, such as antibiotic-associated diarrhea, traveler's diarrhea, acute pediatric diarrhea, diarrhea in the elderly, and HIV-associated chronic diarrhea. It counteracts the effects of the bacterium *Clostridium difficile,* which causes many cases of diarrhea and intestinal inflammation. In human's, this friendly yeast interferes with the toxins given off by pathogens, stimulates the immune system, promotes intestinal health, and helps to restore normal intestinal microflora.

Although *Saccharomyces boulardii* is not a resident of the normal gut flora, it can survive in the lower gastrointestinal tract. It does not cause disease, while maintaining an excellent safety profile. Taking this probiotic orally will create high concentrations in the intestine usually within three to four days. These high levels will last as long as you take the supplement. Within four to six days after you discontinue *Saccharomyces boulardii,* it will disappear.

In order for some pathogens to cause disease they must first attach themselves to specific receptor sites located on the lining of the intestinal tract. Sometimes the pathogen does not directly attach, but produces toxins that attach instead and cause disease. *Saccharomyces boulardii* can inhibit this attachment. It is not only effective as a probiotic, but offers unique advantages over traditional drugs because it does not promote antibiotic resistance.

Yeast are usually hardier than bacteria, so it makes good sense to use a friendly yeast as a probiotic. It probably works by lowering the pH of the fecal stream making it more acidic. This in turn creates a favorable environment for the acid-loving beneficial bacteria to return. If you are suffering from reactive arthritis or other disease states characterized by an hyperimmune response, this yeast is not recommended. If you have chronic yeast infections, you should avoid this probiotic.

In one study, *Saccharomyces boulardii* was added to the feed of a group of chickens. The chickens were then given the pathogen *Salmonella*. Only 5 percent of the chickens became colonized with *Salmonella*, whereas 70 percent of the chickens that were not given the *Saccharomyces boulardii* had *Salmonella* in their intestines. *Saccharomyces boulardii* also inhibits the growth of other pathogenic bacteria in the intestinal tract such as *Yersinia enterocolitica, Staphylococcus aureus, Pseudomonas aeruginosa,* and the yeast *Candida albicans.*

If you decide to try *Saccharomyces boulardii* as a probiotic, be aware that as the pH of the gastrointestinal tract becomes more acidic, it may create more intestinal gas. The best plan is not to increase the amount of this probiotic too quickly. Another plus is that it does not have to be refrigerated, making it ideal for traveling.

STREPTOCOCCUS FAECIUM OR ENTEROCOCCUS FAECIUM

This very hardy organism, previously known as *Streptococcus faecium,* is important to mention because it is often a contaminant or added to formulas of probiotics. There is concern because of antibiotic-resistant strains and because there may be harmful immune cross-reactions in susceptible individuals, which is more likely to happen in people with rheumatoid arthritis and fibromyalgia.

Usually, this bacterium is not a big problem for most healthy people, but *Enterococcus faecium* can be difficult to get rid of if it does begin to cause symptoms. If you begin having symptoms after taking any probiotic product, such as fever or bloody urine, this may be the reason why. Try switching brands to see if the symptoms go away. If you have a compromised immune system, it might be best to select a different product in the first place.

Check the label on your probiotic to see if this bacterium is present. Since *Enterococcus faecium* has been found as an unlisted ingredient in a large number of probiotic products sold in health food stores, you might want to check with the manufacturer to see if each batch is assayed for all the common contaminants and if *Enterococcus faecium* is present. Because of its relationship to an antibiotic-resistance strain, the wisdom of its use as a probiotic today is questionable.

Several reports of hospital acquired infections, due to an antibiotic-resistant strain of *Enterococcus faecium* has been reported. It has been responsible for outbreaks in Europe, Australia, and even the United States. This has important consequences because one strain is resistant to the antibiotic vancomycin. Vancomycin is usually held in reserve for bacteria that cannot be killed by other antibiotics. Also, there may be a link between this organism and cases of chronic arthritis, Crohn's disease, and ulcerative colitis. In specific populations, notably in liver transplant patients and patients with malignancies of the blood, this strain can cause serious and often fatal disease.

STREPTOCOCCUS THERMOPHILUS

Streptococcus thermophilus is found in kimchee, buttermilk and fresh, homemade sauerkraut. It is only present in fresh refrigerated sauerkraut instead of canned or jars that have been heated in the process of manufacturing. The high heat of pasteurization kills the bacteria.

CHAPTER 17

Herbal & Nutritional Supplement Therapies

THE WORD *DRUG* comes from the Dutch word *droog*, meaning to dry, since it was common to prepare medicinal herbs by drying them first. Many compounds derived from plants have pharmacological activity and have been used as medicines by practically every ancient civilization. Hippocrates found uses for over three hundred herbal remedies. The botanical books of the First-Century Greek physician, Dioscorides, and of the second century Roman, Galen, set standards for botanical medicine for more than fifteen hundred years. This knowledge was maintained throughout the Middle Ages by religious orders in monasteries.

Despite the fact that synthetic medicines began to be developed by the late 1800s, the eclectic physicians (similar to modern day naturopathic physicians) kept herbal and other "alternative" traditions alive until the 1930s. That's when herbal medicines were dropped from the official U.S. pharmacopoeia, largely because of disuse. Then slowly, herbs resurfaced in health food stores through the 1950s and 1960s, and increased to extraordinary levels of use through the 1990s. Today, about half of the American population have used herbal and supplemental remedies.

With the emergence of antibiotic-resistant strains of bacteria, natural products take on a greater importance. Even if new antibiotics are developed, in time there will likely emerge infectious bacteria that are resistant to them. The complex chemistry of herbal medicine renders them potentially more therapeutic against a wide variety of microorganisms for which pharmaceutical drugs may be impotent. It is important to look at what Mother Nature's pharmacy has brought us. For centuries, devastating illnesses have been cured with nature's remedies and proper diet.

Western medicine, on the other hand, has shunned diet, nutrition, homeopathy, and herbs, as not having a place in scientific medicine. Even though many drugs originally came from herbs, they are now changed into substances that are so toxic that they have to be tightly regulated. Drugs do not promote health, but are used once you are diseased.

According to statistics from the American Poison Control Center the average deaths per year from medication poisoning are from the following:

- 140,000 died from FDA approved prescription drugs
- 320 deaths from nonprescription drugs
- 1,000 deaths from aspirin
- 3 deaths from vitamins, minerals, or amino acids
- 0 deaths from herbs and herbal extracts when not standardized.

An alarming report in *U.S. News & World Report* indicates side effects of prescription drugs cause over two million patients to be hospitalized. The FDA placed thirty drugs on its monitoring list because of these problems. Back in 1995, the FDA reported that prescription drugs caused $20 billion in side effects and avoidable hospitalizations. It must be much worse today.

Standardized Herbs—Are They Better?

When you see the word "standardized" in reference to an herb it means that there is a guaranteed amount of a certain botanical constituent in the product. Examples would be like having St. John's wort standardized to contain so much hypericin, ma huang for its ephedrine, and milk thistle for its silymarin content. Just because an herb is standardized does not necessarily mean that it is better or stronger.

In a whole plant that comes from nature there may be hundreds of active constituents. By concentrating on only one component, it is possible to lose synergistic compounds that could improve the effectiveness and lessen adverse reactions. As herbs become more standardized, there may be problems with obtaining a specified amount of a particular constituent from a plant. Manufacturers typically use chemical solvents such as hexane, benzene, acetone, and methyl chloride, in the preparations of standardized extracts. Residues of these chemicals are found in the finished product and may be something you do not want added to your body.

What if the company or person researching and preparing a particular standardize herb does not understand which constituent is beneficial for clinical use? In the case of ginseng, the ginseng leaves do not have the same properties as the roots. In the South Pacific, locals all use the kava roots, but the German pharmaceutical companies use the stems to standardized their kava products.

One of the downfalls of the herbal/natural supplement industry is that each batch of herbs may have different amounts of medicine. One batch of crude herb may have a very low level of active constituents, and another batch a high level. Because of the lack of standardization, it was felt that it was necessary to isolate and purify the active constituent. The problem with this process is that it increases the toxicity of herbs as a result of purification. Toxicity was less a factor when using the crude herb because over consumption usually resulted in minor symptoms and seldom severe side effects and death.

I suspect that the main reason that companies are rushing to standardize herbs is because they can patent the product or somehow have exclusiveness over it, meaning more profits. Herbs that come directly as nature made them cannot be so controlled. Traditional herbalists seldom use standardized products. Standardized extracts tend to be more expensive and there is little evidence that they are more effective than using the whole herb. Herbalists will continue to recommend herbs in their more natural state, which include water and alcohol extracts, teas, and pills that do not contain standardized herbs.

Even some nonstandardized herbs can reach toxic levels and cause symptoms if not taken correctly. Just because it comes from nature does not mean it is entirely safe. The dosage a person should take depends on many factors such as age, vitality, and seriousness of the health condition. Therefore, self-treating is not a substitute for being guided by a qualified healthcare practitioner trained in herbal medicine. I suggest you seek one out.

Herbal/Natural Supplements for Bacterial Overgrowth

It is important to do everything you can to increase the healthy function of your immune system and improve the body's internal environment. The following is a list of the many products that can help, but in practicality, it must be tailored to each person's specific needs in order to maximize the desired effects and limit unnecessary treatment.

ACACIA (ACACIA SPP.)

This plant is not well-known in the United States, but is helpful for ulceration in any part of the gastrointestinal tract. It is used for excessive mucus, diarrhea, dysentery, and even for parasitic infestation. Researchers have found antibacterial activity by every member of this genus that has been tested. Acacia has properties to treat *Staphylococcus aureus, Pseudomonas aeruginosa, Salmonella spp, Shigella dysenteriae, Escherichia coli,* and *Proteus mirabilis.* It is used for sore inflammations in the gastrointestinal tract from the mouth to the anus. This includes a painful intestinal tract from dysenteric disease. It coats and soothes as well as provides antimicrobial action.

ACTIVATED CHARCOAL

This substance is commonly sold in pharmacies and health food stores to decrease gas in the intestinal tract. It has also been found to stifle bacterial growth, but not as well as bentonite clay. It can also absorb nutrients, and should be taking away from the time you take other supplements.

ALKYLGLYCEROLS

These compounds found in specially processed shark liver oil are thought to boost the immune system in general and aid in heavy metal detoxification. These are fats that stimulate the production of white blood cells to normal levels and encourage the growth of antibodies, boost platelet counts, and inhibit bacteria and fungi. Alkylglycerols serve as a primary food for the immune system. It is also one of the immune system's chief agents thought to specifically target and weaken cancer cells.

ALOE BARBADENSIS

Most of us know the plant aloe vera, but this is another specie. Aloe vera usually does not contain an important ingredient that makes this plant better for treating the immune system. This particular plant has a remarkable ability to normalize many damaging processes. By doing this, it enhances immune system function. Aloe is a potent anti-inflammatory agent, neutralizing many of the enzymes responsible for damaging the walls of the intestinal tract. This can decrease "leaky gut" and reduce the absorption of allergy-causing proteins. Aloe not only has some antibacterial properties, it also has the ability to reduce the viral and fungal load on the body.

The healing powers of aloe have been know for centuries. Today it is still important in restoring and maintaining health, especially on the gastrointestinal and immune systems, which are intricately related. This particular aloe contains the greatest concentration of acetylated mannan, which is also the most active form. This active ingredient is mostly present in cold-processed, whole leaf aloe.

Aloe barbadensis, when used internally at too high a dose, can cause cramps, nausea, vomiting or diarrhea. The urine may be colored red and kidney inflammation may occur if taken on a continuing basis. It works best on the lower bowel, but if small bowel irritation increases, it would be best to discontinue this plant.

AMINO ACIDS

The amino acids leucine, isoleucine, proline, arginine and histidine strongly stimulate the major white blood cells to gobble up the pathogenic bacteria. People who are deficient in these amino acids also have increased risk of infections.

ANTIOXIDANTS

A person's antioxidant status and stomach acid output appears to be the answer to why everyone infected with H. pylori does not get ulcers or stomach cancer. Antioxidants such as SOD (superoxide dismutase), CAT (glutathione peroxidase), beta-carotene, vitamins A, C, and E, gamma oryzanol, and combinations of these substances, can be protective in preventing and healing the lesions caused by H. pylori.

ASHWAGANDHA (WITHANIA SOMNIFERA)

This plant is not known well in Western herbal medicine, but has great value in strengthening the immune system. It has been found effective against Staphylococcus aureus, Pseudomonas aeruginosa, and Salmonella spp. Its best feature is its reputation as a strong immune tonic and stress protector. It is also used as a nerve sedative in people who are highly stressed. As with most immune tonics this herb works best when taken over time. It might take six weeks to six months before you see the results that this herb can give.

Ashwagandha is not suggested for use during pregnancy since it is used as an abortifacient in India. Use caution when taking in large doses since it from the Solanaceae family, which many relatives have narcotic effects. Its use as folk medicine is considered safe in therapeutic doses. The plant does have a fairly high amount of nicotine. This may be considered contraindicated if you are trying to quit smoking.

ASTRAGALUS MEMBRANACEOUS

This particular herb is one of the best herbs to enhance the immune system and support thymus function. It promotes healing and tissue regeneration. Astragalus is known for its support of T-cell function and as an overall immune tonic. T-cells (also known as killer cells) are the white blood cells of the body that attack the invaders that cause disease in the body. The use of Astragalus increases the level of interferon and antibodies, helps to eliminate toxins, and supports liver and spleen function. In supporting the liver, it protects it against chemical damage caused by chemotherapy.

Astragalus appears to be particularly useful in cases where the immune system has been damaged by chemicals or radiation. It also combats fatigue by nourishing exhausted adrenals. It is a good herb for the bladder because it reduces the potential for infections. It increases the flow of bile and digestive fluids therefore enhancing digestive function. Other medicinal uses include the prevention of infection. It is used for chronic bacterial infections, chronic fatigue, and autoimmune diseases. Astragalus is not recommended in acute infections. No toxicity has been noted. This is one of the best herbs to use to restore a depressed or damaged immune system.

BENTONITE CLAY

Bentonite clay binds toxins and prevents their systemic absorption. This clay has a greater ability to bind toxins than Kaopectate or activated charcoal. Bentonite clay absorbs numerous types of toxins, endotoxins, and bacteria. Its value may be from lowering the overall toxin load in the intestinal lumen. Because of its binding ability, it is important to take this substance away from other supplements and food.

BERBERINE-CONTAINING HERBS

Goldenseal (*Hydrastis canadensis*) was used for years in the treatment of gastrointestinal disorders to inhibit the growth of numerous pathogenic bacteria. It used to be quite effective against most of the harmful bacteria encounter in the intestinal tract. That has all changed. Over the past few years, goldenseal is less effective against harmful bacteria as it once was. As with any antibiotic, even herbal ones, the longer a substance is used the more likely pathogens will become resistant. Other plants containing berberine include barberry (*Berberis vulgaris*), and Oregon grape (*Berberis aquifolium*).

Pathogenic bacteria now resistant to berberine are species of *Pseudomonas, Klebsiella, Citrobacter, Proteus,* and some species of *Vibrio. Staphylococcus aureas* has also been found to be resistant. If you do decide to include goldenseal in your treatment plan, it might be best not to rely on just this one herb, but include others in the treatment mix. Berberine and berberine-containing plants are generally nontoxic when used in therapeutic doses. They should not be used for more than a couple of weeks at a time and do not use during pregnancy.

The antimicrobial activity of berberine increases with intestinal pH. At a pH of 8.0 its antimicrobial activity is typically two to four times greater than when it is 7.0, which is one to four times greater than a pH of 6.0, etc. This suggests that a more alkaline system will improve its chance of working, especially in the treatment of urinary tract infections. See "Uva Ursi" for more information on achieving an alkaline pH.

BERBERINE SULFATE

This compound is widely distributed in nine plant families and has been known to have significant activity against a variety of bacteria in the gut such as *E. coli, Shigella,* and some species of *Vibrio* and *Staphylococcus.* Many gram-positive bacteria may still be susceptible to berberine sulfate, if the concentrations are high enough. The efficacy of berberine sulfate also increases with the increase in pH. Even some of the highly resistant *E. coli* yielded when the pH was more alkaline. *Salmonella* and *Pseudomonas spp.,* and some of the *E. coli* strains are now highly resistant to berberine sulfate.

BETA GLUCAN

Beta glucan increases the ability of immune cells to destroy bacterial, viral, and fungal organisms. It increases the production of blood cells in the bone marrow. This is where both white and red blood cells originate. Beta glucan works by activating the immune cells known as macrophages, which trap and consume foreign substances in the body. It is also a powerful antioxidant (a free radical scavenger) and helps with the regeneration and repair of damaged tissue.

This natural compound is found in products such as shiitake mushrooms and kombucha tea. It is also extracted from the cell membranes of baker's yeast and young rye plants. Beta glucan is completely safe and nontoxic. It has no known adverse effects. Since it is a pure isolate, even when it is extracted from yeast, it does not contain any yeast proteins that could cause an allergic reaction.

BLACK WALNUT (JUGLANS NIGRA)

This herb is an antiseptic and is useful in healing bacterial infections and overgrowths. The active constituent, juglong, has significant activity against many bacteria including species of *Klebsiella* and *Salmonella*, and *E. coli*. Black walnut has traditionally been used to treat illnesses of the intestinal tract, especially parasites and yeast.

Herbalists have traditionally used the husks of black walnut as a nutritional aid for the intestinal system. The green husks have a high iodine content that makes them antiseptic and useful in healing. Its properties are useful in all sorts of cleansing programs, especially in expelling parasites. It also has the ability to rid the body of toxins.

BLUE GREEN ALGAE

This supplement may be a problem for some people who have a history of dysbiosis. Cyanobacteria were present in the stool cultures of people who regularly consume this type of algae. Safer sources containing similar nutrients would be various kinds of sea kelp and marine algae. The easily absorbed trace minerals in seaweed are valuable in building immunity by increasing the body's natural killer cells. Another substance found in seaweed has the ability to chelate heavy metals out of the body.

BREWER'S YEAST OR SACCHAROMYCES CEREVISIAE

Brewer's yeast may act by binding the toxin of pathogens, altering the intestinal microflora, or by increasing the intestinal immune system. Three people with *Clostridium difficile* diarrhea who had relapsed after conventional antibiotic treatment were given brewer's yeast (three tablets three times a day for fourteen days) without additional antibiotics. In each case, the diarrhea resolved within three to five days and did not recur. Previous studies show that brewer's yeast prevents antibiotic-induced diarrhea. A one-week course of treatment costs very little, whereas a course of some antibiotics can cost close to $100 for the same amount of time. Anyone sensitive to yeast may have a problem taking brewer's yeast.

BROMELAIN

This compound is a pineapple extract that could prevent traveler's diarrhea. This enzyme is found in the stems of pineapples and temporarily prevents *E. coli* from attaching to the intestinal tract lining and causing disease, but it only acts for about thirty hours. After this time, the bacteria's activity resumes unless other treatments are included. Bromelain may also interfere directly with the toxins that some bacteria release.

BURDOCK ROOT (ARCTIUM LAPPA)

This is the plant that produces those annoying burrs matted in dogs' fur. Burdock root has a long and safe history of use as a food that provides deep strengthening to the immune system. One of the conditions it is best known for is eczema because it tends to correct the underlying defects in the inflammatory mechanism and immune system. Burdock has antimicrobial activity that helps control the bacteria *Staphylococcus*. In other parts of the world, burdock is used for abscesses, joint pain, respiratory infections, cancerous tumors, skin conditions, venereal disease, and bladder and kidney problems. It also eliminates waste products from the body caused by bacterial toxins. It is a food commonly eaten in Japan and believed to be safe.

BUTYRATE

Butyric acid, or butyrate, plays a beneficial role in nourishing and maintaining healthy colon cells. Adequate butyrate lowers the stool pH, which is associated with protection against colon cancer and enhances an environment that does not support many pathogenic bacteria. The principal food source that produces colon butyrate is the fermentation of soluble fiber by friendly colon bacteria. After many years of testing, I find that the level of butyrate in the colon is often too low, putting a person at risk for colon dysfunction. Butyrate is also reported to help increase the immune system of the digestive tract.

CABBAGE JUICE

Fresh cabbage juice is a traditional treatment for ulcers caused by *H. pylori*. In recent studies, a quart (liter) per day of freshly made cabbage juice resulted in ulcers healing in about ten days. Green cabbage is best, but red cabbage is also useful. The cabbage can be mixed with celery and carrots to make a tastier drink.

CALCIUM D-GLUCARATE

This form of calcium keeps the toxins produced by pathogen bacteria from reabsorbing back into the body. Calcium d-glucarate is a nontoxic compound found in certain fruits and vegetables. It is also a normal constituent found in body tissues and body fluids. The suggested adult dosage is one to three capsules with meals three times daily. I have used this product, along with quercetin (one capsule three times a day with meals), and found it very effective for counteracting the side effects of a food intolerance and the overgrowth of bacteria in the intestinal tract.

Start out taking this product along with quercetin as suggested above. After several weeks of taking these substances, you can start reintroducing small amounts of formerly forbidden foods and see how you tolerate them. You may find that you can tolerate foods that you have not been able to eat for years.

CALCIUM ELENOLATE

This form of calcium has shown bactericidal effects, at least on all the bacteria against which it has been tested. In animal studies, there have been problems knowing when to give this substance so that it will be the most effective. The problem appears to be that calcium elenolate rapidly binds to proteins in the blood. Once bound, it is essentially taken out of action and becomes ineffective. Independent researchers have discovered a method of formulation that could remove the protein-clinging properties, yet leave the bactericidal properties intact. If you are considering taking calcium elenolate as an antibacterial agent, you will need to ask if this problem of binding to proteins has been remedied? As of this writing, it has not been able to do this.

CATECHIN

The bioflavonoid, catechin, can successfully hinder histamine release in human stomachs. This is the same way that drugs work for ulcers. Oral doses of 1,000 mg per day may be needed. Catechin also has antioxidant properties and promotes healing.

CHLORELLA

Chorella is an algae harvested from freshwater sources. It has one of the highest chlorophyll contents of all known plants, twenty times the chlorophyll content of alfalfa. This makes chlorella valuable not only as a nutritional supplement, but possess immune properties that fight bacteria and viruses. Chlorella has also become helpful in the removal of heavy metals such as mercury, cadmium, and lead, from the body.

Its many systemic benefits include healing gastrointestinal ulcers, protection of the liver from environmental pollutants, digestive regulation, healing damaged tissues, protection against radiation, cleansing and building blood cells, and the elimination of body odors. It also has the ability to repair damaged DNA and RNA, and other genetic material. Chlorella increases macrophage activity. Macrophages are white blood cells that consume or digest tumor cells, pathogenic bacteria, and other substances that should not be in the body. Chlorella is effective in breaking down cholesterol deposits. It also improves brain function and memory due to chlorella's capacity to carry more oxygen to brain cells and is a rich source of iron and zinc.

CHLOROPHYLL

Chlorophyll has long been associated with the healing of ulcers. It has preventive and healing properties. Their high chlorophyll content may explain why barley grass and alfalfa herbs work well to heal ulcers.

COLOSTRUM

Colostrum is the pre-milk fluid produced from the mammary glands of mammals during the first twenty-four to forty-eight hours after giving birth. It provides essential growth and immune factors that insure the health and vitality of the newborn. Now, even adults can obtain the benefits that colostrum offers. The product should be from pasture-fed cows that are hormone and antibiotic free.

Research shows colostrum to be a powerful, broad-spectrum substance. It is known to boost the immune system, accelerate healing of all types of injuries, increase vitality and stamina, and improve gastrointestinal performance, especially of the small intestine. It improves the ability to fight pathological bacteria and fungi. These effects may improve the healing of a damaged intestinal lining and consequently reverse difficulties associated with various degrees of malabsorption. Colostrum supplements are known for their protective effects on infants against diarrhea-causing bacteria.

COLLOIDAL SILVER

Colloidal silver has strong antibiotic properties against both the bad and the good bacteria. This is why colloidal silver should only be used for short-term use; that is, about ten days. Since colloidal silver has become so popular as an antibacterial agent, it is now commonly used as a component in water filters. I suspect these properties could affect beneficial bowel flora if used on a continuous basis.

One colloidal silver product was tested to be effective against all three bacteria commonly found in urinary tract infections: *Escherichia coli,*

Klebsiella pneumoniae, and *Proteus mirabilis.* All colloidal silver products are not the same. One lab conducted experiments using five different products and found that each one affected the bacteria *Staphylococcus aureus* differently. In fact, one of the colloidal silver products did not inhibit this staph germ at all while the others had some level of effectiveness.

COENZYME Q10

Coenzyme Q10 (often shortened to "coQ10") is an antioxidant essential for optimal immune function. Current studies support the argument that coenzyme Q10 supplementation may increase antibody production and offer extra protection against infection, especially for immune-compromised individuals. It may be necessary to also take adequate vitamin B6 to insure the maximum production of coQ10, especially among those with compromised diets and the elderly.

DEGLYCYRRHIZINATED LICORICE (DGL)

A special licorice extract, deglycyrrhizinated licorice (DGL) is used in the treatment of ulcers and *H. pylori* infection. Rather than hinder the release of stomach acid the way antacids do, DGL stimulates the body's normal defense mechanisms that prevent ulcer formation in the first place. DGL improves both the quality and quantity of the protective substances that line the intestinal tract; increases the lifespan of the intestinal cell; and improves blood supply to the intestinal lining. DGL is extremely safe and inexpensive. A recent study indicates that the flavonoids contained in DGL were shown to inhibit *H. pylori.*

In order to be effective in healing ulcers, it appears that DGL must mix with saliva. The capsule form of DGL has not been shown to be effective. It is best to buy the chewable tablets and take them at least twenty minutes before meals. Chewing DGL after meals has given poor results. Depending on the response, you may need to take DGL for eight to sixteen weeks.

DIGESTIVE ENZYMES

These supplements aid in the digestion of foods when your own body's enzymes are deficient. Whatever is not properly digested can provide a substrate for the overgrowth of pathogen bacteria, yeast, and parasites. Our bodies are not maintained by what we eat, but rather by what we digest, absorb, and assimilate. Every food must be broken down by enzymes for access by the villi in the intestines, transported by the blood to interstitial fluid, and finally assimilated by individual cells.

Specific digestive enzymes as well as beneficial microflora and minerals manage this biochemical process.

As we age and continue to eat overly cooked and processed foods, we put higher demands on different organs to keep manufacturing digestive enzymes. This ultimately puts more stress on the pancreas since it is only able to build its enzymes from those raw food enzymes we eat. The digestive enzymes that the pancreas produces is largely responsible for keeping the small intestine free from disease-causing bacteria, protozoa, yeast, and intestinal worms. When pancreatin enzymes and other digestive enzymes are reduced or lacking, it puts people at risk of having an intestinal overgrowth of undesirable organisms.

The pancreas secretes digestive enzymes that digest fat, protein, and starch. There are other organs that can adequately digest starch and fat, but the pancreas is critical for protein digestion. If protein is incompletely digested a number of problems are created for the body. Some of them could be allergies and the formation of toxic substances produced during putrefaction. Some of the common symptoms of pancreatin insufficiency include: abdominal bloating and discomfort, increased gas, indigestion, and the passing of undigested food in the stool. A nonenteric coated enzyme preparation will out perform an enteric-coated product for digestive purposes if given prior to a meal.

Another important digestive enzyme, hydrochloric acid, may be taken in capsule form to supplement a deficiency in the stomach. Symptoms commonly reported as stomach acid distress often prove to result from reduced stomach acid not an over abundance. Two forms are available, betaine or glutamic hydrochloric acid. You may find that you tolerate one form better than the other. Taking the correct dosage of hydrochloric acid may be all that is needed to correct bowel microflora ecology.

Other digestive enzymes such as plant enzymes or pepsin might help to lessen the digestive load. I recommend that you seek help in determining which digestive enzyme or enzymes you need. There are many types available and some may not be of any benefit to you. The correct digestive enzyme can make a big difference in how you digest your food and reduce the overload of harmful bacteria in your digestive tract.

Another important body system that becomes stressed in the absence of digestive enzymes is that of the immune system. Immune function relies on proper and complete digestion of food. In the absence of adequate digestive enzymes the body's immune enzymes are drawn from their normal posts and transported to the digestive tract by white blood cells to insure adequate digestion. This pattern leaves the immune system unguarded against invading pathogens.

D-MANNOSE

D-mannose can be used to treat urinary tract infections if the cause is from the bacterium *E. coli*. You may want your doctor to collect a urine sample to test before starting D-mannose because this product is not effective unless the bacterium is *E. coli*. Foods that naturally contain D-mannose are cranberry and pineapple juice. Unfortunately, they do not contain the high amounts needed to treat urinary tract infections.

For adults, it usually takes 1/2 teaspoon every two to three hours to be effective. Many urinary tract infections occur after having sex because of the transference of *E. coli*. Then it may be helpful to take 1/2 teaspoon of D-mannose one hour prior to and just after intercourse. To prevent urinary tract infections take 1/4 teaspoon of D-mannose once a day and eat a healthy diet. D-mannose does not appear to cause any problems with the normal microflora and is even safe for pregnant women and very small children. It is safe even if taken long term.

ECHINACEA (ECHINACEA ANGUSTIFOLIA OR PURPUREA)

Echinacea is a natural antibiotic used by millions of people around the world to prevent illness caused by harmful bacteria. Echinacea stimulates white blood cells to engulf bacteria and viruses. It also helps detoxify and pull waste residues out of the lymph glands. Echinacea contains caffeic acid, which has a wide range of antibacterial activities against bacteria such as *Staphylococcus aureus*, *Clostridium diphitheriae*, *Proteus vulgaris*, and *Mycobacterium tuberculosis*.

Echinacea inhibits an enzyme that many pathogens secrete. It is important to block these enzymes because they allow harmful bacteria to become more invasive. This ability helps echinacea to maintain the integrity of the intestinal surfaces and create a better defense barrier against infection. Use echinacea at the very beginning and throughout the course of an illness to support the immune system. Many studies have found that substances found in this plant can increase antibody production, raise white blood cell counts, and stimulate the activity of key white blood cells. It is assume that this process helps the immune system.

Most varieties of echinacea possess similar properties, but there are some differences. Echinacea appears to be safe even when taken in very high doses, but it is a stimulant. Continued immune stimulation when there is immune depletion may not be the best choice. This herb should not be used if you are getting sick often.

ESSENTIAL OILS

These beneficial oils are used internally and topically as antimicrobials. Essential oils are enjoying a bit of a renaissance among those looking for natural ways to combat bacteria. In addition to their rich mood-enhancing aroma, essential oils are highly antibacterial without the dangerous side effects frequently associated with antibiotics. Pathogenic bacteria are usually anaerobic (exist without oxygen), while beneficial bacteria are usually aerobic (exist where there is oxygen). Essential oils oxygenate cells and reinforce the immune system, while creating a less hospitable environment for harmful bacteria and other pathogens to flourish. An additional benefit is that bacteria are not showing resistant to essential oils.

One of the most popular, especially as a topical antibiotic, is tea tree oil. Made from the leaves and fronds of a shrub-like tree called *Melaluca alternifolia*, this plant has been used for centuries to heal wounds. Tea tree oil was the antiseptic of choice during World War II by Australians and British soldiers, but lost popularity to penicillin and other drugs. Starting in the 1970s, interest returned because of renewed production of this herb. Tea tree is nontoxic when used externally as an antiseptic. It sterilizes on contact and continues to prevent microbial growth for hours. Drinking an ounce or more can cause adverse symptoms such as nausea, confusion, seizures, respiratory depression, and coma.

Tea tree has such a complicated chemical structure that it would be unlikely that microbes would develop resistance. It has been effective against several bacteria including *Clostridium, E. coli, Pseudomonas, Staphylococcus,* and *Streptococcus.* If applied immediately to the skin, it has prevented microbes, such as spirochetes released during tick bites, from entering the body.

Oregano oil also has promise as natural broad-spectrum antimicrobial agents as well as thyme and rosewood oils. These oils are effective against *Streptococcus pneumonia* and *E. coli.* The best source is Greek oregano. Avoid *Oregano vulgare* because it does not have as much of the effective essential oils. Both rosacea and eczema have been helped by using oil of oregano, which tells us that these conditions are probably caused, at least in part, by an infectious agent.

One company has developed a product brought back from the English archives and based on the oils used by thieves in the 16th century. They would rub these essential oils on themselves for protection while robbing the dead bodies of plague victims. Included in the formula are high concentrations of cinnamon, one of the most antimicrobial of the essential oils.

FATTY ACIDS

Various polyunsaturated fatty acids (PUFAs) may be able to reduce the growth of *H. pylori*. Using increasing doses of olive oil and oils such as sunflower oil and fish oil, they found that the growth of *H. pylori* could be reduced by over 30 percent. Linoleic acid, an omega-6 fatty acid, produced even more dramatic results: inhibiting *H. pylori* growth anywhere from 60 to 95 percent, depending on the concentration used. The body depends on a wide range of fatty acids, as well as a proper balance between specific oils. Supplementing with only one type of oil does not sufficiently ensure proper fatty acid nutrition and metabolism.

FIBER

Fibers found in psyllium husks, oat bran, or flaxseed, helps to absorb toxins and promote their elimination from the body. Fiber also increases the rate of transit thought the gastrointestinal tract. It is important to eat adequate dietary fiber each day because it improves all aspects of colon function. One of the most important factors is its role in maintaining suitable intestinal microflora and making the area less hospitable to pathogens, such as *H. pylori*.

Fiber acts in a mechanical fashion like a broom. It decreases transit time and enhances detoxification through various mechanisms, including direct binding of toxins. Another good reason to take fiber is that the intestinal microflora break it down to produce butyrate and other substances, which provides an important energy source for the intestinal cells. Butyrate is the preferred substrate for energy metabolism in the colon and decreases the risk of colon cancer.

There has been controversy about the effect of fiber on mineral absorption. It now appears that large amounts of supplemental fiber, especially hemicelluloses, may result in the impaired absorption of minerals. Fiber found in food does not appear to cause this problem.

An interesting study with animals showed that adding fiber (cellulose powder) to a liquid diet decreased the incidence of bacteria that crossed the intestinal barrier and got into systemic circulation. The incidence decreased from 60 percent down to 8 percent. The best source of dietary fiber is from whole foods, although supplements have their use in the treatment phase of specific diseases. Even if a diet is high in fiber, if it is also high in refined carbohydrates, many of the beneficial effects of fiber are greatly reduced.

Fiber in the form of psyllium seed husks is an excellent source of fiber providing bulk as well as soothing the intestinal lining with its mucilaginous properties. To regulate the intestines, take one to three teaspoons of psyllium husks once a day with a large glass of water. If you have a sensitive digestive tract or a tendency towards bloating, you may want to start with a teaspoon and build up gradually to the full amount over a period of a few weeks. For some people psyllium seed husks causes too much bloating and gas. Perhaps they would do better taking flaxseed or some other form of fiber.

FLAVONOIDS

Flavonoids may limit damage to arteries caused by bacteria-induced inflammation. Bacterial toxins derived from gram-negative bacteria mediate this damage. Hesperitin, a major citrus flavonoid, as well as genestein, rutin, quercetin, and catechin, reduce the toxic effects of bacteria.

GAMMA ORYZANOL

This is a rice bran component that has been found effective for people with chronic gastritis and ulcers. The standard dose is 300 mg of gamma oryzanol per day for four weeks. It decreases symptoms of stomach aches, nausea, heartburn, belching, bloating, and loss of appetite. Gamma oryzanol works to normalize stomach acid.

GARLIC (ALLIUM SATIVUM)

Garlic has had widespread use since ancient times as a broad-spectrum, natural antimicrobial agent and is still one of the cheapest agents to use against many harmful bacteria. During World War I, garlic was the major battlefield wound dressing. A garlic paste was made and wrapped around wounds. After antibiotics were developed, many effective herbal preparations were virtually forgotten by the general population, including garlic. Renewed interest surfaced about ten years ago when researchers screened over two hundred natural plant substances for antimicrobial activity and determined that the allicin from garlic was a potent sulfur-containing antimicrobial.

The effects of garlic have been used against *Escherichia coli*, *Klebsiella pneumoniae*, *Clostridium perfringens*, *Salmonella spp*, and even *Staphylococcus aureus*. Garlic also appears to be very active against *Helicobacter pylori* (*H. pylori*). Fortunately, garlic is not harmful against most of the beneficial organisms needed in the digestive tract.

Garlic has the ability to inhibit bacteria by disrupting their whole enzyme system, which is responsible for cell replication. Here is an antimicrobial substance that is antiyeast and antifungi, and effective against many forms of bacteria. It also kills rotavirus infection, which is responsible for many cases of diarrhea. Garlic does not seem to cause the bacterial resistance that is appearing so often among antibiotics today. Taking garlic is also helpful in mercury and other heavy metal detoxification due to its high sulfur content.

Researchers from Sweden decided to investigate ways of decreasing the risk of tick and other insect bites. They note that recent studies have suggested that the frequency of insect bites may be linked to different body odors (*Lancet* 1996). According to the researchers, there was significant reduction in tick bites when consuming garlic. They suggested that garlic be considered as a tick repellent for those at high risk for tick bites, rather than other agents that might have more adverse effects.

Allicin is the primary antimicrobial agent that results when you crush a garlic clove. It may be better to use the whole clove rather than trying to extract out just one active ingredient, such as the allicin. The Allium group of plants that includes garlic also lists onions, but the largest concentration of antibacterial agents are found in garlic.

If you want to use a garlic clove, first peel it very carefully without nicking it. You will notice that there is very little smell. As soon as you crush it, you get an instantaneous smell of garlic. This is when allicin is produced. When you eat garlic it is important to compress the garlic with a spoon prior to swallowing it, if you are not going to juice it. If you swallow the clove whole you will not convert the garlic to its active ingredient. The active ingredient is destroyed within several hours after the garlic is smashed. To be sure that you are getting active allicin, the garlic must be fresh and raw.

Most people tolerate a few cloves a day without producing a "socially offensive" odor. Otherwise you can decrease the amount of garlic until there is no odor present. There are commercial preparations designed to offer the benefits of garlic without the odor. These preparations are made in such a way that allicin is not formed until the enteric coated tablet is delivered to the intestines. If you take more than the recommended daily dose, even these products may result in a detectable garlic odor. Be sure that the product you select produces active allicin.

Some brands of garlic are imported from China because the soil is very rich in sulfur, which contributes to increase activity. First, the garlic is hand peeled. Then they freeze it very quickly and remove any moisture. With the moisture removed, the allicin is inactive. If garlic were processed with the moisture present, the allicin would disappear in a few days. When the garlic is eaten, it is rehydrated as it makes its way down the digestive track and becomes active allicin again. Many products on the market today have no allicin left after processing.

Garlic is a safe product to use. You would have to eat a trunk load of garlic to have any toxic effect. Some people do get some digestive upset and possibly nausea and vomiting. Garlic is exceptionally pungent and acrid in any quantity as a raw herb or as juice. Care should be taken when consuming it in large quantities. The juice from one bulb of garlic combined even with 24 ounces of water or carrot juice can cause immediate vomiting for some people. It is better to start with a small amount and increase only as the body shows no signs of adverse reactions. One way is to start with 1/4 to 1 teaspoon of garlic juice in 16 ounces of tomato juice each hour as an antimicrobial agent. Most people do better when taking garlic in capsule form. Avoid garlic if you are a nursing mother since it affects the taste of breast milk.

GERMAN CHAMOMILE (MATRICARIA RECUTITA)

Chamomile has been described in medical writings since ancient times. A number of plants have chamomile as part of their name, but German chamomile is the medical chamomile considered here. It is one of the most important medicinal plants obtained from cultivation, being used as a medicinal tea, gargle, cream, ointment, and as an additive for sitz baths or vapor baths.

A chamomile extract helps to heal weeping wounds after having tattoos. This herb can kill and inhibit the growth of bacteria, and be used as an anti-inflammatory for the stomach and intestines. It is also effective against bacterial skin diseases including those of the mouth and gums. Chamomile has two specific fields of action. First, it calms the nervous system; second, it decreases irritation of the gastrointestinal tract. Chamomile extracts taken orally can relax the intestines and reduce inflammation. The wound healing activity of chamomile is closely linked to its anti-inflammatory properties.

Antimicrobial activity has been noted in chamomile oil against *Staphylococcus aureus, Bacillus subtilis* and the yeast *Candida albicans*. Chamomile extracts gives similar activity against *E. coli*. It inhibits *Streptococcus mutans*, group B *Streptococcus*, and *Streptococcus salivarius*. The extract also showed strong antibacterial activity against *Bacillus megatherium* and *Leptospira icterohaemorrhagiae*.

This plant is generally regarded as safe. Some people have experienced skin reactions such as a rash from topical use. People can mistaken German chamomile with "dog chamomile" because of a similar appearance, The later is highly allergic to some people. Chamomile also contains naturally occurring coumarin compounds that can act as blood thinners. Anyone taking prescription anticoagulants should avoid this plant.

GRAPEFRUIT SEED EXTRACT (CITRUS PARADISI)

Grapefruit seed extract (GSE) is becoming the plant of choice against minor bacterial infections and overgrowths. It is a natural extract derived from the seeds and pulp of grapefruit. Use it to fight infections from bacteria, parasites, viruses, and fungi. GSE is nontoxic and does not suppress the immune system the way antibiotics can, nor does it destroy the beneficial bacteria necessary for good health.

GSE is recommended against infections caused by *H. pylori*, the bacteria implicated in ulcers. It is useful when there are sore throats, nasal and skin infections, poison oak, and fungal infections of the nails, scalp, and other areas of the skin. Animals, both house pets and livestock, can benefit from GSE's antimicrobial action. You can add it to their food or water, or apply it topically since it is a great surface disinfectant. Add it to laundry or the dishwater and it will disinfect clothing, linens, and eating utensils. You can use it as you would use a spray-on, wipe-off cleaning solution, since it provides killing action against bacteria. It does not have the toxicity inherent in harmful chemicals. Chlorine bleach is a disinfectant that will work to kill most organisms, but it is irritating and toxic when inhaled.

Tests show that GSE is even more effective than colloidal silver, iodine, tea tree oil and Clorox bleach when tested against the five following common microorganisms: *Candida albicans, Staphylococcus aureus, Salmonella typhi, Streptococcus faecium,* and *E. coli.* GSE proved effective down to just 10 parts per million. The other substances tested were less effective than the GSE and several of them had to be used at full strength before they were as effective. GSE is also effective against species of these organisms: *Vibrio, Streptococcus, Listeria, Shigella, Chlamydia* and many forms of yeast and molds, as well as protozoa and viruses. Many other gram-negative and gram-positive bacteria will be affected by this wonderful product.

To effectively kill most of the bacteria and yeast in about thirty minutes GSE needs to be used at a concentration greater than 100 ppm. When you use a concentration of 500 ppm you can kill most of these microbes in ten minutes. This product is more effective than even alcohol and surgical soap when used as a skin disinfectant. There needs to be skin contact for at least a minute. It is a superior facial cleanser. It prevents mold growth in humidifiers when twenty to thirty drops of GSE are added to a gallon of hot water for thirty minutes.

The liquid concentrate is the most useful because it is compact and easy to carry. When diluted and applied correctly it has a variety of external and internal uses. The only time it is used full strength is to treat warts. It can be used internally similar to an antibiotic or externally as a skin wash or soaking solution. There exists a commercial and professional strength product called Citricidal that makes an excellent food wash when used as directed. Keep a bottle in the kitchen to clean fruits and veggies. Information comes with this product so that you would know the correct dose for GSE's many uses.

GSE is inexpensive and small concentrations of the product can be used with beneficial results. Tablets and capsules offer convenience and a palatable alternative. Use GSE at least three to four times each day for minor bacterial and fungal infections. Each 100 mg tablet is equivalent to four to five drops of the liquid. The usual dose required in pill form is 600 to 1,600 mg a day. It is important to know that this product has a very low chance of toxicity, whereas most disinfectants currently used in both animal and human environments have moderate to high levels. If you use GSE at high doses, expect some intestinal irritation or diarrhea.

GSE is a safe and simple way to disinfect drinking water when camping and backpacking or in an emergency situation where safe drinking water is questionable and boiling is not possible. To treat water, filter it first if possible. At least let suspended particles settle. Retain the clear water and add ten or more drops of GSE for each gallon of water. Shake well or stir vigorously and let it sit for an hour. A slightly bitter taste may be noticed.

Several people have told me that using GSE has kept them from getting sick with diarrhea when camping. Enjoying the great outdoors, even in what appears to be pristine environments, has increased our exposure to parasites and bacteria. Going to places abroad does not have to mean that most of the time you will spend it in the bathroom with traveler's diarrhea. GSE has proven to be exceptionally effective. Use as little as three to five drops in a glass of water each day as a preventative for Montezuma's revenge. If you already have symptoms after eating those strawberries from the roadway stand, you can take two drops in a glass of bottled water at noon and again at bedtime to kill whatever was picked up. Continue this treatment until after the diarrhea stops.

Medical researchers recently discovered that bacterial infections in the mouth might lead to blood clots that can bring on heart attacks and strokes. GSE is very useful for oral hygiene care. Since many pathogens find their way into the body after first entering the mouth, it makes sense to start there. GSE has many uses in all sorts of health conditions such as for colitis, diarrhea, flu, colds, sore throat, nasal infections, vaginal yeast infections, ear infections, warts, acne, athlete's foot, poison oak, fungal infections of the nails, and scalp infections.

GSE is becoming more common in environmentally friendly cleansers and antiseptics. You can use it as a food and dish wash at home as well as a disinfectant for your drinking water. GSE must be diluted before using. Undiluted it can cause skin and digestive irritation. The most negative problem with GSE is that it can kill off intestinal or skin bacteria that are beneficial to the body much like a broad-spectrum antibiotic would do. Perhaps using it all the time is not a good thing to do, but save it for those times that you suspect you are being contaminated with harmful organisms.

GREEN TEA (CAMELLIA SINENSIS)

Green tea, when applied to different strains of *Staphylococcus aureus*, made the bacteria more sensitive to the antibiotic penicillin. This particular bacterium can cause skin infections and abscesses. It is also showing up more often as an overgrowth in the intestinal tract. What makes drinking green tea different from black tea? It is in the processing. Green tea leaves are lightly steamed and dried at higher temperatures, whereas black tea leaves are exposed to more air. This results in a higher content of polyphenols with potent antioxidant properties. Most of the population and studies on tea have focused on the cancer-protective aspects. In addition to exerting antioxidant activity, green tea may increase detoxifying enzymes in the small intestine, liver, and lungs.

Green tea is not associated with any significant side effects or toxicity, but it does inhibit the absorption of non-heme iron (plant-derived) as distinguished from heme iron, which is derived from animal blood. Therefore, it could promote iron deficiency in susceptible people. It is possible that eating foods high in vitamin C or taking a vitamin C supplement would reverse the effect of green tea on iron absorption. Since this is a caffeine-containing beverage, over consumption may produce nervousness, insomnia, anxiety, irritability, etc. Usually this does not occur.

GUM

Gums that contains xylitol, a substance that comes from the bark of the birch tree, contains a bacteria-fighting substance that reduces the risk of a bacterium called "mutans streptococci." This bacteria lives around the teeth and gums and causes tooth decay. Xylitol gum appears to suppress oral bacteria levels. A study (*Journal of the American Dental Association* July 2000) revealed that bacteria levels rose in people chewing aspartame gum or in those who did not chew gum at all.

HYDROGEN PEROXIDE (H2O2)

Hydrogen peroxide can destroy the beneficial anaerobic (live without oxygen) bacteria that are normal to the colon. This is why it is best to avoid the rectal use of hydrogen peroxide by colon hydrotherapist, or when having an enema. If you do use hydrogen peroxide, follow up with rectal replacement of probiotics, especially the beneficial bifidobacteria. Since the bacteria in the upper small bowel are partially aerobic (can live with oxygen), it is fine to use hydrogen peroxide as an oral wash.

Hydrogen peroxide is approved for agricultural use, which includes the drinking water for animals and to spray on crops. Hydrogen peroxide can help to restore the beneficial soil bacteria destroyed by the overuse of pesticides and fertilizers. It can be used as a bath for fresh vegetables instead of chlorine to remove pesticide residues, but only buy "food-grade" hydrogen peroxide. See the section on food washes for more information.

LACTOFERRIN

Lactoferrin is the second most abundant protein in human colostrum, which is the first milk secreted naturally in the milk of mammals. It has a positive influence on the composition of the intestinal microflora of infants and plays a role in the development of a healthy and functional immune system. This helps to fight off infections by being highly effective against a broad range of bacteria such as *Escherichia coli, Staphylococcus epidermidis, Streptococcus pheumoniae, Streptococcus aureus, Vibro cholerae, Pseudomonas aeruginosa, Klebsiella pneumoniae,* and the yeast *Candida albicans*. It does not seem to harm most beneficial bacteria, and even promotes the growth of bifidobacteria in the colon.

MASTIC GUM

Mastic oil comes from the sap of a rare cousin of the pistachio tree. Until recently, mastic was hard to find because the bushy *Pistacia lentiscus* tree grew only on the island of Chios, in the Mediterranean. For centuries, people of this region have cooked with the tree's oil. They have also chewed gum made from its resin to freshen breath and soothe stomach pains. Mastic disappeared from medicine for many centuries because when universities were established, the knowledge about herbal medicine was not included. Now, researchers are beginning to confirm that mastic kills *Helicobacter pylori*, but this treatment is still virtually unknown in the United States.

The *New England Journal of Medicine* (December 1998) discussed the positive effects of mastic gum on *H. pylori*. The *London Times* recently reported that mastic gum was a remedy in the treatment of ulcers, and that the herb has recently been hailed for its potent antibacterial properties. Laboratory tests indicate that this substance can kill at least seven strains of *H. pylori*.

A course of treatment is four to eight 250 mg capsules a day for four weeks. When 70 percent of these people were re-examined, the ulcers were completely replaced by normal cells, and there were not any side effects reported. The article went on to say that even the small number of ulcers that are not caused by *H. pylori* were still helped by mastic gum. This substance appears to have protective and healing effects on damaged tissue caused by the use of aspirin and nonsteroidal anti-inflammatories.

MINERALS

Minerals are responsible for cellular and enzymatic functions throughout the body, including the activation of vitamins. Trace minerals primarily function as activators of enzyme substrate complexes where they serve as cofactors to influence the reactions that keep the body healthy. A deficiency in any one of them keeps the immune system from functioning properly. An example of what minerals can do is found in the following information. Some minerals can be harmful at times, especially iron.

Iron reduces the body's ability to fight off bacteria since nearly all bacteria require iron to transform nutrients into energy. Without this mineral, bacteria cannot grow and multiply. One of the body's defense mechanisms is to reduce plasma iron in order to limit bacterial growth.

When the body's temperature is raised to fever levels the growth of bacteria is inhibited, but not if the iron levels are too high. The obvious conclusion is that iron supplementation is not a good idea during acute infections and is probably just as detrimental when there is a chronic overgrowth of bacteria in the body.

Yet, iron deficiency is a common encounter especially in women and causes immune dysfunction in about twenty million people in the United States. A marginal iron deficiency can influence the immune system, even if the anemia is mild. In these cases, energy usually improves after taking twenty milligrams per day. Too much calcium and magnesium block iron absorption. It is best absorbed after eating, with the addition of a small quantity of vitamin C (100 to 500 mg). Too much iron in the body reduces zinc absorption, which also weakens the immune system. Iron interferes with the absorption of manganese and molybdenum and destroys vitamin E. If you do not have an iron deficiency, avoid taking iron in your supplements because you may be doing more harm than good.

Other minerals such as manganese and selenium provide help for the immune system. Manganese increases natural killer cell activity through increased interferon production. Selenium is associated with depression of the immune system when it is deficient. It also has a role as an antioxidant giving it a protective effect against free radical damage to the thymus and lymph system and other immune dependent organs.

A deficiency in zinc increases susceptibility to infection. Zinc not only functions as part of the immune system response, but in digestion, detoxification, and taste bud effectiveness. Zinc is also protective against free radical damage. A lack of stomach acid, which may be caused by infection or acid-lowering medication, also interferes with zinc absorption. One way to insure that you are getting enough of these important elements is to take a quality hypoallergenic multivitamin and mineral supplement each day.

MUSHROOMS

Different species of mushrooms have been known for thousands of years to hold healing powers. In Asia, Russia and Europe, mushrooms are sought for medicinal purposes, especially for use as antibacterial agents. Their resistance to microbial attack is apparent from their hardiness in dark, moist environments where they thrive, unaffected by viruses, bacteria, and even other fungi. The lower fungi (molds) were the first sources of antibiotics such as penicillin, erythromycin, and tetracycline.

The higher fungi (mushrooms) make potent antibacterial and antiviral compounds to protect themselves against microbes that would otherwise compromise their growth. The mushrooms that contain some of the best health benefits for the immune system include maitake (*Grifola frondosa*), shiitake (*Lentinus edodes*), and reishi (*Ganoderma lucidum*). The active ingredient that they have in common is beta glucan, but not all beta glucans are the same. They vary by their chemical structure.

The beta glucan obtained from maitake mushrooms has a unique and complex chemical structure that may make it more potent than other medicinal mushrooms. Due to its strong ability to enhance immune activities it may be useful in any chronic immune deficiency. Maitake contains properties to protect the liver from damage and may reverse some damage that has already occurred.

Shiitake is probably the most popular of all the exotic mushrooms. It has been a major contributor to Asian medicine for thousands of years, especially in China and Japan. The shiitake mushroom is full of nutritional value. Part of the healing properties of this mushroom is its ability to stimulate the production of white blood cells that ingest foreign invaders and increases the activity of the immune system allowing the body to heal itself.

Reishi has healing properties that cleanses the blood, supports the immune system, strengthens the circulation, and supports the body when it is under stress. Reishi also has great nutritional values that help strengthen the nervous system and helps with stress related conditions. There are many varieties of reishi, but they all contain some health benefits. The liver is essential for a healthy body and this mushroom can be helpful in strengthening this organ. It aids the adrenal glands, which may be how it helps with allergies. Reishi has the ability to exert an overall normalizing effect on the body, as well as preventing and treating infection and restore normal immune function in autoimmune diseases.

Since maitake and shiitake are edible mushrooms that can be eaten as food or made into tea, it is believed that they are safe to use as medicine as well. Reishi is also consider very safe. It is unknown if all of these claims are true, but these mushrooms certainly have enough healing power to be considered adaptogens, which are capable of helping the body to resist stress of all kinds.

Another substance to consider is kombucha (*Fungus japonicus*), which is actually a combination of yeast and bacteria. Though not technically a mushroom, kombucha contains many similar healing properties. One of these is its ability to detoxify the body. It helps clean toxins from the entire body and increases the function of the immune system.

MSM (METHYLSULFONYLMETHANE)

This compound is a natural organic sulfur found in all living things and normally found in food, but destroyed by cooking, processing, storage, and preserving. MSM is one of the main sources of bioavailable sulfur and is as necessary in the diet as vitamin C. Sulfur plays an indispensable role in human nutrition. It is radically different from the harmful sulfurs that include sulfa, sulfate, sulfite, and sulfide.

MSM participates in detoxification and in enzymatic pathways of human metabolism, as well as an antioxidant. MSM can help with some digestive complaints, allergies, and pain. It appears to be generally nonallergic and nontoxic, and enhances tissue flexibility and resilience. It also has a normalizing effect on the immune system. Other uses have been to reduce inflammation, improve peristalsis and therefore decrease constipation, reduce muscle spasms, and reduce scar tissue. MSM can be antiparasitic, particularly if the infestation is from the protozoan *Giardia*.

N-ACETYL CYSTEINE (NAC)

NAC is a nutrient with previously unforeseen benefits for cell growth protection, general detoxification, quenching free radicals, and promoting immune function. It appears to help with the neutralization of some heavy metals such as mercury, cadmium, and lead. NAC not only has the ability to eliminate intestinal toxins, it is an excellent resource for aiding detoxification of other toxic substances foreign to the body. The suggested use of NAC may range from 600 to 1800 mg per day.

N-ACETYL GLUCOSAMINE (NAG)

Glucosamine is an important nutrient for intestinal function. It is a major constituent of the barrier layer that protects the intestinal lining from digestive enzymes and other potentially damaging intestinal content. For this barrier layer to be adequately maintained, its rate of replacement must match or exceed the rate at which it is being worn away. The integrity of the digestive tract is a prerequisite for healthy digestion and absorption, as well as for normal discrimination between self and nonself. Alcohol and nonsteroidal anti-inflammatory drugs (NAIDS), including aspirin and other salicylates, can adversely affect this barrier layer. The overgrowth of pathogen bacteria, bacterial infections, and parasites, will further compromise intestinal integrity.

OLD MAN'S BEARD (USNEA SPP)

In some cases this lichen is as powerful as penicillin. Over 50 percent of the *Usnea* species tested contained antibiotic properties. It is effective against gram-positive bacteria such as *Streptococcus* (strep throat), *Staphylococcus* (impetigo), and *Mycobacterium* tuberculosis (TB). It has little effect on gram-negative bacteria such as *Salmonella* and *E. coli* that inhabit the digestive tract. This may be good news for the *E. coli* that is part of the normal microflora of the human digestive tract. This strain of *E. coli* does not usually cause harm, but may be disturbed when a broad-spectrum antibiotic is used.

In Europe, many antibacterial and antifungal creams contain *Usnea*. This lichen is often effective against lupus, an autoimmune disease. The most widely researched commercial preparation is called "Usno," made in Finland. It is effective against a wide range of bacteria and also some fungi that cause athlete's foot and ringworm. When taken internally, it primarily helps the urinary tract, respiratory system, and the gastrointestinal tract. For any infection, inside or out, consider using *Usnea*, especially when the pathogen is a gram-positive bacterium.

The alcohol tincture is the strongest form of the herb, since the active constituent is not water soluble. Other active ingredients are not alcohol soluble unless prepared by being mechanically ground first, but dissolve better in water. An alcohol/water combination is probably the best form to get the most medicine out of this lichen. Externally, apply full strength with a cotton swab for small cuts, especially if infected. Put a dropperful in water and gargle several times a day for sore or strep throat. Put drops of the tincture in water, fill a plastic spray bottle, and squirt a small quantity up the nasal passages several times daily for sinus infections.

As a preventative or for immune stimulation take thirty to sixty drops of the tincture up to four times a day. For acute bacterial infections, 1 teaspoon up to six times a day. It can be used as a vaginal douche for infections. Add 1/2 ounce tincture to 1 pint water. Douche twice a day for three days. Usnea tincture can be irritating to the mucous membranes of the mouth and throat. It should be diluted in a glass of water or other liquid before taking it. This is not considered a toxic plant in humans.

OLIVE LEAF (OLEA EUROPEA)

Olive leaf has as one of its active components, calcium elenolate, which has extraordinary effects against some bacterial pathogens. It directly stimulates the white blood cells that gobble up the bacteria. Many chronic infections can be treated with olive leaf extract because it is reported to be effective against the whole spectrum of organisms that cause disease.

Many olive leaf products give disappointing results because they are made from inferior ingredients. This is one time that the source is everything. The best source is the original species from Italy, *Olea europea,* and not the hybrid American varieties. You want the olive leaves to come from trees grown in rich, toxic-free soil, not near polluted cities with toxic water irrigation. It is also important that the leaves and buds are processed properly. A bitter compound from the leaf, called oleuropein, gives the trees powerful disease-resistant properties. Oleuropein is present throughout the olive tree, but is eliminated when the olives are cured.

At the dose of four caps daily, recurrent bladder infections were eliminated and did not recur even after six month. I frequently hear my patients comment about an increase in energy after taking olive leaf extract. Many continue to take the product even after their illness is gone. Since fatigue seems to be the number one problem facing many people today, taking a couple of these capsules a day may offer something safe, effective, and energizing for a tired person.

Some of the conditions olive leaf is successful against are sinus and bladder infections. It is also responsive to mouth infections including tooth or gum disease. Start with two capsules followed by another capsule every four hours. For more serious infections, take at shorter intervals. Olive leaf extract is not a panacea. Use it in connection with other holistic treatment programs that include dietary changes, nutritional supplements, exercise, and stress control. A comprehensive program will lead to greater success.

This plant's antibacterial properties have been used against the following bacteria: *Bacillus cereus*, *H. pylori*, *E. coli*, *Pseudomonas*, *Corynebacterium*, *Bacillus subtilis*, *Staphylococcus aureus*, and others. It is also effective against many respiratory diseases of bacterial origin. Olive leaf may prevent food poisoning if you are already taking it when eating contaminated food. Take some with you when you travel if you are concerned about the quality of the food and water.

Olive leaf is extremely safe and nontoxic even at high doses. You may need to find the optimum dosage for you. No known studies have been conducted with regards to pregnancy or nursing mothers, or any interaction with pharmaceuticals. Russian olive leaves, or species other than the domesticated European olive leaf, may make you ill.

OSHA ROOT (LIGUSTICUM PORTERI)

Osha root used in tincture form has successfully treated strep throat when several different antibiotics have already failed. *Streptococcus* is the gram-positive bacterium that causes strep throat. Osha is frequently recommended for use at the first sign of a respiratory infection. Although there have not been any double-blind studies to verify this, osha does seem to inhibit the growth of various bacteria. Like other bitter herbs, this plant tends to improve symptoms of indigestion and increase appetite. Osha tends to be safe, but it has not been tested in young children, nursing women, or those with severe liver or kidney disease.

PANCREATIC ENZYMES

Digestive enzymes produced by the pancreas is largely responsible for keeping the small intestine free from disease-causing bacteria, as well as protozoa, yeast, and intestinal worms. When pancreatin enzymes and other digestive enzymes are reduced or lacking, it puts people at risk of having an intestinal overgrowth of undesirable organisms.

PEPPERMINT OIL (MENTHA PIPERITA)

Peppermint has been used for thousands of years for its medicinal benefits. It helps to relieve pain in both children and adults suffering from stomach and intestinal disorders. It is used as a digestive aid and eases gas, burping, and bloating after eating. It may be used for gripping pain in the intestines as well as for nausea, diarrhea, flatulence, and inflammatory bowel disease. Peppermint is a gastric stimulant and tends to stimulate the flow of stomach digestive fluid necessary for healthy digestion. It strengthens and tones the stomach and is specific for irritable bowel syndrome. Peppermint oil may not be a cure for some digestive problems, but it comes in handy in the meanwhile.

PHENOLIC ACIDS

Acids such as ferulic acid and caffeic acid are present in certain foods and inhibit the activity of bacterial enzymes. Tomato juice is a major source of ferulic acid. It is known that bacteria can produce compounds capable of forming chemical alteration that lead to mutations and cell damage. This may be where information about the anticancer effects of tomatoes came from. Ferulic acid is also a common ingredient in fruits, vegetables, and whole grains. Honey is another food high in ferulic acid, as well as caffeic acid. When honey was tested against twenty-one different bacteria and two different types of fungi, it was found to limit microbial growth.

PROBIOTICS

Most cases of *H. pylori* are related to an imbalance of bacteria in the intestinal system. This is easily repaired with the use of *Lactobacillus acidophilus* and *L. bifidus*. Taking megadoses of probiotics would be the equivalent of using probiotics as an antibiotic. It may take four to five months to get rid of *H. pylori* this way. The dose of probiotic needs to be around 500 billion colony-forming units (cfu) per day. It would be better to have a plan and to use several substances discussed here. See Chapter 16 in this section for more information on probiotics.

PROPOLIS

This supplement was recommended for the healing of wounds and ulcers as far back as 300 B.C. by Hippocrates. This yellow-brown sticky resin is collected from plants by some species of bees. It is the bee glue used to repair and coat the inner surfaces of their hives, as well as inhibit the growth of microorganisms within the hive. Bees also use propolis to embalm the carcasses of hive invaders. The meaning of the word *propolis* is derived from the Greek to mean "for or in defense of the city." In Europe, propolis is usually collected from the buds of poplar, birch, elm, conifer, and horse chestnut trees.

Caffeic acid has a wide range of antibacterial activities and is thought to be one of the active factors in propolis. One study showed propolis' ability to inhibit *Bacillus subtilis*, *Proteus vulgaris*, and *Bacillus alvei*. It is thought to be active against the tuberculosis bacilli, *Mycobacterium*. It was not as effective against many *Salmonella species* and *E. coli*, or *Klebsiella pneumoniae*.

The alcohol extract of propolis may increase the effects of certain antibiotics. In some cases the effects were increased ten to one hundred fold. Antibiotic-resistant strains of *Staphylococcus aureus* became sensitive to erythromycin, tetracycline, penicillin, streptomycin, and cloxacillin, when these drugs were used in combination with propolis.

Some of its external uses are to heal and soothe bedsores, cold sores, shingles, and acne. Propolis is being included in toothpaste and mouthwashes. It can be found in other products used to treat chronic oral cavity problems such as gingivitis and periodontal disease. Topical use on surgical wounds, burns, and skin ulcers healed 80 percent faster when compared to conventional healing methods. The alcohol tincture is best applied undiluted as paint. If this causes excessive discomfort, it can be diluted with a minimum quantity of water. If an alcohol tincture of propolis is placed on the skin, it leaves a yellow stain that is not readily removed by water.

Caution: Anyone sensitive to balsam of Peru or poplar bud should avoid the use of this substance as well. The properties are similar. No studies have been performed on the use of propolis during pregnancy or lactation. Be aware that there has been an increase use of this substance in skincare products and may cause skin rashes in some sensitive people.

RICE VINEGAR

Similar to all types of white vinegar, rice vinegar is a powerful antiseptic. It kills dangerous bacteria on contact. This includes bacteria such as *Salmonella* and *Streptococcus*. The sushi industry is largely dependent on vinegar's ability to prevent germs from growing on raw fish. Japanese housewives add a little rice vinegar to summer rice to prevent it from spoiling. Apple cider vinegar has also been effective against bacteria and parasites.

White vinegar can kill bacteria on vegetables intended for eating. Leave it on your vegetables in a vinegar solution for fifteen minutes. In

Ethiopia, vinegar is being tested as an agent to kill foodborne parasites. Early results show vinegar is doing a good job. Heinz U.S.A. has introduced a white vinegar intended just for cleaning, being twice as strong as conventional vinegar. It promises to make cleaning and disinfecting easier, but should not be used for cooking or as a dietary supplement.

ROBERT'S FORMULA

Usually, herbs are used in combinations instead of just one at a time. One classic example of such a combination is Robert's formula. It contains marshmallow root (*Althea officinalis*), spotted cranebill (*Geranium maculatum*), goldenseal (*Hydrastis canadensis*), echinacea (*Echinacea angustifolia*), slippery elm (*Ulmus fulva*), and cabbage powder. Robert's formula has soothing properties that help to heal ulcers in the stomach or further down the digestive tract. These herbs also have antibiotic properties and can stimulate the immune system.

SARSAPARILLA (SMILAX OFFICINALIS)

Sarsparilla has been used historically all over the world. Evidence seems to support sarsaparilla as an endotoxin binder. Endotoxins are cell wall constituents of bacteria that are absorbed from the gut. Normally, the liver plays a vital role by filtering these toxins before they reach the general circulation. If the amount of endotoxins absorbed are excessive, or if the liver is not functioning adequately, the liver can become overwhelmed and endotoxins will spill into the bloodstream. If endotoxins are allowed to circulate, they can be responsible for much of the inflammation and cell damage that occurs in many diseases, including gout, arthritis, and psoriasis. It has also been used for fevers, digestive disorders, and other skin diseases.

It is common for individuals with psoriasis to have high levels of circulating endotoxins. Binding of endotoxins in the gut is associated with improved symptoms. Sarsaparilla also exhibits some antibiotic activity, but this is probably secondary to its endotoxin-binding actions. Because sarsaparilla reduces the stress on the liver and bloodstream, this is probably why it has been used historically as a tonic and blood purifier. Although no adverse effects have been reported, it is possible that problems could arise if large doses were used over a long period.

SIBERIAN GINSENG (ELEUTHEROCOCCUS SENTICOSUS)

I have included this plant because of its ability to increase nonspecific resistance in humans against numerous pathogens by enhancing the immune system. This includes an increase in white blood cells that protect us against germs. It is also known to help us withstand adverse conditions, increase mental alertness, and improve performance. Many people report that after taking Siberian ginseng they have fewer illnesses. In traditional Chinese medicine, this plant was sought for its ability to restore vigor, memory, good appetite, and increase longevity. This plant is thought to produce cumulative results. The longer you use it, the better it works. It may take six weeks to six months or longer to see results, especially in people who have very depressed immune systems. Siberian ginseng is also indicated in people with fatigue and a lack of vitality and vigor. It is an immune enhancer and helps to restore the immune system to optimum functioning. This plant is considered a nontoxic herb even when used in large doses.

Although Siberian ginseng shares some of the pharmacological properties of Chinese ginseng, it is not from the same plant family. Do not confused it with American ginseng either, because they have different uses. Also, the Chinese and American ginseng should not be used in self-treatment by anyone under the age of forty because of their hormone affects.

SPICES

Some spices may be lethal against some bacteria. The Institute of Food Technologists released a report that researchers at Kansas State University made an interesting discovery. They inoculated apple juice samples with about one million of the pathogen E. coli 0157:H7 bacteria. Then they added one teaspoon of cinnamon. It killed 99.5 percent of the bacteria in three days at room temperature. This amount of bacteria is one hundred times the number typically found in contaminated food. If using certain spices prove to be antibacterial in unpasteurized juices and other foods, it could replace other methods and preservatives for keeping foods safe.

If cinnamon can be effective against one of the most virulent foodborne pathogens today (E. coli 0157:H7), it may have the same effect on other common pathogens such as *Salmonella* and *Campylobacter*. Cinnamon, as well as clove and garlic, may be powerful antimicrobial agents. Unfortunately, they did not work as well in raw ground beef and sausage as they did in liquids such as apple juice. Liquids may be a better medium to kill pathogens since there are no hiding places.

According to *Herbal Antibiotics* by Stephen Buhner, herbs have been used in our foods for years for protecting us from infectious and pathogenic disease. A group of researchers at Cornell University examined traditional food preparations for the effectiveness of spices. They found that as the local climate increases its temperature the number of spices used in food also increases. The hot climates uses lots of spices and the cold climates seldom use any.

The spices most commonly used all possessed powerful antimicrobial activity. The most powerful were garlic, onion, allspice, and oregano. They also discovered that combining spices often were more effective at killing germs than using them alone. These multiple spice combinations became the most effective when combined with salt and when lemon or lime juice was added during cooking.

THYME (THYMUS VULGARIS)

Thyme appears to inhibit *Helicobacter pylori* (*H. pylori*). This bacterium is now recognized as a common cause of chronic gastritis, peptic ulceration, and gastric cancer. The highest activities were demonstrated by the use of a water extract of thyme and to a lesser degree from an alcohol extract. A dried thyme water extract at a concentration of 4.5 mg/ml was sufficient to completely inhibit the growth of *H. pylori* in a laboratory sample. Thyme is a powerful antiseptic that helps destroy fungal infections, skin parasites, and kills intestinal worms. It also stimulates the immune system and aids in digestion. Thyme has been used for fungal and bacterial skin disorders and as a mouthwash to reduce oral bacteria.

The antibacterial and antifungal activity of the essential oil of thyme is well recognized. Thymol is one component of the essential oil. Brief exposure to low concentrations of thymol rapidly killed pathogenic bacteria in the mouth. Components of thyme oil were effective against seven strains of gram-positive and gram-negative bacteria. Thyme oil and thymol decreased the growth of *Salmonella typhimurium*, and was antibacterial against *Staphylococcus spp.* and *Sarcina spp.* A broad spectrum of activity was observed for thymol against bacteria causing upper respiratory tract infections. A significant amount of this oil is excreted in the urine, making it slightly useful as a urinary antiseptic. Another plant that contains 60 percent thymol is horsemint (*Monarda punctata*).

The ability of thymol to kill microorganisms is significantly reduced by the presence of proteins. There are no known contraindications or special precautions, but thymol is a powerful disinfecting agent and can cause irritation to the tissues. Some people have been known to get a skin rash if the essential oil is used on the skin. Internally there have not been reports of overdoses when taken in therapeutics amounts. It would take a significant amount of plant material to obtain enough oil to become toxic levels. There have been reports of poisoning when doses of 0.2 to 1 ml of pure oil has been consumed at one time.

TRACE MINERALS

In general, trace minerals aid in the repair and healing of body tissues. Zinc and manganese are especially important for tissue repair and mucus production. Having an adequate supply of trace minerals inhibits the development of ulcers and has therapeutic effects as well. You do not have to take these nutrients separately, but are available in a good multiple vitamin-mineral supplement.

TRANSFER FACTOR

Transfer factors are components in colostrum, a substance that rapidly defends an infant's immature immune system. Otherwise, when a baby is born, invading microorganisms could rapidly overcome and destroy the new life. Immunity is established rapidly if the baby is allowed to nurse. Infants who are not breastfed consistently show a greater susceptibility to infections and allergies.

Transfer factors can be used by other species other than the source from where it came, which is usually cows. Transfer factors are small immune messenger molecules whose role is to transfer immune recognition signals between immune cells. They assist in educating naive immune cells about a present or potential danger, such as identifying pathogens as hostile invaders. With the presence of this substance, an immune system is capable of recognizing an infection and fighting it off before it can do any significant damage. An immature immune response may take ten to fourteen days to fully develop. Such a delay may be too late to help with an acute illness. Transfer factors can induce an immune response in less than twenty-four hours.

The process used in preparing transfer factors removes lactose from the final product resulting in little risk of milk allergies or lactose intolerance. Transfer factors are equally effective whether administered by injection or taken orally. The immunity provided is long lived and can help people of all ages who are suffering from a variety of ailments. Infants and the elderly are the two groups especially at risk for infections. Taking this substance appears to be very safe.

There have been claims that transfer factor has been successful in the treatment of fibromyalgia and chronic fatigue syndrome, as well as Lyme disease. These and other illnesses caused by infectious organisms may benefit from substances such as this. Since some of these illnesses result from new bacterial strains, as well as known strains that have developed resistance to antibiotics, it is important to find more alternatives to drug therapy for combating these pathogens.

TURMERIC (CURCUMA LONGA)

Turmeric is a popular herb familiar to many of us as the orange-yellow spice responsible for the color and distinctive taste of curries. India produces nearly the whole world's crop and uses 80 percent of it. This herb is highly toxic to *Salmonella* in the presence of visible light, but not to *E. coli*. This phototoxicity potential might be useful in the treatment of skin disorders such as psoriasis and in skin infections cause by bacteria.

Some of the properties of turmeric are anti-inflammatory, antioxidant, and the ability to decrease liver cholesterol. An alcoholic extract of turmeric, its essential oil and curcumin inhibited the growth of gram-positive bacteria, but much weaker than conventional antibiotics. The essential oil of turmeric has significant antifungal activity at the proper dilutions. The essential oil also increases bile secretion.

Turmeric is listed as generally safe for its intended use as a spice, seasoning, and flavoring agent. No adverse effects are expected when consumed within the recommended dosage. In high doses, it may cause minor discomforts, such as heartburn or stomach upset. Combining this herb with bromelain may enhance its absorption and activity. High doses should not be given to people taking antiplatelet or anticoagulant drugs. If using topically, cautioned should be used against excessive exposure to sunlight. Care should be given in women who wish to conceive or if complaining of hair loss.

UVA URSI (ARCTOSTAPHYLOS UVA URSI)

Uva ursi commonly known as bearberry or uva ursi, has a long history of use for urinary tract infections, but is often overlooked as a great herbal medication for the overgrowth of many intestinal organisms. Researchers usually focuses on the active constituent, arbutin, but using the combination of all the constituents working together gives uva ursi its urinary and intestinal antimicrobial properties. This herb's antibacterial components work most effectively in an alkaline environment.

The following pathogens are sensitive to the medicinal properties of uva ursi: *Klebsiella, Proteus vulgaris, Ureaplasma urealyticum, Mycoplasma hominis, Pseudomonas aeruginosa, Enterococcus faecalis,* and *Citrobacter.* This herb also has active properties to fight *Staphylococcus aureus* and *Escherichia coli* infections, and many types of yeast.

The pH of urine produced by a healthy individual on a meat and fish diet is 4.5—6.0; a vegetarian diet will be more alkaline. If the urine pH during a urinary tract infection is above 7, this usually indicates the release of ammonia and implicates the following bacteria. *Proteus spp., Klebsiella spp.,* some *Citrobacter spp.,* some *Haemophilus spp., Bilophila wadsworthia*, the yeast *Cryptococcus neoformans* and several other bacteria and fungi. Infections with these organisms should respond to treatment with bearberry. Treatment will be more effective if the urine is made even more alkaline with a buffering agent such as sodium bicarbonate, sodium citrate, citric acid and tartaric acid.

Another method of alkalinizing the urine is to take a multimineral formula where the minerals are chelated to citrate, malate, fumarate, or succinate. You could also make the urine alkaline by taking 1/2 teaspoon of baking soda or a tablet of Alka Seltzer Gold. This increases the potency of the herb. Uva ursi should not be taken with any substance that causes the urine to be acidic, since this reduces the antibacterial effect. An alkaline pH can be maintained by consuming a diet rich in vegetables, fruits and fruit juices, potatoes, etc.

Uva ursi should not be used long term because the high tannin content may irritate the stomach or cause cramping, nausea, vomiting and constipation. The high tannin levels can also cause various nutrients to be malabsorbed. It is to be avoided in pregnant or lactating women or children less than twelve years. Sometimes the diuretic action of uva ursi keeps people up at night with frequent visits to the bathroom. It may be best to take this herb earlier in the day.

VITAMIN A

Vitamin A is the "anti-infective" vitamin and stimulates or enhances numerous immune processes. This vitamin helps the thymus work better and can actually promote thymus growth. Since vitamin A is fat-soluble, a person who cannot digest fat will also have a problem getting enough of this vitamin. The health of the gut and adequate stomach acid production makes a difference in how well vitamin A is metabolized by the body.

Besides being converted into vitamin A, beta-carotene functions as an antioxidant and quenches free radicals. Since the thymus gland is very susceptible to free radical damage, taking beta-carotene may enhance the immune system even more than vitamin A.

VITAMIN B6

A deficiency of vitamin B6 results in the depression of the immune system in general. Factors that predispose a person to a deficiency of vitamin B6 are excessive protein intake, consumption of yellow dyes, alcohol use, taking oral contraception, and low dietary intake.

Vitamins: Natural vs. Synthetic

Since 1939, as dictated by federal law, all refined flour, grain, and rice products, as well as many processed foodstuffs, are "spike," or fortified, with synthetic vitamins. Some breakfast cereals contain particularly high doses of synthetic vitamins as well as inorganic minerals. For all these years, people of the U.S. have had a daily ration of synthetic vitamins put into their foods.

One of the worse deceptions is passing off on a gullible public synthetic vitamins, or crystalline-pure fractions of vitamin complexes, and saying that the body does not know the difference. Counterfeit supplements can seriously impair the most important of body functions by contributing to biochemical imbalances. Synthetic vitamins are reverses or mirror images of natural vitamins. Because the structure is reversed, a left-handed molecule cannot take part in a chemical reaction meant for a right-handed molecule any more than a left hand can fit in a right-handed glove. This odd geometry would prevent it from being metabolized properly by the body and therefore properly utilized.

A synthetic vitamin can be utilized for its drug or pharmacological effect, but the body requires real vitamins to repair tissues and cells and to restore the body's approximately twenty-four billion cells that break down each day. In most instances, the body needs vitamins in their natural form and all of the minerals in an organic form to maintain health.

Natural vitamins carry with them trace mineral activators. The body cannot work properly without them and fail the body when synthetically manufactured. They also fail when derived by refining or isolating them, even from natural sources. Whole foods, especially fruits and vegetables, pack disease-preventing clout. They harbor hundreds of phytochemicals giving the body a source of extraordinary protection. Examples of what vitamins can do for you are discussed in this chapter.

VITAMIN B12 AND FOLIC ACID

Deficiencies in vitamin B and folic acid result in improper white blood cell production and abnormal responses of the immune system. Folic acid deficiency is common in the United States. Not having enough of both of them can lead to impairment by the body to kill pathogen bacteria. This goes for the other B vitamins as well. Folic acid also plays a very important role in the healthy development of fetuses.

VITAMIN C

This popular vitamin plays a big role in enhancing the immune system. Depletion of this vitamin also destabilizes the integrity of the liver's ability to detoxify. It has been shown to be antibacterial mainly by making the body more resistant to disease. It is important that bioflavonoids be taken as the same time since these compounds raise the effects of vitamin C.

Natural ascorbic acid is derived from citrus fruits, ascerola cherries, rose hips, green peppers, and other fruits and vegetables. However, most of the ascorbic acid vitamin C on the market is synthetically produced from corn sugar. Even when it is synthetically manufactured, it can be called natural and organic, because corn sugar comes from corn and corn is found in nature. In this case, the term natural is misleading and rendered meaningless.

VITAMIN E

Vitamin E not only increases a healthy response of the immune system, but also prevents free radical induced damage. Vitamin E doses of 300 IU per day have been shown to inhibit bacteria's activity in test tubes, but it is not known if this occurs in the body.

CHAPTER 18

Treating Bacterial Overgrowth with Homeopathy

DURING ITS 170 years of existence, homeopathy has been opposed by orthodox medicine. It was developed in Germany by the research of Dr. Samuel Hahnemann (1755–1834), who was an experienced physician and a competent chemist, mineralogist, and botanist, and an able translator of eight different languages. His research stemmed from dissatisfaction with the standard medical practices of his time.

As far back as Hippocrates (460–377 B.C.) it was mentioned that cinchona (an extract of quinine bark) could be used as a treatment for swamp fever because of its value as a stomach tonic, but Hahnemann disagreed. He decided to take a course of cinchona extract himself. To his surprise, he developed a set of symptoms remarkably similar to those of swamp fever. All the symptoms disappeared when he stopped taking the herb. From this event Hahnemann produced the first axiom of homeopathy, which is "like cures like," and this became known as the Law of Similars.

Hahnemann's approach to medicine represented a dramatic move away from the established method of the day, which was by the use of opposites. For example, an illness that produces fever and diarrhea would call for the combined use of medicines that were antifever and anticonstipation. Orthodox medicine works to suppress symptoms. The results are seen in the inhibitory medicines produced by antihistamines, antibiotics, and antacids.

In order to prove the Law of Similars, it is first important to test a substance for medicinal use by giving it to healthy volunteers and carefully noting the symptoms it produces. For example, a substance that produces a runny nose, watery, red eyes and repeated sneezing would be of great value in treating hay fever. The common onion produces just those symptoms and makes a good remedy for this type of allergy. It is important that the symptoms match closely before onion will have a therapeutic effect. The most effective results will come from the most similar remedy.

The second thing that must be observed in treatment is the "Law of the Minimal Dose." This states that the effective dose for a disorder is the minimum amount necessary to produce a response. The process is known as potentization, and involves a sequence of progressive dilutions and a rhythmic shaking called succussion.

It is interesting that one of the very earliest laws of pharmacology, known as the Arndt-Schulz Law expresses the homeopathic effect. Formulated by Arndt in 1888, the law states that for every substance small doses stimulate, moderate doses inhibit, large doses kill. Homeopathic medicine begins at the stimulatory end of the curve and moves to smaller and smaller doses. Its emphasis is on the stimulation of the body's natural balancing mechanisms. Because of the use of very diluted doses, the toxicity of homeopathy is very low. The medicines are regarded as acting more strongly as the dilution increases.

Homeopathic Remedies For Food Poisoning

Food poisoning is the frequent source of sudden and violent abdominal pain along with nausea, vomiting, cramping pains, and explosive diarrhea. There are different kings of food poisoning. Some forms are the result of eating poisonous plants, fish toxins, shellfish poisoning, and bacteria-tainted meats, fruits, and vegetables. Most of the causes of bacteria caused food poisoning is because of improperly cooked, handled, stored or refrigerated foods.

Most common food poisonings are usually short in duration and self-limiting. The onset usually begins with acute intestinal distress and then nausea, vomiting, and profuse diarrhea. Although some potentially fatal forms of food poisoning exist, such as botulism, fish and shellfish poisoning, most forms are merely exceedingly unpleasant but seldom fatal.

It is impossible to list all the available homeopathic remedies that can be used for cases of digestive upset and diarrhea. I have listed the most commonly used ones for cases of food poisoning. Homeopathy is a wonderful way to treat many health concerns and I recommend that you educated yourself with the many books available. Perhaps start with the ones on first aid and emergency care.

ARSENIUM ALBUM

Take 6x–30x potency every two to four hours, as required.

This is the most common remedy for food poisoning. Arsenium is especially good for poisoning from tainted meat, but is usually the remedy of choice in any case of food poisoning, especially if you do not know which one to use.

Diarrhea: severe diarrhea usually associated with vomiting, frequent bouts of offensive smelling and burning diarrhea

Stools: small in quantity, highly offensive in odor and dark in color, painless but burns once touches the skin

Vomiting: burning vomit that irritates the throat

Chills: chilly, person feels worse from the cold

Thirst: thirsty, but only for small sips of water at a time, prefer hot or warm drinks

Worse: symptoms become worse after midnight

Better: warm drinks may be soothing

Restless: constant changing of positions, especially in bed, cannot get comfortable

Stomach: burning pains that are worse from most foods or drinks, especially cold foods or drinks, which are quickly vomited, abdomen is swollen and painful with gnawing and burning pains

Miscellaneous: feel very weak and the person cannot bear the sight or smell of food, great debility and prostration on the slightest exertion, especially in the extremities, sudden and profuse sweating, intolerance to pain, anxiety is present, for intestinal colic from food poisoning or for travelers with "turista"

IPECACUANHA (IPECAC)

Take 3x–6x potency taken every two to four hours.

This is a remedy for persistent nausea, which nothing relieves. Vomiting doesn't relieve, just as sick as before.

Stool: constant call to stool and cannot get off the toilet, very slimy stools

Vomiting: severe and continuous with salivation and persistent and constant vomiting, nausea is not relieved by vomiting, griping pains in the intestines, with or without vomiting, vomiting of food several hours after eating, vomiting of slimy white mucus

Miscellaneous: tongue is clean, even though stomach is disordered

NUX VOMICA

Take 6x–30x potency every two to three hours or as needed.

Nux vomica is good remedy to use in cases of digestive upset or for travelers with "turista." It is one of the most characteristic remedies for diarrhea in infants. A keynote symptom is "they want to, but can't."

Diarrhea: alternates with constipation

Stools: frequent stools with small evacuations; much urging to stool, stool may contain slime and blood, temporary relief after passing stool

Vomiting: vomiting with much retching after eating, feel better after vomiting, bloating and gas along with nausea

Chills: they are chilly and irritable

Worse: usually in the AM and after a big meal

Miscellaneous: They want to but can't. This is a keynote of Nux vomica whether the condition involves vomiting, moving bowels, or urinating. The person is wakeful after 3 a.m., falls asleep toward morning, and awakens feeling wretched.

PYROGEN

Take 12x–30x potency every two to four hours, as required.

This is one of the preeminent remedies in most forms of common food poisoning. Together with Arsenicum, Pyrogen most frequently comes to mind in intestinal distress. It is indicated in what is called "Camp diarrhea," which is the result of eating under less than sanitary conditions outdoors where cooking supplies are left with rancid oil or grease or drinking contaminated water or food.

Diarrhea: very offensive, brown-black stools that are painless and involuntary

Stools: large, black, and with carrion-like odor, or small and passed in black balls

Vomiting: there is vomiting, water is even vomited almost as soon as it is drunk, resembles coffee grounds

Stomach: abdomen is bloated and sore with intolerable cutting, cramping pains

VERATRUM ALBUM

Take 6x–30x potency every two to four hours or as needed.

Profuse rice water stools may indicate this remedy. A keynote symptom is "cold sweat on the forehead."

Diarrhea: very loose and profuse in quantity, acute diarrhea is accompanied by vomiting and icy cold sweat, alternates between vomiting/diarrhea
Stools: great prostration follows the stool, stools are forcefully evacuated
Vomiting: there is profuse and violent retching and vomiting; vomiting being the most characteristic symptom
Thirst: great thirst for large quantities of cold or iced fluids
Better: fresh air
Miscellaneous: cold sweat breaks out on the forehead and even over the entire body, collapse is possible, symptoms of cramps in the extremities and continued retching, do not feel restless

Nosodes

Nosodes are homeopathic dilutions of pathological organs or tissues, or weakened or killed bacteria, fungi, parasites, virus particles, or yeast. Sounds awful, but homeopathic nosodes can assist the body by desensitization and stimulation. Nosodes help the immune system recognize a disease-causing entity and assist the elimination of the pathogens naturally. They provide a template to the immune system, thereby making an indirect attack on disease by stimulating the immune system and white blood cell production.

Nosodes can be of great value in the treatment of certain diseases. They are used not only to break up the lingering effects of a disease, but also to prevent the disease from occurring in the first place. Other non-nosode remedies may be more helpful following a nosode, but it may take a nosode to prevent the disease.

Nosodes have been used throughout homeopathy's history and are recognized in all homeopathic pharmacopeias throughout the world. Historical references exist as early as 800 B.C. For example, the Chinese practiced a type of preventive vaccination where the secretions from pox lesions were sniffed. Hippocrates referred to the use of vomited material to cure vomiting. In the fifteenth century, Paracelsus wrote about the healing effect of pathological products. Because of these teachings, tuberculosis patients were treated with dilutions of their sputum and cured.

Around 1820, a German veterinarian, Wilhelm Lux, introduced homeopathy into veterinary medicine. He first worked with the blood and nasal discharge of diseased animals making them into homeopathic remedies.

The famous American homeopath, Constantin Hering, began using pathological products around 1831. He is credited with the origination of the term "nosode" from the Greek word for sickness. Hering is responsible for the expansion of information about nosodes and continued to experiment with them. He recommended the use of potentized watery excrement of cholera, the black vomit of yellow fever, the desquamated skin of malignant scarlet fever, etc. He was the first to propose that the nosodes could be used for the prevention of infectious diseases. This research was confirmed by the work of Baron von Boenninghausen who used Variolinum for the prevention of smallpox.

With the discovery and isolation of bacteria, the number of specific nosodes grew. Today, these remedies can treat a wide variety of conditions. You should not try to treat yourself with nosodes, but seek the help of someone trained in their use, since nosode therapy should be used with care. Typically an individual will become worse before improving. This worsening is a sign of how harmful the pathogen is and the level of the body's vital force response.

If someone possesses a healthy immune system, they are good candidates for nutritional, botanical, or homeopathic therapy. A person with an overwhelmed immune system, or if they are infected with a pathogen of stealth capability, then it may necessitate more drastic measures. If a person has a condition that has deteriorated into a degenerative state, they may not possess sufficient vital energy to respond to a homeopathic nosode.

Homeopathic nosode remedies, including remedies prepared from microorganisms, also work according to the "Law of Similars." This is somewhat similar to taking a vaccine. It heightens the immune response to a particular organism, such as found in the bacterial overgrowth of *Salmonella, Pseudomonas,* or *Citrobacter.* Recently, the nosode for *Mycoplasma* has become available. Usually, nosodes can be given along with other indicated homeopathic remedies.

The use of homeopathic drainage remedies (liver, lymph, etc.) in low potency are highly recommended when using nosodes. The drainage remedies enhance excretion from the body of the pathogen or its toxins. Nosodes are to be given orally ten drops under the tongue three times a day, except in the case of highly sensitive or immune compromised individuals. Then it is best to just rub into vascular areas of the skin for a few weeks, followed by gradually increasing the drops orally once a day, until you work up to the full dose.

Nosodes made from many of the pathogenic bacteria discussed in this book are now available from a naturopathic physician or from a person trained in homeopathy. This includes *Pseudomonas, Citrobacter, Klebsiella, Proteus, Mycoplasma,* and others. Even the bacteria that cause food poisoning can be found in the form of a nosode such as for botulism, *Listeria,* and *Salmonella.* With the discovery and isolation of more bacteria, and other pathogens overgrowing in the intestinal tract, even more nosodes will become available.

Severe and live-threatening illnesses such as pneumonia, meningitis, tuberculosis, and bone infections should not be treated by the inexperienced. These conditions may require conventional treatment and the expertise of a knowledgeable practitioner. If your condition continues to reoccur, this is really not an acute disease and should be treated with homeopathic care that is far more involved.

In the possible case of bioterrorism, there are homeopathic nosodes that could be helpful, if not necessary for the prevention and treatment of illnesses such as anthrax, smallpox, and cholera. The nosode for anthrax is Anthracinum. As far back as 1831, Anthracinum was used to treat anthrax. We owe it to J.W. Lux for the first known preparation and therapeutic use of Anthracinum. Two of the first that were treated were workers on a farm affected by anthrax on the hands. Both were cured.

Variolinum is the nosode for smallpox. The first preparation was made about 1830 by Dr. G. A. Weber, and applied with astonishing success in the cattle plague. He is quoted as curing every case with it and also cured men poisoned by this contagious disease. His report was published in 1836 but few people paid any attention to it. One person who did, Dr. P. Dufresne of Geneva, the founder of the *Bibliotheque Homoeopathique,* used it and prevented the spread of the disease in a flock of sheep and cured the shepherds as well.

There are reports from old writings that giving Variolinum to people during a smallpox outbreak prevented them from getting the disease. In one family, where the father already had smallpox, it was given as a prophylactic and no one else got it even though they had not been vaccinated. Another nosode may be also helpful. It is Vaccinotoxinum, which is collected by scraping the eruption of the smallpox vaccine. Also, there are reports of success using Vaccininum 6x in water several times a day with a strict diet, repeated for eight days. In more severe cases the 200th potency was used.

There is some thought that *Brucella melitensis* was used to derive a more dangerous organism such as the genetically engineered *Mycoplasma* that exists today. This species of *Brucella* is also available in the form of a nosode. Another name for the disease that is caused by this organism is brucellosis or undulating fever.

Cholera should be mentioned in case prompt action is called for and efficient medical aid is scarce. The symptoms appear in a person in apparent health who is suddenly struck down and seized by the most violent symptoms of vomiting, diarrhea and cramps. It is important to be treated quickly. There is a nosode for cholera, but three other types of homeopathic remedies could be helpful; they are Camphora,

Cuprum metallicum and Veratrum album. They are best used in the 200th potency for one or two doses or in the 30th potency every quarter to half hour until improvement sets in.

- Camphors are indicated when there is an extreme degree of prostration, surface is icy cold, complains of burning in abdomen, with desire to be uncovered.
- Cuprum metallicum is indicated when cramps are very marked, icy cold all over wants to be covered, not sweating.
- Veratrum album is indicated when they are drenched in a cold sweat, especially on the brow, marble coldness of surface of the body, violent diarrhea and vomiting.

Nosodes for botulism (*Botulinum*) and the plague (*Yersinia pestis*) are available through licensed health practitioners. Also available are nosodes for dengue fever, Legionnaire's disease, tularemia, *E. coli* and others.

APPENDIX A

Food Poisoning Agents and Their Symptoms

FOODBORNE ILLNESSES are common worldwide. Such illnesses can be caused by pathogenic bacteria, toxins produced by the bacteria growing in the food before consumption, toxins produced by the bacteria overgrowing in the intestinal tract, or a wide variety of viral and parasitic infections. *Campylobacter* and *Salmonella* are probably the most common causes of food poisoning today. Other sources of foodborne diseases include *Shigella, Listeria,* and *E. coli.* The following list contains information on the bacteria most responsible for food poisoning today:

AEROMONAS HYDROPHILIA

Aeromonas is a bacterium that is present in all freshwater environments and in brackish water. Some strains are capable of causing illness in amphibians and fish, as well as humans who become infected through open wounds or by eating or drinking enough bacteria in food or drink. Not much is known about the other species of *Aeromonas,* but they are also aquatic microorganisms and have been known to cause human disease.

Digestive symptoms are possible in people, even in healthy people. If someone has an impaired immune system or some forms of cancer, then there may be a general infection in which the bacteria spread throughout the body. The infectious dose is unknown, but SCUBA divers have become ill after drinking small amount of seawater. Only recently has there been efforts attempting to tract the incidences of infection. Most cases have been sporadic rather than associated with large outbreaks, but increased reports have been reported from several clinical centers.

Aeromonas hydrophilia is found in fish and shellfish, as well as meats (beef, pork, lamb) and poultry. Little is known about the virulence of this organism, but it is believed that not all strains cause disease, since this bacteria is commonly found in the environment. The diarrhea may be watery (rice and water) or a dysentery-type illness containing blood and mucus. On rare occasions the diarrhea is severe and may last for several weeks. People at most risk for severe infections are those with leukemia, carcinoma, and liver disease. Other people at risk are those treated with immune suppressive drugs or who are undergoing cancer chemotherapy. Infected children usually have diarrhea.

BACILLUS CEREUS

This gram-positive, bacterium is usually of low virulence being widespread in air, soil, water, dust, and animal products. *Bacillus cereus* deserves special mention because it is the specie most likely to cause opportunistic infection. It will not always cause symptoms and is usually a transient visitor, but consider it a possible pathogen in any amount. A *Bacillus* specie may be isolated from the stool in 15 percent of healthy individuals. The spores were also found in pork pancreatin glandulars, a vital nutritional component of many nutritional programs.

What you see and smell may provide some clues to the food's safety, but it is how the food was handled and stored that is most important. In 1997, a teenage boy and his father became ill after eating spaghetti with homemade pesto that they had prepared four days earlier. The pan used to reheat the pasta was only wiped clean with a paper towel. This allowed bacteria remaining in the pan to contaminate the leftovers. They developed abdominal pain, vomiting, and diarrhea, within thirty minutes of eating the food. The spaghetti had been left out at room temperature for more than an hour several times before it was reheated. The father recovered, but the boy died two days later of liver failure.

Doctors identified the cause of the illness as *Bacillus cereus*. Only three other deaths from *Bacillus cereus* have ever been reported, and this is the first known case that produced liver failure. Incidents like this one make the medical literature because of their rarity, and it is extremely unlikely that a typical case of food poisoning would become this severe. This case is brought up here because it does point out some important lessons about food safety.

Eating food that has been kept at room temperature after cooking permits the growth of bacteria. Food poisoning from this bacterium has been most associated with rice, but vegetables and meat dishes mishandled after cooking are also responsible. Leftovers should be refrigerated immediately. The spore of this bacterium survives boiling for varying periods and is sufficiently resistant to heat. When you are ready to eat leftovers, be sure to heat them thoroughly at a high heat. Unfortunately, reheating the food during preparation may kill the bacteria, but it does not eliminate the activity of the heat-stable toxin that could be present.

This organism causes two distinct types of food poisoning, one causing diarrhea and one causing vomiting. Diarrhea is associated with a wide range of foods including meats, milk, vegetables, and fish. The strain that causes vomiting usually grows on rice. It is the most likely one encountered if you get sick immediately or a few hours after eating cooked rice in Asian restaurants. This is often the result of leaving rice in a cooking wok overnight and reheating it the next day.

The vomiting type has occurred after eating other starchy foods such as potato, pasta, and cheese products. Food mixtures such as sauces, puddings, soups, casseroles, pastries, and salads have frequently been incriminated. Additional symptoms could include abdominal cramps and/or diarrhea. Duration of symptoms is generally less than twenty-four hours. The rapid onset time, along with eating rice, is often sufficient to diagnose this type of food poisoning. The symptoms do parallel those caused by *Staphylococcus aureus*.

The symptoms of the diarrhea type of food poisoning mimics those of *Clostridium perfringens*. The onset of watery diarrhea, abdominal cramps, and pain occurs six to fifteen hours after eating contaminated food. Nausea may accompany the diarrhea, but vomiting rarely occurs. Infection is usually self-limiting and persists no longer than twenty-four hours. Some people do not show any symptoms, but if they are present, they are usually mild. Rarely do symptoms become severe.

Most laboratories will not look for this organism or its toxins unless it is specifically requested. It may be found in the food, vomit, or feces of the infected person. If antibiotics are going to be used, sensitivity testing is needed because susceptibilities to penicillin, cephalosporin, and tetracyline are not predictable. Other species of *Bacillus* have been known to also cause food poisoning and have been isolated from lamb and chicken.

CAMPYLOBACTER JEJUNI

Before 1973, this gram-negative bacterium was not recognized as a cause of human disease, but primarily an animal pathogen, especially in sheep and cattle. It is relatively fragile and sensitive to environmental stresses, drying, heating, disinfectants, and acidic conditions. The toxin that is produced is destroyed by heat. *Campylobacter* may be part of the normal and healthy bowel flora in some animals such as chickens. Now, this bacterium is recognized as one of the most prevalent foodborne pathogen in the United States, accounting for nearly 2.5 million cases of infectious diarrhea each year. It causes more diarrhea illness than *Shigella* and *Salmonella* combined.

Outbreaks of *Campylobacter* are common among troops stationed in the U.S. and abroad. Usually, outbreaks only affect small groups, but one case in Bennington, Vermont, involved about two thousand people after the town temporarily used a nonchlorinated water source. Several outbreaks occurred when children drank raw milk. Another one happened after eating raw clams. However, most infections are associated with either eating inadequately cooked or recontaminated chicken meat or handling chickens.

There are estimates that almost 100 percent of retail chickens contain *Campylobacter*. This is not surprising since many healthy chickens carry these bacteria in their intestinal tracts. The bacteria are often carried by healthy cattle and by flies on farms. Nonchlorinated water sources, such as streams and ponds, may also be a source of infections. Properly cooking chicken, pasteurizing milk, and disinfecting drinking water will kill the bacteria.

The U.S. Department of Agriculture conducted a survey in 1996 and 1997 and found that more than 90 percent of turkeys tested positive. This foodborne pathogen is also found in raw eggs, unpasteurized dairy products, and raw meat. In agribusiness, chickens are routinely fed antibiotics causing further overgrowth of this organism Usually, cattle and poultry are the sources of human infection, but puppies, kittens, pigs, sheep, rodents, and birds, may also serve as carriers.

One way to pick up *Campylobacter* is by eating foods that were placed on contaminated cutting boards and counter tops. Many people use poor hygiene practices by trimming raw poultry on a cutting board, transferring it to a plate, taking it to the barbecue, cooking it, and then placing it back on the same unwashed plate or cutting board. Only cooking to the proper temperature of 160°F gets rid of it.

During Thanksgiving and Christmas, millions of turkeys will be purchased and prepared for eating. It is important to follow proper cooking instructions to avoid spending time in the emergency room. It is unfortunate that these unwelcome guests come home with you from the grocery store along with the turkey. Turkeys should be double-wrapped in plastic bags while in the refrigerator or freezer. Anything that touches a raw turkey should be scrubbed with warm, soapy water. Use a meat thermometer to ensure that the turkey is cooked to 180°F and the stuffing cooked inside the turkey reaches 165°F. In addition, use pasteurized egg substitutes in dessert and eggnog recipes that call for raw eggs. Avoid raw cider because it may contain nasty bacteria.

Campylobacter contamination is increasing in shellfish, such as oysters and clams. It poses serious health risks, especially if eaten raw. Shellfish do not usually harbor this pathogen, but acquire them by filtering water through their systems. Without killing the shellfish, the bacteria concentrate in their meat. The reason there is an increase in poisonings is because shellfish often reside in estuaries where fecal runoff from sewage can pollute the water. Researchers tested several bays and rivers in Oregon and North Carolina and found *Campylobacter* in 10 to 15 percent of the clams and oysters there.

Each state regulates its own oyster farms, but most states only require the water to be tested for *E. coli*, not *Campylobacter*. Since this bacterium concentrates in the meat, testing the water is not that predictable. The best way to test for contamination is to test the meat. *Campylobacter* species can survive for days in meat products, as well as fresh and salt water.

People who travel to Asia and those who eat pre-packed sandwiches and cold meat are among those at highest risk of infection with *Campylobacter* according to a report out of London. It is estimated that around forty-four thousand people in the United Kingdom (UK) are infected with this organism each year. Because so many people are being infected by this bacterium, it prompted officials to investigate the sources of infection.

One in five subjects had traveled outside the UK in the weeks prior to diagnosis. A large proportion of these individuals had traveled to Asia, especially to India and Pakistan. There was also a high incidence of infection among backpackers who traveled to places such as Bali. One in eight had traveled within the UK. These findings suggest that doctors should obtain a full travel history from patients if they present with symptoms.

The study also found that the source of infection within the UK was most often linked with the consumption of cold meat. Almost one in three people had eaten pre-packed sandwiches, 21 percent had eaten paté, while 20 percent had eaten meat. Recent contact with animals, in particular domestic pets, also increased the risk of infection. More than half of those diagnosed with the bacterium had reported being in contact with animals and 45 percent said they had had contact with pets, particularly cats and dogs.

Symptoms typically begin with lower abdominal pain and may be severe enough to mimic acute appendicitis. The abdominal pain is followed by diarrhea containing blood and pus. Diarrhea may be watery or sticky and the color of the blood may not be red, but hidden by the color of the feces. Fever and nausea are commonly present. Symptoms may include headache and muscle pain.

Usually, the onset of symptoms appears within two to seven days and commonly lasts up to two weeks. Sometimes it can take two to four weeks after becoming infected before symptoms appear. Generally, most people will recover completely within a few days without treatment, but about 25 percent of cases relapse. Drink plenty of fluids to reduce the chances of dehydration. *Campylobacter* is though to cause death in one per one thousand cases. Fatalities are rare in healthy people and usually occur in cancer patients or in the otherwise debilitated. Children under five years and young adults (fifteen to twenty-nine) are more frequently affected than other age groups.

Human studies suggest that it only takes about four to five hundred bacteria to cause illness in some people. A person's immune system and their inner terrain dictate just how many organisms it will take to cause symptoms.

In more severe cases, antibiotics such as erythromycin or fluoroquinolone can be used to shorten the length of time you are sick, if they are given early in the illness. This organism is generally not killed by penicillins and cephalosporins and is beginning to build up a resistance to other antibiotics. Adequate actions for control are strongly needed in both animal and human medicine. The public health issue of resistance in *Campylobacter* has global dimensions because of ever-increasing international trade and travel.

This organism can also become a permanent resident in the intestines causing chronic illness and gastrointestinal problems. It is often necessary to rid the body of this organism in order to address rheumatic disorders including ankylosing spondylitis, and colitis arthritis. *Campylobacter* has been linked to temporary paralysis and a neurological disease called Guillain-Barré syndrome. It is also associated with Reiter's syndrome and people with HIV.

It is difficult to tell pathogenic from nonpathogenic strains. *Campylobacter* requires special laboratory culture procedures, which a physician would need to request, but most clinical laboratories are equipped to test for this organism. It is difficult to isolate *Campylobacter* from food because the bacteria are usually present in very low numbers.

CLOSTRIDIUM BOTULINUM

Some foodborne outbreaks in the U.S. are cause by toxins from *Clostridium botulinum*. Foodborne botulism (as distinct from wound botulism and infant botulism) is a severe type of food poisoning caused by the ingestion of foods containing the potent neurotoxin formed during the growth of this bacterium. Food poisoning from this organism does not happen frequently, but there is considerable concern because of its high death rate, if not treated immediately and properly. Most of the ten to thirty outbreaks that are reported each year in the U.S. are associated with home-canned foods, but occasionally commercially produced foods are involved.

Almost any type of food that is not very acidic (pH above 4.6) can support growth and toxin production from these bacteria. The most common foods involved are canned soups, smoked/salted or luncheon meats, sausages, seafood products, vegetables, fruits and condiments, but beef, milk products, pork, poultry, and other foods have been involved. The proper canning and adequate heating of home-canned food before serving is essential. Canned foods showing evidence of spoilage should be discarded; so should swollen or leaking cans. Pets may become ill from botulism poisoning after eating the same contaminated food.

In recent years, non-canned foods such as foil-wrapped baked potatoes, chopped garlic in oil, and patty melt sandwiches, have caused outbreaks in restaurants. Other foods involved were sautéed onions and potato salad made from baked potatoes. Baked potatoes have been responsible for a number of outbreaks. Two separate outbreaks of botulism have occurred involving commercially canned salmon.

This bacteria's spores (dormant stage) are highly heat-resistant and may survive boiling for several hours at 212°F. However, exposure to moist heat at 248°F for thirty minutes will do the job. Toxins produced by these bacteria are readily destroyed by heat when cooked at 176°F for thirty minutes. Toxin production can occur inside a refrigerator at temperatures as low as 37.4°F. This organism does not require strict oxygen-free conditions.

It doesn't take much of the toxin to cause symptoms. It primarily affects the nervous system. Onset is often abrupt, occurring as soon as two hours or as late as eight days after eating contaminated food. Early signs of intoxication consist of marked lassitude, weakness, and dizziness, usually followed by double vision and progressive difficulty in speaking and swallowing. There may be a dry mouth, nausea, vomiting, abdominal cramps, and diarrhea. Difficulty in breathing, weakness of other muscles, abdominal distention, and constipation, may also be common findings. Major complications include respiratory failure caused by paralysis. It can take weeks to months to resolve these symptoms. In infants, the first symptoms are usually constipation, general weakness and a weak cry.

Infant botulism was first recognized in 1976 and affects children under the age of one year. After the child has eaten honey containing the spores of C. botulinum, these bacteria colonize and produce toxin in the intestinal tract. The digestive system of very young children has not matured enough to protect itself from botulism organisms sometimes found in raw, uncooked honey. Once the digestive and immune systems have a chance to mature, they can protect the child from this organism. To be safe, do not feed honey to children less than two years old.

Symptoms may begin as constipation or diarrhea. This is followed by lethargy, weakness, weak or altered crying, poor sucking ability, decreased gag reflex, pooling of oral secretion, an expressionless face, and problems breathing. There may also be loss of head control. The recommended treatment is primarily supportive care. Antibiotics are not recommended. Botulism may be confused with other illnesses and is diagnosed by finding the toxins and the organism in the infant's stool.

Some cases of botulism involving adults have come from undetermined sources. It is suggested that these cases are the result of intestinal colonization of the bacteria. Some of these overgrowths occurred after the person had surgery of the gastrointestinal tract or was given an antibiotic. It seems that these procedures altered the normal gut microflora and allowed *C. botulinum* to colonize the intestinal tract. Often, the symptoms are similar to those seen in infant botulism.

Finding *C. botulinum* toxin or organisms in the feces establishes the diagnosis, but you have to suspect this organism and request the test. Otherwise, no one will test for it. An antitoxin is available through state health departments. Antitoxin should be given as soon as possible after the diagnosis, since it is less likely to be of benefit if given more than seventy-two hours after the onset of symptoms.

Two popular brands of infant formula are being recalled in the United Kingdom because of a possible link to a recent case of botulism in a five-month old infant. The batches were made three years ago so it is unlikely that this formula remains on store shelves, but may still be in some homes. There is no way to prove that these products caused the child's illness, but it reminds us of how vulnerable we are when foods are contaminated with bacteria.

In January 2001, there was a botulism outbreak linked to eating fermented food in a southwest Alaska village. Fourteen people had eaten fermented beaver tail and paw and approximately twenty hours later symptoms suggestive of botulism included dry mouth, nausea, blurry vision, and general weakness. Three people developed severe symptoms and almost died. Beaver is hunted in southwest Alaska and certain body parts often are fermented and eaten later. In this outbreak, the tail and paws had been wrapped in a paper rice sack and stored for up to three months in the entry of a house.

Alaska's foodborne botulism rates exceed those in any other state and are among the highest in the world. From 1950 to 2000, Alaska recorded 226 cases of foodborne botulism from 114 outbreaks. All were Alaska natives, and all were associated with eating fermented foods. Alaska continues to have high foodborne botulism rates because fermented foods are part of the Alaskan native culture.

CLOSTRIDIUM PERFRINGENS

Clostridium perfringens poisoning is a commonly reported foodborne illness in the United States with an estimate of about ten thousand cases annually. At least ten to twenty outbreaks are reported each year and this has been going on over the past two decades. Dozens or even hundreds of person are affected at a time. Many outbreaks probably go unreported, especially when few people are affected. This specie of *Clostridium* is a gram-positive anaerobic bacteria (grows without oxygen). It is widely found in the environment and frequently occurs in the intestines of humans and animals. The spores (dormant stage) of these bacteria can persist in the soil where there is fecal pollution. It takes a large number of these bacteria to cause illness.

It is the bacteria themselves, not toxins, that seem to cause symptoms. Institutional feeding (such as school cafeterias, hospitals, nursing homes, prisons, etc.) where large quantities of food are prepared several hours before serving is the most common circumstance of *C. perfringens* poisoning. The young and the elderly are the most frequent victims. In most instances, the actual cause of poisoning is by temperature abuse of prepared foods. Small numbers of the organisms are often present after cooking and multiply to food poisoning levels during cool down and storage of prepared foods. Meats, meat products, and gravy are the foods most frequently implicated. Inadequate refrigeration and insufficient reheating of foods causes most of the outbreaks. A typical example is a gravy that has been prepared twelve to twenty-four hours before serving, been improperly cooled, and reheated shortly before serving. The longer the reheating period, the less likely the gravy will cause illness.

Symptoms include intense abdominal cramps and diarrhea, which begin eight to twenty-two hours after eating foods containing large numbers of those bacteria. The illness is usually over within twenty-four hours, but less severe symptoms may persist in some individuals for one or two weeks. A few deaths have been reported as a result of dehydration and other complications. There is a more serious type of food poisoning caused by *Clostridium botulinum*, but usually this strain is more commonly ingested. Poisoning is diagnosed by the symptoms and the typical onset of illness. Diagnosis is confirmed by detecting the toxin in the feces or finding large numbers of these bacteria in suspected foods.

ENTEROCOCCUS SPP.

Enterococci are common bacteria present in the gastrointestinal tract of animals and humans. Although usually harmless, these bacteria sometimes cause serious gastrointestinal, urinary, abdominal, and bloodstream infections in surgical or immune compromised people if they gain access to parts of the body (eg, wounds) outside their normal habitat.

Enterococci have received worldwide attention, thanks to their ability to be resistant to all penicillins and also to the important antibiotic vancomycin. These resistant bacteria threaten to compromise effective treatment caused by multi-resistant gram-positive bacteria. This is especially true in seriously ill patients where other antibiotics have failed. See Chapter 16 for more information.

ESCHERICHIA COLI 0157:H7 (E. COLI)

The digestive tract of animals and humans is an ideal habitat for the growth of bacteria. Most gut bacteria are harmless types and can even provide essential nutrients to their host. When animals consume contaminated food, the native bacteria compete with the invaders and provide at least some protection against foodborne illness. *Escherichia coli* (*E. coli*) is usually a harmless bacterium in the human gastrointestinal tract, and outnumbered by other types. Some strains of *E. coli* are not people-friendly, and these highly virulent forms can cause acute illness or even death.

It all began in the 1950s when antibiotics were used in farm animals for the purpose of faster weight gain with less feed, not for the purpose of disease control. By 1963, the World Health Organization warned that there was a possibility of resistant pathologic bacterial strains being produced from this practice. The warning was not taken seriously. In 1981, it finally happened. We were faced with the appearance of a mutant and very dangerous form of *E. coli* that causes severe internal bleeding in the intestines and kidneys. It was called *Escherichia coli* 0157:H7.

Outbreaks began occurring more often in the U.S. by 1982 and have continued to escalate since then. In 1994 over five hundred people developed serious food poisoning after eating at a Jack-in-the-Box. Of those infected, fifty developed internal bleeding problems and four small children died. This strain of *E. coli* is becoming more common and more opportunistic.

Undercooked or raw ground beef (hamburger) has been the primary cause in most cases of food poisoning. Raw milk transferred these bacteria to school children in Canada. In the Pacific Northwest, *E. coli* is thought to be second only to *Salmonella* as a cause of bacterial diarrhea. Blame has been placed on fast food restaurants and on meat packing plants, but often the meat being delivered to them is already tainted. Currently, testing for this deadly strain of *E. coli* is not done until after the beef is processed.

According to the CDC, last year there were 285 reported cases of illness from *E. coli*, 108 were caused by alfalfa sprouts, 20 by tainted ground beef, 52 from person to person contact, and 17 from wading pools. These days, it may be risky to eat raw alfalfa sprouts. *E. coli* outbreaks in the United States are usually caused by eating undercooked food, particularly ground meat; swimming in a public pool where someone defecated; and drinking water contaminated by farm animal excretions. This organism can be transmitted between people by the fecal-oral route, and especially among infants in diapers.

Antibiotic-resistant *E. coli* is commonly spread from animals to people according to a report in the June 2001 issue of the *Journal of Antimicrobial Chemotherapy*. Investigators analyzed turkeys and chickens commonly given antibiotics, as well as chickens infrequently treated with antibiotics. Then they examined fecal samples from people who had contact with these animals. They found that people who had contact with animals given antibiotics were more likely to get antibiotic-resistant bacteria from these same animals.

Infection can occur in people of any age, but severe infection is most common in children and the elderly. The symptoms usually begin acutely with severe abdominal cramps and watery diarrhea that may become very bloody within twenty-four hours after eating or drinking contaminated food, water, or unpasteurized milk. Some people report diarrhea as being all blood and no stool, which has given rise to the term hemorrhagic colitis. There may also be stomach rumblings, gas, nausea, cramps, and vomiting. Fever is usually absent or low grade, but may occasionally reach over 102°F. The diarrhea may last one to eight days in uncomplicated infections.

Victims finding profuse, visible blood in the diarrhea would probably seek medical attention, but less severe cases are probably more numerous. About 5 percent of the cases become more complicated and may or may not have diarrhea. The more severe symptoms typically develop in the second week of illness. They include a rising temperature and white blood cell count. This is more likely to occur in children less than five years old or in adults over the age of sixty. This illness can be so severe as to cause death. This one, and similar strains of *E. coli*, produces high levels of potent toxins that are indistinguishable from *Shigella* dysenteriae type 1.

The mainstay of treatment is supportive care. Fluid replacement is important. Generally, antibiotics are not recommended when there is the absence of fever or blood in the stools, since they can alter intestinal flora adversely and promote resistant organisms. For more severe diarrhea, antibiotics may be indicated, especially if vomiting, abdominal cramps, fever, or bloody stools are present. When there is diarrhea, the best diet is one of liquids and bland foods. Anyone at high risk should be taken to a doctor. Anyone developing complications is likely to be hospitalized.

If you are traveling, you should eat at restaurants with a reputation for safety and avoid foods and drinks from street vendors. Consume only cooked foods that are still hot, fruits that can be washed and peeled, and bottled beverages without ice, unless you know the ice was made from safe water. Uncooked vegetables should be avoided. The proper disposal of feces from infected people, good hygiene, and careful hand washing with soap helps limit the spread of infection.

Cooking and pasteurization will destroy E. coli bacteria. If the bacteria are on the outer surface of a steak or chop, cooking easily destroys them. If they are in hamburger, the bacteria may be concealed deep within the ground meat. Hamburgers having any "pink" meat can still harbor live E. coli. Anyone eating an undercooked hamburger these days is really putting themselves at risk for illness.

Currently, the diagnosis of individual cases of E. coli requires a culture of the diarrhea. Not all labs have the proper testing equipment. Negative results do not exclude it. E. coli 0157:H7 may produce colon lesions indistinguishable from those of ulcerative colitis. This bacterium should be considered and tested for in acute cases of colitis and even chronic inflammatory bowel disease. Anyone infected should require two negative stool cultures before being considered "cured." Report known outbreaks of bloody diarrhea to public health authorities.

Here are some examples of previous outbreaks:

- Recently, day-care facilities and nursing homes found contamination as the vehicle for person-to-person infection. Swimming pools and water parks are sources of contamination.
- The most likely source of the outbreak that sickened elementary school students in Wisconsin recently was an infected classmate who handled items at the school's self-serve food bar, which spread the bacteria to his classmates.
- During the spring and fall of 2000, outbreaks occurred among school children in Pennsylvania and Washington. They were associated with school and family visits to farms where children came into direct contact with farm animals.
- In 1996 there was an outbreak associated with Odwalla brand apple

juice products. There was also a non-food-related outbreak thought to be waterborne.

- In 1995 there were reports from Georgia and Tennessee of an outbreak. A community outbreak occurred in southern Australia.
- In New Jersey, 1995, there was sporadic infections, as well as an outbreak at a summer camp. An outbreak was reported in Washington and California associated with dry-cured salami.

Some strains of *E. coli* do not cause harm, such as the ones that are part of the natural bowel flora in humans. Strains, other than *E. coli* 0157:H7, may only cause mild cases of illness. The most frequent symptoms of these less virulent strains include watery diarrhea (sometimes bloody), abdominal cramps, low-grade fever, nausea and malaise. Infants in less developed countries and visitors to these areas are at greater risk. Usually, these organisms are not considered a serious disease hazard in countries having high sanitary standards and practices. Water contaminated with human sewage or an infected food handler may lead to contamination of foods. Some foods, especially raw beef and chicken are more likely to be contaminated. Symptoms are usually self-limiting. Infants and debilitated elderly people may become dehydrated and need appropriate electrolyte replacement therapy if they have had diarrhea for several days. Be sure not to use the local water when traveling, especially when making up infant formulas.

LISTERIA MONOCYTOGENES

This gram-positive bacterium has long been recognized as an important foodborne pathogen causing around two thousand five hundred serious illnesses and five hundred deaths each year. Some studies suggest that anywhere from 1 to 10 percent of the human population may be carriers. It is found in at least thirty-seven species of mammals, both domestic and wild. This includes at least seventeen species of birds and possibly some species of fish and shellfish. It is also found in the soil and other environmental sources. Most of the cases are sporadic, making links to food very difficult.

The popularity of queso fresco, a Mexican-style fresh soft cheese made from unpasteurized milk, has resulted in several outbreaks in Hispanic communities since the 1980s. In 1985, an outbreak of abortions attributed to *Listeria monocytogenes* occurred among Hispanics in Los Angeles and Orange counties, California. It killed forty-eight adults, newborns and fetuses. It sickened nearly one hundred others. Because queso fresco in these communities is produced in private homes, food safety regulations are difficult to enforce. Education of milk and cheese producers and consumers about the increased risk for acquiring infections from consuming unpasteurized milk, or fresh soft cheese made from unpasteurized milk, can be challenging because of language and other social barriers.

Then the federal government stepped up its monitoring program for *Listeria*, resulting in a significant drop in food-related illnesses. Before this event most of us had never heard of *Listeria*, much less knew how to avoid it. Another outbreak of food poisoning caused by *Listeria* sickened more than thirty-five people in nine states and killed four. In 1999, four deaths, three instances of miscarriage or stillbirth, and more than a dozen other cases of illness possibly linked to tainted, ready-to-eat turkey products were reported.

From October 24, 2000 to January 1, 2001, twelve cases of *Listeria* food poisoning were identified in North Carolina. Most victims reported eating queso fresco bought at local Latino markets, in parking lots, or from door-to-door vendors. All twelve patients were Hispanic. Ten were pregnant women resulting in five stillbirths, three premature deliveries, and two infected newborns. The eleventh woman had meningitis caused by these bacteria. The only male patient presented with a brain abscess. All eleven women reported symptoms that included fever, chills, headache, abdominal cramps, stiff neck, vomiting, and eyes that were disturbed by bright light.

As a result of this outbreak, North Carolina health authorities stopped the sale of raw milk and educated storeowners that it is illegal to sell unregulated dairy products. The FDA requires pasteurization of all dairy products sold across state lines except cheese made from raw milk that has to be aged a minimum of sixty days. Despite North Carolina laws prohibiting the sale and consumption of raw milk products, this practice persists in some communities.

Following a *Listeria* outbreak in Yakima County, Washington, an education program was introduced to train grandmothers, the primary cheese producers in that community, in the safe production of soft cheeses. Twenty-eight states permit the sale of raw milk directly from farmers to consumers. Until all states prohibit such sales, outbreaks associated with eating queso fresco and other unpasteurized dairy products may continue despite efforts to educate consumers, especially those who do not speak or read English and whose cultural dietary habits favor such products.

In 2000, public health officials in Ohio, Tennessee, Connecticut, and New York, noticed a suspicious surge in the number of people made ill by *Listeria* found in processed meats, including hot dogs and cold cuts. It is thought that dust kicked up when maintenance work was being done at the plant spewed *Listeria* onto meat that had already been pasteurized. The death toll from this epidemic reached fifteen adults and six fetuses. At least eighty others became sick. Recently, reported cases of food poisoning were transmitted by contaminated rice salad in one outbreak. In other outbreaks, it was chocolate milk, cold corn, and tuna salad. It is not unusual to find the rated of infection to be 72 percent in people exposed to foods contaminated with *Listeria*.

The government testing program does not catch all the processed meats heading to grocery stores. Food companies are not required to do their own checks for this organism, although some do it voluntarily. As a result, it may be too easy for a batch of contaminated food to slip through the regulatory cracks. This could be particularly unsettling if you are someone that buys cold cuts and hot dogs and other ready-to-eat products. Pathogens present in foods that do not require reheating can flourish and cause illness in unsuspecting people eating them.

This is a very hardy bacterium and resists the effects of freezing, drying, and heat remarkably well. Thorough cooking typically destroys this offending organism. It can survive refrigeration at temperature as low as 30°C. The difficulty with the detection of *Listeria* is that it can take up to thirty days before symptoms begin to manifest. The most common foods associated with *Listeria* are raw and unpasteurized milk and their products such as soft-ripened cheeses and ice cream. Also avoid soft cheeses such as brie, feta, and blue cheese.

Other foods at risk are smoked seafood, hot dogs, and some foods from deli counters such as sliced turkey, raw vegetables, fermented raw-meat sausages, raw and cooked poultry, raw meats of all types, and raw and smoked fish. Consumers at high risk of getting this bacterium can protect themselves against illness by avoiding these foods. The hard cheeses, as well as cottage cheese, cream cheese, and yogurt are usually safe.

It is thought that it may only take about one thousand organisms to cause disease in susceptible people. The high-risk groups include the elderly, people with cancer, diabetes, kidney disease, AIDS, or those who take immune suppressive medications because of organ transplants. In this group, these bacteria can be life threatening. Taking antacids also put people at a higher risk of illness because it reduces normal stomach acid that usually kills this organism. An outbreak in Switzerland involving cheese suggested that even healthy uncompromised individuals could develop the disease, especially if the food was heavily contaminated with the organism.

One of the greatest dangers of this bacteria is its ability to survive and multiply inside certain white blood cells called phagocytes giving it access to the brain or to an unborn fetus. *Listeria* can be very serious for pregnant women since it can migrate through the placenta to the unborn child and cause miscarriage or stillbirth. If treated promptly, some cases can be resolved with antibiotics. The contaminated food harboring *Listeria* and eaten by pregnant women can cause mental retardation and blindness in the unborn child. About one-third of the deaths from *Listeria* involve pregnant women and their fetuses. The woman may not have any symptoms or only symptoms that feel like a mild case of influenza.

Symptoms can appear flu-like including a persistent fever. Frequently reported symptoms are headache, abdominal pain, fever, nausea, vomiting, and diarrhea. The average time between exposure and illness is about twenty-four hours, but can range anywhere from six to fifty hours. These symptoms may precede a more serious form of *Listeria* infection that could progress to meningitis or a blood infection. *Listeria* is fatal in around 20 to 30 percent of the cases, but rarely leads to problems in healthy people with strong immune systems. *Listeria* infection should be considered in any person presenting with acute gastroenteritis.

Listeria is a serious public health concern because it can be life threatening. To ensure food safety and because *Listeria* can grow at refrigerator temperatures, It is advised that all consumers reduce the risk of illness by following the following advice:

- Use as soon as possible any perishable item that is precooked or ready-to-eat.
- Clean the refrigerator regularly.
- Use a refrigerator thermometer to make sure that the refrigerator always stays at 40°F or below. There have been cases of *Listeria* that survived temperatures as low as 37°F.

Since pregnant women, older adults, and people with weakened immune systems are at higher risk for poisoning by this bacterium, the following foods have a greater likelihood of containing *Listeria* monocytogenes and should be avoided:

- Do not eat hot dogs and luncheon meats, unless they have been reheated and steaming hot.
- Do not eat soft cheeses such as feta, brie, and camembert cheeses, blue-veined cheeses, and Mexican-style cheeses such as "queso blanco fresco." Cheeses that may be eaten include hard cheeses; semi-soft cheeses such as mozzarella; pasteurized processed cheeses such as slices and spreads; cream cheese; and cottage cheese.
- Do not eat refrigerated meat spreads, especially from deli counters (e.g., prepared salads, meats, and cheeses). Canned or shelf-stable meat spreads may be eaten.

- Do not eat smoked seafood bought at the grocery store, unless it is added to a recipe to be cooked, such as a casserole. Smoked seafood, such as salmon, trout, whitefish, cod, tuna or mackerel, is most often labeled as nova-style, lox, kippered, smoked, or jerky. The fish is found in the refrigerator section or sold at deli counters of grocery stores and delicatessens. Canned or shelf-stable smoked seafood may be eaten.
- Do not drink raw (unpasteurized) milk or eat foods that contain unpasteurized milk.
- Pregnant women are especially advised not to eat precooked hot dogs and deli meats unless they are heated to steaming level. They should also wear protective gloves when working in the soil or preparing raw meats.

Guidelines for preventing *Listeria* poisoning are similar to those for preventing other foodborne illnesses. The general recommendations are:

- Wash hands and surfaces often. Wash raw vegetables thoroughly before eating. Wash hands, knives, and cutting boards after each handling of uncooked foods.
- Don't cross-contaminate. Keep uncooked meats separate from vegetables. Keep cooked foods separate from ready-to-eat foods.
- Cook to proper temperatures. Cook raw food from animal sources thoroughly (e.g., beef, pork, fish, or poultry)
- Refrigerate promptly.

Listeria can only be positively diagnosed by culturing the bacteria from blood, cerebrospinal fluid, or stool. Unfortunately, detecting *Listeria* from stool is difficult and of limited value. The methods of detecting *Listeria* from food are complex and time consuming. Hopefully, new DNA probes will allow a simpler and faster confirmation of suspected contamination.

Answers to meat-safety questions are available at the USDA meat and poultry hotline, (800) 535-4555. Information about recalls is available at this web address. http://www.fsis.usda.gov/OA/recalls/rec. Consumers, who have recalled meat products, even if they have been stored in freezers, should discard or return them to the point of purchase.

PLESIOMONAS SHIGELLOIDES

This is a gram-negative bacterium found in freshwater fish, shellfish, and many types of animals, including cattle, goats, swine, cats, dogs, monkeys, vultures, snakes, and toads. Infection in humans is suspected to be waterborne. Unsanitary drinking water, recreational water, or contaminated water used to rinse uncooked foods are the likely source. This organism does not always cause illness, but may reside temporarily as a transient member of the intestinal flora. It has been found in people with diarrhea, but it has also been found in healthy individuals without producing any symptoms.

Most *P. shigelloides* infections occur in the summer months along with environmental contamination of freshwater (rivers, streams, ponds, etc.). The usual route of contamination is by drinking contaminated water or eating raw shellfish. Most of the disease-causing strains associated with human gastrointestinal illness have been from people living in tropical and subtropical areas. Since many people travel to tropical areas for vacations, it is important to be aware of this source of food poisoning.

Plesiomonas shigelloides does not occur just in other parts of the world. In 1980, an outbreak in North Carolina followed an oyster roast. Thirty-six out of 150 people who had eaten roasted oysters experienced nausea, chills, fever, vomiting, diarrhea, and abdominal pain beginning two days after the event. This bacterium was recovered from oyster samples and patient stools.

Usually the symptoms are mild and self-limiting with fever, chills, abdominal pain, nausea, diarrhea, or vomiting. Onset may begin twenty to twenty-four hours after eating contaminated food or water. The diarrhea is watery, without mucus or blood. If a person is healthy, the symptoms should be over in one to two days. Infants and children under five years of age may have much more severe symptoms, such as high fever and chills. The diarrhea may be greenish-yellow, foamy, and blood-tinged. Complications can occur in people who are immune compromised or seriously ill with liver disease.

It is thought that there has to be at least a million organisms to cause disease. Because of the self-limiting nature of this illness, few cases have been reported in the United States. Its rate of occurrence therefore is unknown and is probably included in the "unknown" group of diarrhea diseases that are treated with and respond to broad-spectrum antibiotics. Since this a virulent bacteria, it certainly has the potential to cause problems such as gastrointestinal disease.

SALMONELLA ENTERITIDIS

Most states require *Salmonella* outbreaks to be reported to the CDC. They have been tracking infections since 1962, but have not been able to stop the more than 1.4 million cases of diarrhea and more than six hundred deaths that occur each year in the United States. The highest rate of infection occurs in infants about the age of two months. The reason is not known unless it is because of their immature immune system. The elderly are also at a higher risk than the general population. Seasonal peaks occur in July through October.

Salmonella contamination has steadily increased from an official rate of 29 percent of all USDA-approved chicken broilers in 1967 to 37 percent in 1979. The USDA eventually stopped reporting the levels, but some surveys revealed contamination levels at some plants as high as 60 percent. It is the way chickens are raised that cause bacteria to multiply. All that crowding, stress, and the misuse of antibiotics, creates an ideal environment for the growth of *Salmonella*. These gram-negative bacteria are typically harbored in the henhouse contaminating the eggs and the chickens. *Salmonella* is one of the more common causes of food poisoning, especially in the warmer months, with many cases being linked to eating poultry and egg-containing foods.

Food poisoning cause by *Salmonella* occurs worldwide, but most reports come from North America and Europe, with cases on the rise each year. Only a small number of infected people are tested and diagnosed with as few as one percent of the cases reported. It may occur in small, localized outbreaks in the general population. It also occurs in large outbreaks in hospitals, restaurants, or institutions for children or the elderly. For years, food safety experts have warned consumers about the threat of foodborne illness caused by *Salmonella enteritidis*.

Thousands of dirty chickens are bathed together in a chill tank, creating a mixture known as fecal soup, which spreads contamination from bird to bird. Consumers pay for this "soup" when they buy chicken, since up to 15 percent of poultry weight consists of fecal soup. The USDA released a study in 1988 that conceded that washing does not adequately remove *Salmonella* germs left behind by fecal contamination, even after forty consecutive rinses.

Environmental sources include water, soil, insects, factory surfaces, kitchen surfaces, animal feces, and raw meats. Domestic and wild animals can harbor the *Salmonella* bacterium, including poultry, pigs, and cattle. So can pets such as turtles, chicks, dogs and cats. During the 1960s and early 1970s, an estimated 280,000 infants and small children were thought to have been infected by turtles. Prohibition of the distribution of small turtles by the FDA in 1975 may have prevented many cases of turtle-associated infection. The fad of having pet iguanas also caused an increase in *Salmonella* transmission. Since 1986 the popularity of iguanas and other reptiles has been paralleled by an increased incidence of *Salmonella* infection. Animals do not have to have any symptoms to pass these bacteria on to humans. It is found in the natural microflora of their intestinal tract, but thrives when animals are given antibiotics.

A twenty-one-year-old woman had two days of fever, chills, and nausea and three weeks of lower back pain. One year earlier, her doctor found a 1 centimeter ovarian cyst. She reported extensive contact with her roommate's pet turtle, including bathing in the same bathtub where the turtle was kept. She was a strict vegetarian and did not eat animal-based foods that would be contaminated with *Salmonella*. No other household member reported the same symptoms. Cultures from the ovarian abscess grew a specie called *Salmonella hartford*.

Salmonella is common in raw or under-cooked meats, including poultry, clams, shrimp, and fish. Drinking unpasteurized milk and consuming contaminated creams, sauces, and ice cream can also cause illness. Poultry products such as eggs often cause food poisoning. This includes sunny side-up eggs, Caesar salad dressing, or uncooked cookie dough that contain raw eggs. Raw eggs are also commonly used in egg protein shakes and ice cream. Various *Salmonella* species have been isolated from the outside of eggshells as well as from the inside.

Other foods to consider are salad dressings, cake mixes, and cream-filled desserts and toppings. Fecal contamination can contaminate fruits and vegetables as well. Recently, there was a warning about buying certain cantaloupes from Mexico carrying the *Salmonella* bacteria. Any food prepared on surfaces contaminated by raw chicken or turkey can become tainted. Less often, the illness may stem from food contaminated by a food worker. *Salmonella* outbreaks are more likely to occur in places where many people eat the same food such as in restaurants, nursing homes, hospitals, and prisons. The CDC estimates that 75 percent of those outbreaks are associated with the consumption of raw or inadequately cooked Grade A whole shell eggs.

According to ongoing research at the University of Arizona, oysters and clams are becoming increasingly contaminated with *Salmonella* bacteria. Shellfish do not naturally harbor this bacterium, but acquires them by filtering water through their systems that then concentrate in their meat. This is happening because of fecal runoff from sewage that pollutes the estuaries where the shellfish live. Of the oysters tested, the estimated presence of *Salmonella* is 50 to 70 percent. Most states only require the water to be tested for *E. coli*. *Salmonella* species can survive in meat products and in fresh and salt water for days.

Alfalfa sprouts are considered a health food and many people are eating raw sprouts today. Just about every full-sized salad bar has them, or had them before the outbreaks of food poisoning. In five outbreaks more than twenty-two thousand people were calculated to have suffered illness, and two deaths were thought caused by the poisoning. The illness was caused by six different serotypes of *Salmonella enterica*, and one outbreak of *Escherichia coli* 0157.

The outbreaks were traced to three different sprout growers who had not properly disinfected the seeds before sprouting them. It is thought that sources of contamination included rodent infestation of collected seed and irrigation water contaminated with chicken manure fertilizer.

Since current sprout disinfection methods are unreliable, people with high risk of infection, such as those with low levels of stomach acid and the immune compromised, elderly, and very young should avoid raw sprouts. Alfalfa sprouts are often served inconspicuously in salads or sandwiches thereby leading to unrecognized exposure. *Salmonella* can present with a broad array of clinical presentations.

The most common symptoms include fever, abdominal cramps and pain, diarrhea, nausea, headaches, and occasionally vomiting. The onset usually begins anywhere from six hours to three days after being exposed to the *Salmonella* bacteria. Acute symptoms may last a couple of days depending on the health of the person, the different infecting bacterial strain, and just how much exposure occurred. Most people recover without any medical treatment, but some people do end up at the doctor's office. Infants are at risk, as well as the elderly, pregnant women, and anyone with transplanted organs or weakened immune systems. Some people are left with a chronic arthritic condition three to four weeks after the onset of symptoms.

Long-term effects can result in weakened immunity, kidney and cardiovascular damage, and arthritis. It can become a chronic infection in some people who remain symptom-free, yet capable of spreading the bacteria to others. *Salmonella* is an invasive organism that can escape from the intestine and be carried in the blood to other organs. Sometimes *Salmonella* species penetrate the lining of the small intestine or colon and produce microscopic ulcerations, bleeding, and secretion of electrolytes and water. This invasive process and its results may occur whether or not the organism releases any toxins.

It only takes a few *Salmonella* organisms to make a person sick. To prevent the increased growth of these bacteria, always keep your eggs at a temperature of 45°F or lower. It is best to eat eggs immediately after they are cooked. Wash your hands thoroughly after handling eggs and wash any utensil or surface that comes into contact with raw eggs.

Progress in developing a nation-wide inspection system concerning egg farms and egg processing plants does not seem to be happening. A new federal egg refrigeration requirement applies only to eggs until they reach retail locations. It does not cover their handling once on the store shelves and in restaurants. Eggs are a good source of protein and can be a healthy choice to a well-balanced diet. However, they need proper handling so they are not a source of foodborne illness. Once *Salmonella* bacteria enter the bloodstream, they have the unique capability to spread anywhere. They prefer to locate to sites of preexisting abnormalities. This is why it is so important to keep the internal terrain healthy. *Salmonella* infection can be quite variable, with reported intervals of anywhere from four weeks to thirty-five years.

In a 2000 issue of the *New England Journal of Medicine*, researchers describe the first recognized U.S. outbreak of antibiotic resistant (fluoroquinolone) *Salmonella* infection. The outbreak occurred in two nursing homes and one hospital in Oregon, between February 1996 and December 1998. The authors identified eleven nursing home patients who harbored this strain of *Salmonella*. One patient was thought to be the carrier and had acquired the infection during hospitalization in the Philippines. Direct patient-to-patient contact, or contact with contaminated surfaces, were the most likely mechanisms of transmission.

The risk of *Salmonella* infection was significantly increased in patients who were treated with fluoroquinolones in the six months prior to the outbreak. The only other known case of fluoroquinolone-resistant *Salmonella* in the U.S. occurred in a patient in New York. This person had been previously hospitalized in the Philippines as well. With people moving around the world in increasing numbers, infections such as this one will become more common. Those involved in infection control in hospitals, as well as public health authorities, should be aware that fluoroquinolone-resistant *Salmonella* has arrived in the United States.

SALMONELLA TYPHIMURIUM

You now know there is a link between *Salmonella,* undercooked eggs, and contaminated chicken. What you may not know is that you are also faced with a different and more antibiotic-resistant *Salmonella* strain that appears to have made its way into U.S. dairy cows. This strain is called *Salmonella typhimurium* DT 104. It is found among normal bowel microflora, but thrives in animals given antibiotics. DT 104 is becoming more common in raw and under-cooked meats, clams, sushi, sauces, and ice cream. Long-term effects can result in weakened immunity, as well as kidney and cardiovascular damage.

Now that we know that cattle and cattle products are the likely source of DT 104, this strain of *Salmonella* has emerged as a major player in the foodborne illness arena. The incidence of these bacteria has increased thirty-fold since 1990, and experts estimate that DT 104 now causes as many as 165,000 illnesses a year. What is most disturbing about DT 104 is that it resists most treatments normally effective against *Salmonella*. There are still some heavy-duty drugs that can knock it out, but it is only a matter of time before this organism finds a way to outwit the newest treatments. Fortunately, most people who become infected get better even without the help of antibiotics.

Salmonella typhrimurium recently infected four thousand people in Great Britain. This strain is not one of the most dangerous ones, but if it passes its ability to be resistant to 98.8 percent of all antibiotics to other strains, the potential for deadly infections could become more common. Multi-drug-resistant *Salmonella typhimurium* is especially common in India, Vietnam, South Africa, China, and Pakistan. This organism was behind three outbreaks of foodborne illness in the state of Washington and northern California in 1997. More than 150 people, mostly Hispanic children, came down with cramping, diarrhea (sometimes bloody), fever and vomiting. The onset was twelve to seventy-two hours after ingesting these bacteria. Symptoms generally lasted four to seven days. Nineteen people ended up in the hospital, all of which recovered. The source of the *Salmonella* appeared to be a soft Mexican cheese made with raw, unpasteurized milk, presumably taken from cows infected with the DT 104 strain.

Another case occurred in a twelve-year-old boy from Nebraska. The boy's father was a rancher who had treated calves with severe diarrhea two weeks prior to the child's illness. Identical strains of *S. typhimurium* samples were cultured from the boy and from one of the sick calves.

Symptoms to expect are nausea, crampy abdominal pain, followed by diarrhea, fever, and sometimes vomiting. The onset usually appears twelve to forty-eight hours after eating contaminated poultry, eggs, beef, pork, or unpasteurized milk. Antibiotics may be necessary for infants or the elderly who become very ill.

Protect yourself against DT 104 by handling food properly. Thorough cooking usually kills most strains of *Salmonella*. Wash you hands before and after preparing foods. Thoroughly clean any surface and utensils that come into contact with raw meat and poultry. This advice is especially important for those people with weak immune systems.

In 1999 there were three outbreaks of multi-drug-resistant *Salmonella typhimurium* infections in employees and clients of small animal veterinary clinics and an animal shelter. They were in Washington, Idaho, and Minnesota. *Salmonella* infections usually are acquired by eating contaminated food. However, direct contact with infected animals, including dogs and cats, also can result in exposure and infection if there is fecal-oral contact (*Morbidity & Mortality Weekly Report* 2001).

Although most of the estimated 1.4 million *Salmonella* infections that occur each year in the U.S. are transmitted through food, this bacterium is transmitted through exposure to contaminated water, reptiles, farm animals, and pets. What is unusual is that most outbreaks are from large animal facilities, not small clinics.

Even when animals recover from *Salmonella*-caused diarrhea, they can continue to shed fecal *Salmonella* for several months. It is important for people with suppressed immune systems to avoid animals under six months and those with diarrhea. Wash hands before eating and after handling food. All surfaces contaminated with feces should be cleaned and disinfected. No eating should be allowed in animal treatment or holding areas.

SHIGELLA SONNEI

This bacterium is closely related to *E. coli* and produces a similar type of diarrhea. *Shigella* is not a member of the normal bowel microflora, although it may be carried in the intestinal tract for days or weeks, even in healthy individuals. Antibiotic-resistant strains have been emerging since the 1960s. More than 50 percent of the reported cases are now resistant to at least four antibiotics.

Like other infectious causes of diarrhea, *Shigella* is strongly associated with water polluted with human feces. This occurs where there is poor sanitary practices such as improper sewage disposal. In certain cases insect control may be needed, because flies can transmit *Shigella* when open sewage is present. Its fecal-oral mode of spreading can also be from food, hands, or people in close contact with infected cases. Because it takes so few organisms to infect people, it can spread through a population in a short time. Major outbreaks often occurred during military campaigns.

The foods most associated with *Shigella* poisoning are salads (tuna, shrimp, macaroni, potato, and chicken), poultry, milk and dairy products, and raw vegetables. *Shigella* can also be passed in water contaminated with feces to whatever it touches. Unsanitary food handlers also spread these bacteria to an unsuspecting public. It is found in daycare centers where children and the staff are lax when washing their hands. It can be found in the suburbs where wells are drilled too close to septic tanks.

Less than 10 percent of the reported outbreaks of food poisoning in this country are from *Shigella poisoning*. Yet, fifteen thousand to twenty thousand cases are still reported yearly. Since many cases of food poisoning are not reported, it is estimated that the numbers are much higher. Once these bacteria are introduced into a household or a day care center, it doesn't take long before simple hand-to-mouth transfer among toddlers exceeds 50 percent. If left untreated, organisms may still be present up to one month after the initial infection. During this time *Shigella* continues to be infectious.

Shigella is highly contagious and less than one hundred bacteria can start an infection even in healthy people. Not everyone gets sick after consuming *Shigella*. If you are one of those individuals that does get sick, it only takes about twelve hours in the small intestines to start things rolling. Within one to four days, it is invading the large intestine. Disease is caused when *Shigella* organisms penetrate, multiply, and cause destruction of cells lining the colon producing acute inflammation and shallow ulcers scattered along the surface. Some strains produce nasty toxins similar to *E. coli* 0157:H7.

In 1985, a huge outbreak occurred in Midland-Odessa, Texas, involving as many as five thousand people. The contaminated food was chopped, bagged lettuce, prepared in a central location for a Mexican restaurant chain. Several outbreaks occurred on college campuses, usually associated with fresh vegetables from the salad bar. The source was usually traced to an ill food service worker.

Another incident involved sandwiches served on Northwest Airlines flights that had been prepared in one central kitchen. There have been outbreaks on cruise ships where food has been served buffet style and left out for long periods. Most of the time the suspected organism is *Shigella sonnei*. When other species have been implicated, they are more likely to be associated with contaminated water. One specie, *Shigella flexneri*, is now thought to be sexually transmitted.

In Iowa, June 2001, there were sixty-nine cases of diarrhea resulting from a visit to a large city park with a wading pool. An inadequately disinfected wading pool was implicated as the source of the outbreak. Symptoms included diarrhea in all of the victims, but not everyone had the following symptoms: nausea, vomiting, bloody diarrhea, and headache. Several people were hospitalized. The pool was frequented by diaper and toddler aged children and there could be as many as twenty to thirty children in the pool at one time. Inadequate disinfection of this pool combined with heavy use by young children, who are often incontinent, created a favorable environment for the transmission of *Shigella*. A small volume of ingested water can cause infection.

Most cases of *Shigella sonnei* occur in young children. Subsequent to the Iowa wading pool outbreak, a community wide outbreak of *Shigella* involving several local day care centers occurred. The ease with which single outbreaks can expand into community wide outbreaks shows the importance of educating the community about potential modes of transmission such as with child care facilities, food handlers, and swimming. There needs to be prevention recommendations during outbreaks such as thorough hand washing after using restrooms, changing diapers, and before handling/preparing food, removal of children at child care facilities with diarrhea, and the exclusion of people from swimming while ill with diarrhea. Child care facilities should follow strict hygiene recommendations, including supervised hand washing for young children, and could consider refraining from using water play tables and inflatable pools that may lead to the transmission of infectious microbes. In addition, communication with pool operators about ongoing outbreaks may improve vigilance in maintaining disinfectant levels necessary to reduce the risk for transmission among bathers at community pools.

The symptoms are acute diarrhea marked by painful passage of bloody stools with cramping. *Shigella* should be suspected in any person with these symptoms along with fever, toxemia, or other systemic symptoms. The presence of blood and pus in the stool is suggestive, but not specific, since other invasive pathogens such as *E. coli*, *Campylobacter*, and some noninfectious diseases, can also produce these symptoms. In severe cases, there may be dehydration and weight loss.

The disease is almost always self-limiting with symptoms lasting a few days to a month, although most cases recover in less than a week without treatment. If symptoms become severe, or affect people with compromised immune system, it is important to contact a doctor because some strains can become life threatening. *Shigella* bacteria have been associated with Reiter's disease, reactive arthritis, and hemolytic-uremic syndrome.

With this organism, it is important to know that there is the possibility of drug resistance. This can happen when a multi-drug resistance *E. coli* is present simultaneously in the bowel and pass some of its resistant genes to the *Shigella* bacteria. The people most susceptible to the severest symptoms are infants, the elderly, and anyone with a compromised immune system. *Shigella* infection is a common problem in people suffering with AIDS and AIDS-related complex, as well as non-AIDS homosexual men.

It is still hard to find organisms in foods because lab methods are not well developed at this time. Stool specimens or rectal swabs will yield the organisms if the test is done promptly. Specimens collected early in the course of illness are more likely to be positive, because the organisms are much more numerous at that time. Absence of a positive lab test does not necessary mean you do not have *Shigella*.

STAPHYLOCOCCUS AUREUS

Staphylococcus, or better known as just "staph," is suspected of causing 25 percent of all food poisonings, only second to *Salmonella*. This common cause of food poisoning has a high potential for outbreaks. This is because food handlers with staph-causing skin infections contaminate foods left at room temperature. Then the toxins produced by this bacterium are ingested with the food that has been sitting out, usually more than two hours. It is not the bacteria that make you sick, but ingesting the toxins that they produce.

Foods with a high salt or sugar content favor the growth of *Staphylococcus aureus*. Foods implicated in outbreaks include contaminated eggs, tuna, creme filled pastries, milk, meat and poultry, potato and macaroni salads, ham and other salted meat or fish. Usually more than one person is affected. Onset is sudden, usually appearing within one to six hours after eating the poisoned food. The attack is usually brief, often lasting less than twelve hours. The typical features of staph food poisoning are nausea, vomiting, abdominal cramps, non-bloody diarrhea, and occasionally headaches and fever.

Symptoms can be severe in some cases, especially if there is a great loss of fluid and metabolites from the body. This is more likely to occur in the very young, the elderly, or chronically ill people. Rapid IV replacement of electrolytes and fluids often brings dramatic relief. A Gram stain of the vomit may show the organism. Careful food preparation is essential for prevention. People with any skin lesions, wounds, cuts, or broken surfaces, should not prepare food until their skin has healed.

VIBRIO VULNIFICUS AND VIBRIO PARAHAEMOLYTICUS

The most common bacteria to contaminate shellfish (oysters, clams, and crabs) are fecal bacteria from the *Vibrio* family. Because this gram-negative, bacteria is a naturally occurring organism found in warm, coastal waters, it might be present in approved shellfish harvesting waters. It is one of the most abundant microorganisms found in seawater having been isolated from waters off the Gulf of Mexico, Atlantic, and Pacific coasts of the United States, and Hawaii.

The most likely sources are raw mollusk shellfish, primarily oysters. Most reports of illness occur during the warm months of the year, primarily April through October, but there have been reported cases all through the year. The FDA requires that each container of shellfish be tagged to indicate the source. These tags trace the shellfish to a specific area and a particular harvester.

Vibrio vulnificus thrives in the brackish water of Florida. Nearly 50 percent of oysters from Florida estuaries test positive for this organism with increasing reports yearly. Between 1981 and 1993, this bacteria was responsible for 80 percent of reported foodborne deaths in Florida. Deaths caused by *Vibrio vulnificus* have occurred in other states along the Gulf Coast, and in California, Utah, Kentucky, Oklahoma, and Arkansas. Infections in non-coastal regions have been traced to eating seafood derived from Gulf Coast waters.

Shellfish will filter the bacteria from the water and retain them in their tissues, leaving the shellfish unharmed. Unfortunately, it can harm the humans that consume these shellfish raw or undercooked. Through cooking typically destroys these bacteria. *Vibrio* can still be present in cooked foods that have been recontaminated. No major outbreaks have been attributed to *Vibrio vulnificus* in the United States, but sporadic cases are prevalent during the warmer months. Some states require restaurants that serve raw oysters to warn customers of their associated health risks. Currently, only Alabama, California, Florida, Louisiana, and Mississippi, are require to post a placard warning persons with liver disease and immune suppression to avoid eating these foods. In one survey, only 71 percent of restaurants were compliant with this law.

Symptoms of this particular poisoning generally appears within fifteen hours after eating the shellfish, and consist of mild to moderate stomach upset and other digestive symptoms that can last for about three days. Symptoms include fever, chills, lower extremity pain, nausea, vomiting, and diarrhea. Over 70 percent of people poisoned with this specie of *Vibrio* have bulbous skin formations. Usually, this specie of *Vibrio* does not pose a threat to healthy consumers. Some individuals who already have medical problems can develop a severe, potentially fatal blood poisoning. It only takes about one hundred organisms to cause illness in a predisposed person.

Onset of severe illness may be rapid. If diarrhea and vomiting persists consult a physician. This infection can be severe in people with underlying medical conditions and life threatening in someone who is immune compromised. This includes people with liver disease, leukemia, lung cancer, AIDS/ARC, diabetes, or asthma requiring the use of steroids, and people using other immunosuppressive drugs. In these individuals, the bacteria enter the bloodstream, resulting in septic shock, rapidly followed by death in 50 percent of the cases. Because this is a preventable disease, it is important to target people at risk and warn them of the dangers.

Skin infections are caused by penetration of the organism through pre-existing skin lesions or through lesions incurred during seawater-related activities, such as cleaning fish or shucking oysters. Divers should be aware that lacerating part of their body on coral could result in contamination by this organism. Skin infections can become serious and require surgical intervention. Blood infections caused by *Vibrio vulnificus* can be deadly, as can wound infections. Few people die when only the digestive tract is involved. Almost always, eating raw oysters was the common source of the blood infections and digestive symptoms. Associated liver disease was the main reason that people died. Cultures from the stool or wounds can identify this organism if the lab is specifically requested to do so. Unfortunately, many cases of *Vibrio*-associated illness are not recognized and most clinical laboratories do not routinely test for them.

A new and more toxic strain, *Vibrio parahaemolyticus*, was first found contaminating oysters harvested from Galveston Bay, Texas. This strain of *Vibrio* bacteria had never been seen before in U.S. shellfish. Most people get diarrhea, usually within twenty-four hours of eating infected seafood, along with abdominal cramping, nausea, and headaches. Researchers theorized that the rising seawater temperatures (global warming) and salinity levels might have contributed to this large outbreak.

Although oysters from the harvest sites were found to contain well below the allowable limit of total bacteria counts (ten thousand per gram of oyster meat), half of the oysters contained enough *Vibrio* to cause illness. So far, the largest outbreak of food poisoning in North America was caused by *Vibrio parahaemolyticus*. It occurred in the Pacific Northwest with more than two hundred confirmed cases reported in California, Oregon, Washington, and British Columbia. All poisonings were from the consumption of raw or undercooked shellfish, particularly oysters.

Early detection and initiation of treatment of these infections are very important, particularly for high-risk individuals. This requires a heightened awareness by clinicians, laboratory technicians, and epidemiologists. There are at least twelve pathogenic *Vibrio* species recognized to cause human illness. The ones causing the most medical problems include *Vibrio vulnificus*, *Vibrio parahaemolyticus*, and *Vibrio cholerae*.

VIBRIO CHOLERAE

A related organism, *Vibrio cholerae*, is responsible for Asiatic or epidemic cholera. No major outbreaks of this disease have occurred in the U.S. in recent history. However, sporadic cases have occurred suggesting the possible reintroduction of the organism into the U.S. marine and estuarine environment. Probably more sporadic cases have occurred, but have gone undiagnosed or under reported. These sporadic cases were associated with the consumption of raw or improperly cooked shellfish. Some cases were due to recontamination after proper cooking.

Illness is caused after eating food, such as raw oysters, contaminated with *Vibrio cholerae*, which attach to the small intestine and produce the cholera toxin. People consuming antacids or other buffering agents are more at risk because it takes fewer organisms to cause illness; otherwise, it is thought to take about a million bacteria. Remember, these are really small organisms so a million can fit into a small amount of food.

In 1991 outbreaks of cholera in Peru quickly grew to epidemic proportions and spread to other South American and Central American countries, including Mexico. Over 340,000 cases and 3,600 deaths have been reported in the Western Hemisphere since January 1991. Some cases in the United States were brought here by travelers returning from South America or were associated with illegally smuggled crustaceans. It is more common in Japan, where large outbreaks occur with regularity.

Symptoms of Asiatic cholera may vary from a mild, watery diarrhea to an acute diarrhea, with characteristic rice water stools. Onset is generally sudden, with incubation periods varying from six hours to five days. Diarrhea, abdominal cramps, and fever are the predominant symptoms. Some people with also have vomiting and nausea. Others might have blood and mucus in their stools. Diarrhea can be quite severe, lasting for a week. The illness is generally self-limiting. Antibiotics such as tetracycline shorten the course of the illness. Death can occur from dehydration and loss of essential electrolytes. Medical treatment to prevent dehydration prevents all complications. Everyone is susceptible to infection, but individuals with damaged or undeveloped immunity, reduced stomach acid, or malnutrition, may suffer more severe forms of the illness.

Cholera is generally a disease usually spread by poor sanitation resulting in contaminated water supplies. The sanitation facilities in the U.S. are responsible for the near eradication of epidemic cholera. Sporadic cases occur when shellfish harvested from fecal polluted coastal waters are consumed raw. Cholera may also be transmitted by shellfish harvested from nonpolluted waters since this bacterium is also part of the microflora of these waters. *Vibrio cholerae* can cause severe wound infections in both immune compromised and healthy individuals whose wounds are exposed to warm seawater.

Pathogenic and non-pathogenic forms of the organism exist, so suspected foods must be tested for the production of cholera toxin. Data suggests that the majority of infections are foodborne and associated with consumption of raw or undercooked shellfish. Doctors should obtain a travel history when evaluating a patient with acute watery diarrhea, and should consider cholera in the differential diagnosis when a patient has returned from a trip to a country where cholera is known or suspected to be present.

YERSINIA ENTEROCOLITICA

This gram-negative bacterium was unknown until the 1960s. It seems possible that *Yersinia* can persist in a passive state in the tissue of its host. *Yersinia* is yet another bacteria in a growing list of stealth organisms able to enter cells and remain there undetected. There are estimates of seventeen thousand cases of *Yersinia* infection each year in the United States. Places such as Northern Europe, Japan, Scandinavia, see it more often. The rates are much lower here, but that may be because few laboratories routinely screen for *Yersinia*.

The onset of symptoms occurs between twenty-four and forty-eight hours after eating or drinking something contaminated with *Yersinia*, since this is the usual route of contamination. *Yersinia* can be found in meats such as pork, beef, and lamb. They can also be found in oysters, fish, and raw milk. The exact source of the food contamination is unknown, but since it is present in the soil and water and in many wild animals, this offers ample opportunities for it to enter the food supply. Poor sanitation and improper handling by food processors probably contributes to contamination.

Yersinia can cause a type of colitis, usually occurring in children. The symptoms include fever, diarrhea, vomiting, and abdominal pain. Sometimes the symptoms include swollen lymph glands and arthritic pain. Initially, it may be diagnosed as Crohn's disease. What if Crohn's disease is actually caused by the invasion of bacteria? Diarrhea occurs in about 80 percent of the cases with abdominal pain and fever being the most reliable symptoms. There are cases of reactive arthritis due to this organism along with mild intestinal symptoms. The bacteria are usually gone from the feces and cannot be detected there, despite ongoing and sometimes progressive arthritis. That is because the bacteria are now living inside the cells of the body and other types of testing are required to detect them.

The symptoms may also mimic appendicitis and has caused unnecessary removal of some people's appendix. One of the primary symptoms of both is abdominal pain in the lower right quadrant. There may be complications if these bacteria enter the bloodstream. This is usually rare and so are deaths due to *Yersinia* infection. They may also produce symptoms that mimic inflammation of the lymph system, as well as cause infections in wounds, joints, and the urinary tract. Commonly, the very young, the debilitated, the very old, and people subjected to immune suppressive therapy, are going to be the most likely to have complications due to this pathogen.

Yersinia is not part of the normal human bowel microflora. Another specie (*Yersinia pseudotuberculosis*) has been found in the diseased appendix of humans. Both bacteria have been found in animals such as pigs, birds, beavers, cats, and dogs, but only *Yersinia enterocolitica* has been detected out in the environment (ponds, lakes) and in food sources (meats, ice cream, milk). A diagnosis is made when *Yersinia* is isolated from feces, blood, vomit, or from the suspected food. There is some difficulty in isolating *Yersinia* from feces, so it would be better to rely on blood tests. Intracellular persistence of *Yersinia enterocolitica* has been found in the intestinal epithelium by immunofluorescence technique.

Several months after inoculating rats with *Yersinia enterocolitica,* scientists made positive cultures from the liver, the spleen, the lymph nodes and even from the feces. This was at a time when the disease had already disappeared in most rats. Therefore, it seems possible that the triggering microbes persist in a rather passive state in the tissue of the host. This is understandable since it is an intracellular invasive organism able to enter cells and remain there alive and even to reproduce. Several other microbes linked with reactive arthritis such as *Chlamydia* share this same feature. Results have been obtained with long-term antibiotic treatment.

Bibliography/References

Books

Acheson, David WK, and Robin K. Levinson. *Safe Eating.* New York, NY: Dell Publishing, 1998.

Alibek, Ken, et al. *Biohazard: The Chilling True Story of the Largest Covert Biological Weapons Program in the World.* New York, NY: Random House, 1999.

Allen, H.C. *Materia Medica of the Nosodes.* India: B. Jain Publishers Ltd, reprinted 1999.

Baranowski, Zane. *Colloidal Silver: The Natural Antibiotic Alternative.* New York, NY: Healing Wisdom Pub, 1995.

Bove, Mary. *An Encyclopedia of Natural Healing for Children & Infants.* New Canaan, CT: Keats Pub, 1996.

Bratman, Steven, David Kroll. *Natural Health Bible.* Prima Pub, 2000.

Bratman, Steven, David Kroll. *The Natural Pharmacist: Your Complete Guide to Herbs.* A Division of Prima Pub, 1999.

Bricklin, Mark. *The Practical Encyclopedia of Natural Healing,* New York, NY: MJF Books, 1983.

Boericke, William. *Homoeopathic Materia Medica, 9th ed.* India: Indian Books & Periodical Syndicate.

Buhner, Stephen H. *Herbal Antibiotics:Natural Alternatives for Treating Drug-Resistant Bacteria.* Vermont: Story Books, 1999.

Chin, J. *Control of Communicable Diseases Manual, 17th ed.* Washington, DC: American Public Health Association, 2000.

Consumer Reports Complete Drug Reference, 2000 ed. Yonkers, NY: 2000.

Ellingwood, Finley. *American Materia Medica, Therapeutics and Pharmacognosy.* Portland, Oregon: Eclectic Medical Publications, reprinted 1983.

Felter, Harvey. *The Eclectic Materia Medica, Pharmacology, and*

Therapeutics. Portland, Oregon: Eclectic Medical Publication, reprinted 1983.

Garrison, Robert, Elizabeth Somer. *The Nutrition Desk Reference* 3rd ed. New Canaan, CT: Keats Pub, 1995.

Gregory, Scott J. *A Holistic Protocol for the Immune System*. Palm Springs, CA: Tree of Life Pub, 1989.

Bottlieb Bill. *Alternative Cures: The Most Effective Natural Home Remedies for 160 Health Problems*. Rodale Press, 2000.

D'Adamo, Peter J. *Eat Right For Your Type*. New York, NY: GP Putnam and Sons, 1996.

Gibson, Douglas. *Studies of Homeopathic Remedies*. Beaconsfield, Bucks, England: Beaconsfield Pub Ltd, 1987.

Guillory, Gerard. *IBS: A Doctor's Plan for Chronic Digestive Troubles*. Point Roberts, WA: Hartley & Marks Pub, 1996.

Gursche, Siegfried, Zoltan Rona, and Alive Research Group. *Encyclopedia of Natural Healing: A Practical Self-Help Guide*. BC, Canada: Alive Publishing 1997.

Hansen Evie, Cindy Snyder. *Seafood Twice a Week*. Richmond Beach, WA: National Seafood Educators, 1997.

Heumer, Richard P, Jack Challem. *Guide to Beating the Supergerms*. Pocket books, a division of Simon & Schuster, New York, NY, 1997.

Howell, Edward. *Enzyme Nutrition: The Food Enzyme Concept*. Wayne, NJ: Avery Pub Group, 1985.

Igram, Cass. *Killed on Contact*. Cedar Rapids, Iowa: Literary Visions Pub, 1992.

Juemer, Richard P, Jack Challem. *The Natural Health Guide to Beating the Supergerms*. NY, London: Pocket Books, 1997.

Jacka, Judy. *A-Z of Natural Therapies*. Victoria, Australia: Lothian Books, 1995.

Julian, OA. *Materia Medica of Nosodes with Repertory*. India: B. Jain Publishers, revised/reprinted 2000.

Lee, William H. *The Friendly Bacteria: How lactobacilli and bifidobacteria can transform your health*. New Canaan, CT: Keats Publishing, 1988.

Lindlahr, Henry. *Philosophy of Natural Therapeutics*. Kent, UK: 1975.

Lipski, Elizabeth. *Digestive Wellness: Updated 2nd ed*. Los Angeles, CA: Keats Pub, 1996.

Macleod, G. *A Veterinary Materia Medica & Clinical Repertory with a Materia Medica of the Nosodes*. England: The C.W. Daniel Company, 1983.

Mattman, Lida. *Cell Wall Deficient Forms: Stealth Pathogens 2nd ed*. Boca Raton, FL: CRC Press, 1992.

McKenna, John. *Natural Alternatives to Antibiotics: Using Nature's Pharmacy to Help Fight Infections*. Garden City Park, NY: Avery Pub Group, 1996.

Mills, Simon, and Kerry Bone. *Principles and Practice of Phytotherapy: Modern Herbal Medicine.* Edinburgh, NY, Philadelphia, etc: Churchill Livingstone, 2000.

Murray, Michael T, *Natural Alternatives to Over-the Counter and Prescription Drugs.* New York, NY: William Morrow and Co, 1994.

Murray, Michael T, *Stomach Ailments and Digestive Disturbances.* Rocklin, CA: Prima Pub, 1997.

Murray, Michael T, *The Healing Power of Herbs revised 2nd ed.* Rocklin, CA: Prima Pub, 1995.

Murray, Patrick, et al. *Medical Microbiology, 3rd ed.* Missouri: Mosby Publishing, 1998.

Nash, EB. *Leaders In Homoeopathic Therapeutics.* India: B. Jain Publishers, reprinted 1984.

Ritchason, Jack. *The Little Herb Encyclopedia, 3rd ed.* Utah: Woodland Publishing, 1995.

Shepherd, Dorothy. *Homoeopathy In Epidemic Diseases.* Essex, England: Health Science Press. reprinted 1981.

Sherris, John C, et al. *Medical Microbiology: An Introduction to Infectious Diseases,* NY: Elsevier Science Pub Co, 1984.

Spoerke, David G. *Herbal Medications.* California: Woodbridge Press, 1980.

Squire, Berkeley. *Repertory of Homoeopathic Nosodes & Sarcodes.* India: B. Jain Publishers, revised edition 1999.

Tenney, Deanne. *Medicinal Mushrooms.* Utah: Woodland Publishing, 1997.

The Vinegar Book, Canton, OH: Tresco Publishers.

The Merck Manual, 17th ed, Merck Research laboratories, 1999.

Wade, Carlson. *The Home Encyclopedia of Symptoms, Ailments and their Natural Remedies.* West Nyack, New York: Parker Pub Co, 1991.

Webb, Tony, et al. *Food Irradiation: Who Wants It?* Rochester, Vermont, etc: Thorsons Publisshers, 1987.

Weil, Andrew. *Natural Health, Natural Medicine.* Boston: Houghton Mifflin Co, 1990.

White, Linda B, Steven Foster. *The Herbal Drugstore: The Best Natural Alternative to Over-the Counter and Prescription Medicines.* Rodale Press, 2000.

Wright, Johathan V. *Dr. Wright's Guide to Healing with Nutrition.* New Canaan CT: Keats Pub, 1984.

Yiamouyiannis, John. *Fluoride the Aging Factor.* Delaware, OH: Health Action Press, 1986.

Periodicals

Aldridge, KE, et al. "A five year multicentre study of the susceptibility of the Bacteroides fragilis group isolates to cephalosporins, cephamicins, penicillin, clindamycin and metronidazole in the United States." *Diagn Microbiol Infect Dis* 1994;18:235-41.

Amin, AH, et al. "Berberine sulfate antimicrobial activity, bioassay, and mode of action." *Can J Microbiol* 1969;15:1067-1076.

"Among Biological Weapons, Smallpox is in a Class by Itself." *New York Times* October 8, 2001.

"An atlas of Salmonella in the US: serotype-specific surveillance, 1968-98. Atlanta, Georgia: US Department of Health and Human Services, 2001.

"Anthrax vaccine sickens some." *The Register-Guard* (Eugene, OR) Aug 6, 1999.

Backer, HD, et al. "High incidence of extra-intestinal infections in a Salmonella outbreak associated with alfalfa sprouts." *Public Health Rep* 2000;115:339-345.

"Bacteria Switch Identified." *Reuters News* May 11, 1999.

Balaban, N, and A Rasooly. "Staphylococcal enterotoxins." *Int J Food Microbiol* 2000;61:1-10.

Barwick, RS, et al. "Surveillance for waterborne-disease outbreaks-United States, 1997-1998." *CDC surveillance summaries* (May) MMWR 2000;49.

Baseman, Joel, et al. "Mycoplasmas: Sophisticated, Reemerging, and Burdened by Their Notoriety." *Journal of Infectious Diseases* vol. 3, no. 1 Feb 1997.

Bauchner, H. "Parents impact on antibiotic use." *APUA Newsletter* 1997;15(1):1-3.

Bellamy, Wayne, et al. "Identification of the bactericidal domain of lactoferrin." *Biochimica et Biophysica Acta* 1992;1121:130-136.

Bernet, MF, et al. "Lactobacillus acidophilus LA 1 binds to cultured human intestinal cell lines and inhibits cell invasion by enterovirulent bacteria." *Gut* 35:483-89.

Billing, J, and PW Sherman. "Antimicrobial functions of spices." *Quarterly Review Biology* 73;March 1998.

Bjerklie, David, et al. "Shopping for Protection." *Time* October 8, 2001.

Boggi, Velio. "The Neglected Organ: Bacterial Flora has a Crucial Immunostimulatory Role." *Perspectives in Biology and Medicine* Winter 1992;2.

Brazier, JS, et al. "Metronidazole resistance among clinical isolates belonging to the Bacteroides fragilis group: time to be concerned?" *J Antimicrob Chemother* 1999;44:580-1.

Brown, LM. "Helicobacter Pylori: Epidemiology and Routes of Transmission." *Epidemiol Rev* 2000;22:283-297.

Bruun, JN, and CO Solberg. "Hand carriage of gram negative bacilli and Staphylococcus aureus." *BMJ* 1973;2:580-2.

Buhner, Stephen. "Herbal Analogues to Antibiotics." *NFM's Nutrition Science News* August, 1995.

Buts, JP, et al. "Stimulation of secretory IgA and secretory component of immunoglobulins in small intestine of rats treated with Saccharomyces boulardii." *Dig Dis Sci* 1990;35:251-6.

Carey, John. "Are You Prepared for Bioterrorism?" *Business Week* October 1 2001;58-59.

Carroll, Brian. "Lyme causes severe GI symptoms in previously treated patient." *The Lyme Times* July-October, 1999.

"CHDS: chronic Idiopathic- (or Infectious?—or Iatrogenic) Immune Dysfunction Syndrome & Stealth Pathogens." *Candida & Dysbiosis Information Foundation* vol 2, no. 4-5 Feb 1998.

Chandra, Ranjit Kumar, "Effect of Vitamin and Trace Element Supplementation on Immune Responses and Infection in Elderly Subjects." *The Lancet,* Nov 1992;340:1124-1127.

"Children's Infections." *The Eck Institute of Applied Nutrition and Bioenergetics Newsletter* vol. 14 no. 8 Aug 1997.

Chiou L, et al. "A survey of knowledge, attitudes, and practices related to fermented foods known to cause botulism among Alaska Natives of southwest Alaska." [Abstract]. Presented at the 2nd International Conference on Emerging Infectious Diseases, Atlanta, Georgia, July 2000.

Cichoke, AJ. "Maitake-The King of Mushrooms." *Townsend Letter for Doctors* 432, May 1994.

Clark, Alice M, et al. "Antimicrobial Activity of Juglone." *Phytotherapy Research,* vol. 4 no.1 1990.

Clausen, MR, et al. "Colonic fermentation to short-chain fatty acids is decreased in antibiotic-associated diarrhea." *Gastroenterology* 1991;101: 1497-504.

Collins, Drew. "Colon Therapy." *The Encyclopedia of Natural Therapeutics III* 1985;T1-T8.

"Community outbreaks of shigellosis-United States." *MMWR* 1990;39:509-519.

"Congress Pressures FDA For Softer Labeling Of Irradiated Foods." *FDA Week* May 12, 2000.

Cutler, Alan F. "Diagnosing and managing H. pylori infections." *Medical Laboratory Observer* vol. 31 Aug 1999.

Decker, MD, and W Schaffner "Nosocomial diseases in healthcare workers spread by the airborne or contact routes (other than tuberculosis)." *Hospital epidemiology and infection control* 1996;859-82.

Dennis, David T, et al. "Tularemia as a Biological Weapon." *JAMA* 2001;285:2763-2773.

"Dignosis and management of food borne illness, a primer for physicians." *MMWR* 2001;50:RR-2.

Doebbeling, BN, et al. "Comparative efficacy of alternative handwashing agents in reducing nosocomial infections in intensive care units." *N Engl J Med* 1992;327:88-93.

Doube, A, and AJ Collins. "Is the Gut Intrinsically Abnormal in Rheumatoid Arthritis?" *Ann Rheum Dis* 1988;47:627-19.

Drobniewski, FA. "Bacillus cereus and related species." *Clin Microbiol Rev* 1993;6:324-338.

Eichenwald, H, O. Kotsevalov, and LA Fasso. "The cloud baby: an example of bacterial-viral interaction." *Am J Dis Child* 1960;100:161-73.

Elder, RO, et al. "Correlation of enterohemorrhagic E.coli 0157 prevalence in feces, hides and carcasses of beef cattle during processing." *Proc Nat Acad Sci* 2000;97:2999-3003.

Elmer, GW, CM Surawicz, and LV McFarland. "Biotherapeutic agents. A neglected modality for the treatment and prevention of selected intestinal and vaginal infections." *JAMA* 1996;275:870-6.

English, Jim, and Dean Ward. "Lactobacillus GG." *Focus* August 1998.

Epstein, SS, and JW Gofman, "Irradiation of food." *Science* 1984;223:1354.

"Experts Doubt US is Ready for Biowarfare Attack." *Reuters News* September 18, 2001.

Falagas, ME, and S. Siakavella. "Bacteroides, Prevotella, and Porphyromonas species. A review of antibiotic resistance and therapeutic options." *Int J Antimicrob Agents* 2000;15:1-9.

Foca, M, et al. "Endemic Pseudomonas aeruginosa Infection in a Neonatal Intensive Care Unit." *N Engl J Med* 2000;343:695-700.

Frantz, SW, et al. "Chlorhexidine gluconate activity against clinical isolates of vancomycin-resistant Enterococcus faecium (VREF) and the effects of moisturizing agents on CGH residue accumulation on the skin." *J Hosp Infect* 1997;37:157-64.

Frenette, C, JD MacLean, and TW Gyorkos. "A large common source outbreak of ciguatera food poisoning." *J Infect Dis* 1988;158:1128-1131.

Friedman, CR. "Sprouts, salads and ciders: The growing challenge of fresh produce-associated foodborne infections." Program and abstracts of the 40th Interscience Conference on Antimicrobial Agents and Chemotherapy; Toronto, Ontario, Canada; September 17-20, 2000. Abstract 1891.

Friedman, MS, et al. "Escherichia coli O157:H7 outbreak associated with an improperly chlorinated swimming pool." *Clin Infect Dis* 1999;29:298-303.

Galland, Leo, and Stephen Barrie. "Intestinal Dysbiosis and the Causes of Disease." *Journal of Advancement in Medicine.* vol 6, no.2 1993.

"Garlic Keeps the Ticks Away." *Journal of The American Medical Association* August 16, 2000;284.

Gibson, GR. "Dietary modulation of the human gut microflora using the prebiotics oligofructose and inulin." *J Nutr* 1999;129:1438S-41S.

Glynn, MK, et al. "Emergence of multidrug-resistant Salmonella enterica serotype Typhimurium DT104 infections in the United States." *N Engl J Med* 1998;338:1333-8.

Goddard, J. "What's going on with Lyme disease in the South?" *Infect Med* 2001;18:132-133.

Goetz, AM, et al. "Nosocomial Legionnaires' disease discovered in community hospitals following cultures of the water system: seek and ye shall find." *Am J Infect Control* 1998;26:8-11.

Goldin, BR, et al. "Survival of Lactobacillus species (strain GG) in human gastrointestinal tract." *Dig Dis Sci* 1992;37:121-8.

Goldberg, Burton. "What Your Doctor Doesn't Know Can Kill You." *Alternative Medicine,* May 2000:14-16.

Goldstein, Avram. "Health Agencies Step Up Preparations for Biological Attack," *Washington Post* October 5 2001;B01.

Goodwin, C, et al. "Helicobacter pylori infection." *Lancet* Jan 25, 1997;V349:265.

Gordon, Jay N. "Grapefruit Seed Extract Useful for Infant Infections and Candidiasis." *Townsend Letter for Doctors & Patients* July 1996.

Hazenberg, Maarten P, et al. "Are Intestinal Bacteria Involved in the Etiology of Rheumatoid Arthritis?" *APMIS* 1992;100:1-9.

Headrick, ML, et al. "The epidemiology of raw milk-associated food-borne disease outbreaks reported in the United States, 1973-1992." *Am J Public Health* 1998;88:1219-21.

Henderson, Donald A, et al. "Plague as a Biological Weapon." *JAMA* 2000;283:2281-2290.

Henderson, DA, et al. "Smallpox as a biological weapon: medical and public health management." *JAMA* 1999;281:2127-2137.

Higuchi, ML, et al. "Detection of Mycoplasma pneumoniae and Chlamydia pneumoniae in ruptured atherosclerotic plaques." *Braz J Med Biol Res* 2000 Sep;33(9):1023-6.

Hilton, E, et al. "Efficacy of Lactobacillus GG as a diarrheal preventive in travelers." *J Travel Med* 1997;4:41-3.

Hobson, DW, et al. "Development and evaluation of a new alcohol-based surgical hand scrub with persistent antimicrobial characteristics and brushless application." *Am J Infect Control* 1998;26:507-12.

Hughes, Viki L, and Sharon L. Hillier. "Microbiologic Characteristics of Lactobacillus Products Used for Colonization of the Vagina." *Obsterics & Gynecology* 1990;75:233.

Hughes, Bronwyn G, and Larry D. Lawson. "Antimicrobial Effects of Allium Sativum L. (Garlic), etc." *Phytotherapy Research* vol.4 1991;154-158.

Hunter, JO. "Food allergy or enterometabolic disorder?" *Lancet* 338:495-6.

Huwez, FU, MJU Al-Habbal. "Mastic in treatment of benign gastric ulcers." *Gastroenterol Jpn* 1986 Jun;21(3):273-4.

"Hybrid seed mix up causes furor." *The Registar-Guard* (Eugene, OR) May 19, 2000.

Inglesby, Thomas V, et al. "Anthrax as a Biological Weapon." *JAMA* 1999; 281:1735-1745.

"Irradiation compounds vitamin loss from cooking." *Food Chemical News* November 1986;42.

Iskao, K, et al. "Gastric Juice Levels of Lactoferrin and Helicobacter pylori Infection." *Scan J Gastroenterol* 1997;32:530-534.

Isolauri, E, et al. "A human Lactobacillus strain (Lactobacillus casei sp strain GG) promotes recovery from acute diarrhea in children." *Pediatrics.* 1991;88:90-7.

Jansson, E, et al. "An 8-year study on mycoplasma in rheumatoid arthritis." *Ann Rheum Dis* 1971;30:506-508.

Jernigan, B, et al. "Outbreak of legionnaires' disease among cruise-ship passengers exposed to a contaminated whirlpool spa." *Lancet* 1996;347:494-9.

Johnson, R, and EC Jong. "Ciguatera: Caribbean and Indo-Pacific fish poisoning." *West J Med* 1983;128:872-874.

Kassir, Z. "Endoscopic controlled trail of four drug regimens in the treatment of chronic duodenal ulceration." *Irish Medical Journal* June 1985;78,6:153.

Klauder, JV, and BA Gross. "Actual causes of certain occupational dermatoses. A further study with special reference to effect of alkali on the skin, effect of soap on pH of skin, modern cutaneous detergents." *Arch Dermatol Symp* 1951;63:1-23.

Klovdahl, A, et al. "Tuberculosis: an undetected community outbreak involving public places." *Soc Sci Med* 2001;52:681-94.

Kolata, G. "Cipro isn't the only drug that can be prescribed, anthrax experts say." *New York Times* October 17, 2001.

Kramer, JM, et al. "Campylobacter contamination of raw meat and poultry at retail sale: identification of multiple types and comparison with isolates from human infection." *J Food Protect* 2000;63:1654-1659.

Larson, E. "A causal link between hand washing and risk of infection? Examination of the evidence." *Infect Control Hosp Epidemiol* 1988;9:28-36.

Larson, E, et al. "Assessment of alternative hand hygiene regimens to improve skin health among neonatal ICU nurses." *Heart Lung* 2000;29:136-42.

Layton, Marcelle, et al. "Smallpox as a Biological Weapon." *JAMA* 1999;281:2127-2137.

LeDuc, JW, and J Becher. "Current status of smallpox vaccine." *Emerg Infect Dis* 1999;5:593-4.

Levy, SB. "Antimicrobial resistance: bacteria on the defence." *BMJ* 1998;317:612-613.

Levy, SB. "Multidrug resistance: a sign of the times." *N Engl J Med* 1998;338:1376-1378.

Lewis, MJ. "Water fit to drink? Microbial standards for drinking water." *Rev Med Microbiol* 1991;2:1-6.

Lewis, R. "The rise of antibiotic-resistant infections." *FDA Consumer* Sept 1995.

Lind, K. "Manifestations and complications of Mycoplasma pneumoniae disease: a review." *Yale J Biol Med* Sep-Dec 1983;56(5-6):461-8.

Linnan, MJ, et al. "Epidemic listeriosis associated with Mexican-style cheese." *N Engl J Med* 1988;319:823-8.

Maki, DG. "The use of antiseptics for handwashing by medical personnel." *J Chemother* 1989;1(Suppl):3-11.

Marx, LJ. "Spriochete Bacterial Infections." *Townsend Letter for Doctors & Patients* April 1999.

Maugh, Thomas H. "Spreading a new idea on disease:mounting evidence may link viruses and bacteria to everything from gallstones to Alzheimer's." *Times Medical Writer,* reprinted from the *Los Angeles Times* April 22, 1999.

McFarland, LV. "Epidemiology, risk factors and treatments for antibiotic-associated diarrhea." *Dig Dis* 1998;16:292-307.

Mead, PS, et al. "Food-related illness and death in the United States." *Emerg Infect Dis* 1999;5:607-625.

Meers, PD, and GA Yeo. "Shedding of bacteria and skin squames after handwashing." *J Hyg* (Camb) 1978;81:99-105.

Milbank, Dana. "U.S. Warns More Terrorism Likely." *Washington Post* October 1, 2001;A01.

Mines, D, S Stahmer, and SM Shepherd. "Poisonings: food, fish, shellfish." *Emerg Med Clin North Am* Feb 1997;15(1):157-77.

Moneysmith, Marie. "Why Green Tea is Better." *Great Life* Nov 2000; 54.

"More Missing Diagnoses than just Candida albicans." *APIC* position statement. vol. 2 no. 3 Jan 1997.

Murray, BE. "The life and times of the enterococcus." *Clin Microbiol Rev* 1990;3:46-65.

Murray, HW, et al. "The protean manifestations of Mycoplasma pneumoniae infection in adults." *Am J Med* 1975;58:229-42.

Murray, Michael T. "The Natural Approach to Ulcers." *Health Counselor,* 1997.

"New ProcessingTechnique Unleashes the Killing Power of Olive Leaves on Viruses and Bacteria." *ACCM* April 1997.

"National Antimicrobial Resistance Monitoring System 1999 annual report." Atlanta, Georgia: US Department of Health and Human Services, 1999.

"New Radioactive Dumpsites: gardens and farms." *The Natural Activist* Sept/Oct 1997.

Nicholson, GL. "Doxycycline treatment and Desert Storm." *JAMA* 1995;273:618-619.

Nicholson, Garth. "Diagnosis and Treatment of Persian Gulf War Illness: identification of Cell-Invasive Mycoplasma Fermentans (incognitus strain) and its Successful Treatment with Antibiotics." *AAEM* Conif, Boston, 1996.

Nicholson, G, and Nancy Nicholson. "Chronic Fatigue Illness and Operation Desert Storm." *J Occup Environ Med* 1996;38(1):14-16.

Nicholson G, and NL Nicholson. "Diagnosis and treatment of mycoplasmal infections in Gulf War illness-CFIDS patients." *Intl J Occup Med Immunol Toxicol* 1996;5:69-78.

Ostrom, CM. "Antibiotics dangerously overused, group warns." *Seattle Times* October 17, 2001.

"Outbreaks of Escherichia coli O157:H7 infection associated with eating alfalfa sprouts—Michigan and Virginia." *MMWR* 1997;46:741-4.

Parry, MF, et al. "Gram-negative sepsis in neonates: a nursery outbreak due to hand carriage of Citrobacter diversus. *Pediatrics* 1980;65:1105-9.

Paton JC, and AW Paton. "Pathogenesis and diagnosis of Shiga toxin-producing Escherichia coli infections." *Clin Microbiol Rev* 1998;11:450-479.

Patterson, JE, and MJ Woodburn. "Klebsiella and other bacteria on alfalfa and bean sprouts at the retail level." *J Food Sci* 1995;45:492-5.

Phillips, PE. "Evidence implicating infectious agents in rheumatoid arthritis and juvenile rheumatoid arthritis." *Clin Exp Rheumatol* 1998;6:87-94.

Piccioni, R. "Food irradiation: contaminating our food." *Ecologist* 1998;18(2):48-55.

Pollack, Andrew. "New Ideas in the War on Bioterrorism." *New York Times* October 9, 2001.

Preuss, HG. "Oregano oil may protect against drug-resistant bacteria." *Science Daily* October 11, 2001.

Quale, J, et al. "Experience with a hospital-wide outbreak of vancomycin-resistant enterococci." *Am J Infect Control* 1996;24:372-9.

Rabbani, GH, et al. "Randomized contolled trial of berberine sulfate therapy for diarrhea due to enterotoxigenic E. coli and Vibrio cholerae." *J Inf Dis* 1987;155:979-984.

Radetskuy, Peter. "Last Days of the Wonder Drugs." *Discover* Nov 1998.

Rees, JC, and KD Alten. "Holy water: a risk for hospital-acquired infection." *J Hosp Infect* 1996;32:51-5.

Reid, G, et al. "Is there a role for lactobacilli in prevention of urogenital and intestinal infections?" *Clin Microbiol Rev* 1990;3:335-44.

Reid, G, et al. "Adhesion of three Lactobacillus strains to human urinary and intestinal epithelial cells." *Microbios* 1993;75:57-65.

Ricken, Karl-Heinz. "Clinical Treatment of Functional Dyspepsia and Helicobacter pylori Gastritis." *Biomedical Therapy* vol. 15 no. 3 1997.

Rotter, ML, et al. "A comparison of the effects of preoperative whole-body bathing with detergent alone and with detergent containing chlorhexidine glucontate on the frequency of wound infections after clean surgery." *J Hosp Infect* 1988;11:310-20.

Rubin, Daniel. "H. pylori and Vitamin C." *Focus* May/June 1998.

Rudland, S, et al. "The enemy within: diarrheal rates among British and Australian troops in Iraq." *Mil Med* 1996;161:728-31.

Rump, JA, et al. "Treatment of diarrhea in human immunodeficiency virus-infected patients with immunoglobulins from bovine colostrum." *Clinical Investigator* 1992;70(7):588-94.

Russell, AD, SA Hammond, and JR Morgan. "Bacterial resistance to antiseptics and disinfectants." *J Hosp Infect* 1986;7:213-25.

Roels, TH, et al. "Clinical features of infections due to Escherichia coli producing heat-stable toxin during an outbreak in Wisconsin: a rarely suspected cause of diarrhea in the United States." *Clin Infect Dis* 1998;26:1223-1227.

Salminen, S, et al. "Demonstration of safety of probiotics—a review." *Int J Food Microbiol* 1998;44:93-106.

Sasatsu, M, et al. "Triclosan-resistant Staphylococcus aureus [letter]." *Lancet* 1993;342:248.

Sattar, SA, J Tetro, and VS Springthorpe. "Impact of changing societal trends on the spread of infections in American and Canadian homes." *Am J Infect Control* 1999;27:S4-S21.

Scott, Donald W. "Mycoplasma: the linking Pathogen in Neurosystemic Diseases." *Nexus* Sept/Oct 2001;17-22.

Shaffer, N, RB Wainwright, and JP Middaugh. "Botulism among Alaska Natives: the role of changing food preparation and consumption practices." *West J Med* 1990;153:390-3.

"Shigella surveillance: annual tabulation summary, 1999." Atlanta, Georgia: US Department of Health and Human Services 2000.

Smith-Palmer, A, et al. "Antimicrobial properties of plant essential oils and essences against five important food-borne pathogens." *Applied Microbiol,* 1998;26:118-22.

Smith, R, et al. "Neurologic manifestations of Mycoplasma pneumoniae infections: diverse spectrum of diseases. A report of six cases and review of the literature." *Clin Pediatr Apr* 2000;39(4):195-201.

Sniffen, Jason, and Jeffrey P. Nadler. "Bioterrorist Threats: Potential Agents and Theoretical Preparedness." 39th Interscience Conference on Antimicrobial Agents and Chemotherapy, Day 3—September 28, 1999.

Speers, R, et al. "Increased dispersal of skin bacteria into the air after shower-baths." *Lancet* 1965;1:478-83.

Stephen, S, et al. "Botulinum toxin as a Biological Weapon." *JAMA* 2001;285:1059-1070.

Summaries of Salmonella outbreaks associated with Grade A eggs as reported in *MMWR* Aug 19 1988;37(32), and *MMWR* Dec 21 1990;39(50).

Surawicz, CM, et al. "Prevention of antibiotic-associated diarrhea by Saccharomyces boulardii: A prospective study." *Gastroenterology* 1989;96:981-988.

"Stomach Help:Tips for the Traveler." *Your Health* 59, August 1999.

Stouffer, Judy. "Vinegar and Hydrogen Peroxide as Disinfectants." *Science News* vol. 154 August 8, 1998;(6):83-85.

Tarr, P, et al. "Hemolytic-uremic syndrome in a 6-year-old girl after a urinary tract infection with Shiga-toxin-producing Escherichia coli O103:H2." *N Engl J Med* 1996;335:635-638.

Taylor-Robinson, D. "Mycoplasmas in rheumatoid arthritis and other human arthritides." *J Clin Pathol* 1996;49:781-2.

"The use of antimicrobial household products." *APIC News* Nov/Dec 1997;13.

"The Role of the Gut and GI Flora in Unsuspected Chronic Diseases." *Candida & Dysbiosis Information Foundation* vol. 4 no. 1, March 2000.

Tenover, FC, and JE McGowan. "Reasons for the emergence of antibiotic resistance." *Am J Med Sci* 1996;311:9-16.

"The beneficial bacteria that line the intestinal tract may help to prevent the body's immune system from causing inflammation in the gut." *Science* September 1, 2000;289;1560-1563.

"Toxic Bacteria Found in US Oysters." *JAMA* 2000;284:1541-1545.

Tuffnell, DJ, et al. "Methicillin resistant Staphylococcus aureus; the role of antisepsis in the control of an outbreak." *J Hosp Infect* 1987;10:255-9.

Bibliography/References

"Ulcers and Your Health." *Natural Way* Sept/Oct 1998.

US Food and Drug Administration. "Guidance for industry: reducing microbial food safety hazards for sprouted seeds and guidance for industry: sampling and microbial testing of spent irrigation water during sprout production." *Federal Register* 1999;64:57893-902.

US Food and Drug Administration. "Irradiation in the production, processing and handling of food." *Federal Register* 2000;65:64605-7.

US Senate, Ninety-fifth Congress, Hearings before the Subcommittee on Health and Scientific Research of the Committee on Human Resources, Biological Testing Involving Human Subjects by the Department of Defense, 1977; released as US Army Activities in the US Biological Warfare Programs, vol. 1-2 Feb 24, 1977.

Vakil, Nimish. "Guidelines for H.pylori-Induced Peptic Ulcer Disease Treatment." *Drug Benefit Trends* 1996;8(B):21-24,32.

Vanderhoof, JA, et al. "Lactobacillus GG in the prevention of antibiotic-associated diarrhea in children." *J Pediatr* 1999;135:564-8.

Villar, RG, et al. "Investigation of multidrug-resistant Salmonella serotype Typhimurium DT 104 infections linked to raw-milk cheese in Washington state." *JAMA* 1999;281:1811-6.

Wainwright, RB, et al. Food-borne botulism in Alaska, 1947-1985: epidemiology and clinical findings." *J Inf Dis* 1988;157:1158-62.

Wall, PG, et al. "A case control study of infection with an epidemic strain of multiresistant Salmonella Typhimurium DT104 in England and Wales." *Commun Dis Rep* 1994;4:R126-R131.

Walker, Morton. "Olive Leaf Extract." *Explore* vol. 7 no. 4 1996.

Waters, Robert S. "Pseudomonas Infection on Indwelling Catheter Eliminated by Magnet Therapy." Letters to the Editor, *Townsend Letter for Doctors & Patients*, April 1999.

Weiss, Rick. "Bioterrorism: An Even More Devastating Threat." *Washington Post* September 17, 2001;A24.

Weiss, Rick. "Fear of Bioterrorism Attack Spurs Requests for Controversial Shot." *Washington Post* September 29, 2001;A16.

White, DG, et al, "The isolation of antibiotic-resistant salmonella from retail ground meats." *New England Journal Medicine* 2001;345:1147-54.

Williams, RK, and NA Palafox. "Treatment of pediatric ciguatera fish poisoning." *Am J Dis Child* 1990;144:747-748.

Williams, Rocky. "Mysterious Aluminum Contamination of Food Crops and Livestock is Spreading Through 40 States and into US Food System." *Militia of Montana*, PO Box 1486, Noxon, MT 59853.

Yoshitaka, Ohno, and Howard Reminick, "How the Condition of Your Body's Water Affects Bacteria and Its Life-Long Influence on Health and Aging." *Explore* vol. 10, no. 3 2001.

Yound, G, and M McDonald. "Antibiotic-associated colitis: Why do patients relapse?" *Gastroenterology* 1986;90:1098-1099.

Zimecki, Michal, et al. "Immunostimulatory activity of lactotransferrin and maturation of CD4-CD8-murine thymocytes." *Imunology Letters* 30(1991)119-124.

Zimmerman, RK. "Risk factors for Clostridium difficile cytotoxin-positive diarrhea after control for horizontal transmission." *Infect Control Hosp Epidemiol* 1991;12:96-100.

Websites

"Animal Bites and Infection." *Reuters News* February 24, 1999. www.onhealth.com/ch1/in-depth

"Bacteria Linked to Severe Morning Sickness/How to Really Treat Ulcers." www.mercola.com/newpage43.htm

"Bad Bug Book—Ciguatera." US Food & Drug Administration. http://vm.cfsan.fda.gov/~mow/chap36.html

Beller, M. "Botulism in Alaska: a guide for physicians and health-care providers—1998 update." Anchorage, Alaska: Alaska Department of Health and Social Services. www.epi.hss.state.ak.us/pubs/botulism/bot_01.htm

"Biotech Crops Need More Oversight." *Reuters News* April 06, 2000. www.onhealth.com/fitness/briefs/reuters

"Bugs Beat Bugs: Bacteria Reduce Diarrhea in Hospitalized Children." www.gsdl.com/news/connections/vol12/conn20010425.html

Buttram, Harold E. "Vaccine Scene 2000—Review and Update." www.mercola.com/2000/mar5/vaccine_update.htm

Byrnes, Stephen. "Vitamin A—A Vital Nutrient." www.mercola.com/2000/feb6/vitamin_a.htm

Cassel, Ingri. "Does Milk Really Look Good On You?" www.mercola.com/2000/feb27

Chipley, Abigail. "The Killing Fields." *Vegetarian Times* Dec 2000. www.vegetariantimes.com

Ciguatera Fish Poisoning, Quick Guide www.holistichealthlines.one.net.au/HMG/ciguatera.html

"Ciguatera Fish Poisoning." *Public Health Resources.* www.state.hi.us/health/resource/comm_dis/cddcigua.htm

"Ciguatera Poisoning: One Woman's Victory." www.harmonicharvest.com/ciguatera.html

"Contrails—Death Delivered to Your Door." *Christian Media* Issue 3 vol. 6 Fall 1999.

www.contrailconnection.com/sicknessreports/sickness8.htm

www.contrailconnection.com/states/oregon.htm

"Diseases, Disorders and Related topics (Bacterial Infections and Mycoses)."

www.mic.ki.se/diseases/c1.html

"Disinfecting Kitchen Cuts Disease Risk."

www.mercola.com/1998/jun/1/disinfecting_kitchen.htm

"Don't Bring New Bugs Home from the Hospital." *Reuters News* August 07, 1998. www.onhealth.com/ch1/columnist/

Droze, Kim. "Deadly Germ Warfare Target..You!" Jan 6, 2000. www.ediets.com/news/article

"Farmers Shy Away From Biotech Crops." *Reuters News* April 05, 2000. www.onhealth.com/fitness/briefs/reuters

"Genetically engineered foods—are they safe?" *Safe Food News.* www.safe-food.org

"Good Bacteria Block Pathogens Causing Urinary Tract Infections in Women."

www.gsdl.com/news/connections/vol12/conn20010321.html

Green, VW. "Cleanliness and the health revolution." New York: Soap and Detergent Association 1984.

www.sdahq.org/about/order_formjs.html

Hatakka, K, et al. "Effect of long term consumption of probiotic milk on infection in children attending day care centers: double blind, randomised trial." *BMJ* 2001;322:1-5.

www.bmj.com/cgi/content/full/322/7298/1327

"Healthy swimming 2001." CDC

www.healthyswimming.org

"Is Organic Food Truly Organic?" *Reuters News* June 24, 1999.

www.onhealth.com/ch1/briefs

Hanson, Michael, Jean Halloran. "Jeopardizing the Future? Genetic Engineering, Food and the Environment." Policy Institute/Consumers Union.

www.pmac.net/jeopardy.html

"Knowing Enzyme Structure May Reduce Bacteria Resistance." *Reuters News* August 21, 1998.

www.onhealth.com/ch1/briefs

Mann, Denise. "Cut, Bagged Produce Raise Health Risks." Jan 6, 2000

www.ediets.com/news/article

Message to Physicians on Anthrax. *AMA* October 12, 2001.

www.ama-assn.org/ama/pub/article/2403-5382.html

"Monsanto Genetically Engineered Soya has Elevated Hormone Levels: Public Health Threat" Oct. 1997.

www.holisticmed.com/ge/warning.html

"Monsanto's Toxic Roundup" Nov 1996.
www.holisticmed.com/GE/roundup.html
"Molecular Probes for Bacterial Vectors in Ciguatera Sea Food Poisons."
National Center for Environmental Research.
http://es.epa.gov/ncerqa_abstracts/grants/95/minority/minnadat.html
Organic Food Standards Proposed
http://onhealth.com
Otwell, WS. "Ciguatera."
http://vm.cfsan.fda.gov/~ear/CIGUAT.html
Palafox, N, et al. "Successful Treatment of Ciguatera Fish Poisoning
With Intravenous Mannitol."
www.rehablink.com/ciguatera/treat.htm
"Pierced Tongues a Bacteria Haven." *Reuter News* April 18, 2000.
www.onhealth.com/ch1/briefs
"Principles on judicious therapeutic use of antimicrobials." American
Veterinary Medical Association.
www.avma.org/scienact/jtua/default.asp
Report on ciguatera poisoning, October 1998.
http://www.nt.gov.au/nths/publich/cdc/vol5_4/ciguatera.htm
"Scientists synthesize potent antibiotic." *Reuters News* April 06, 2000.
www.onhealth.com/conditions/briefs/reuters
Scott, S. "Ciguatera Fish Poisoning Remedied by New Drug."
http://starbulletin.com/96/08/16/news/oceanwatch.html
"Sweeney, L: Do Divers Dare?"
www.rehablink.com/ciguatera/dare.htm
"Universal Childhood Immunization." *Optimal Wellness Center
Newsletter.* www.mercola.com/2000/feb6/vaccine.htm
'Vaccines and Immune Suppression."
www.mercola.com/article/vaccines_and_immune_suppression.htm
"When Microbes Can't Be Stopped." *Reuters News* June 27, 1995
www.onhealth.com/ch1/in-depth
www.onhealth.com/ch1/briefs
Whistleblowers/USDA records
www.whistleblower.org/index.htm
1999 consumer advisory. US Food and Drug Administration.
www.cfsan.fda.gov/~lrd/hhssprts.html

Internet Medical Journals that May Be Helpful for Current Health Information

American Journal of Clinical Nutrition
www.faseb.org/ajcn
AMA Archives of Internal Medicine, Family Medicine, and Pediatrics & Adolescent Medicine
www.ama-assn.org
Association of American Physicians and Surgeons
www.primenet.com/~snavely
British Journal of Nutrition
www.cabi.org/catalog/journals/primjour/bin/bin.htm
British Medical Journal
www.bmj.com
European Journal of Clinical Nutrition
www.stockton-press.co.uk/ejcn/index.html
Journal of the American Medical Association
www.ama.assn.org
Lancet
www.thelancet.com
New England Journal of Medicine
www.nejm.com
Pediatrics
www.pediatrics.org
Science News Online
www.sciencenews.org
The Medical Tribune
www.medtrib.com

Other Useful Websites for Health Information

Maintained by the US Department of Health and Human Services.
www.healthfinder.gov
National Library of Medicine's consumer focused directory.
www.nim.nih.gov/medlineplus
A searchable medical dictionary with 65,000 plus definitions.
www.graylab.ac.uk/omd
A searchable library from the American Academy of Family Physicians.
www.familydoctor.org

Includes medical dictionary, references, links and news.
www.medicinenet.com

US Centers for Disease Control and Prevention and offers information on diseases, travel health, and other health issues.
www.cdc.gov

Provides information on virtually every licensed medical doctor in the United States.
www.ama-assn.org/aps/amahg.htm

National Center for Complementary and Alternative Medicine.
www.nccam.nih.gov

One of the Internet's biggest collection of peer-reviewed articles.
www.medscape.com

American Association of Retired People's (AARP) health information portal, which includes links to publications, articles, and research.
www.aarp.org/healthguide

Information on prescription drugs, medical devices and food safety including dietary supplements from the U.S. Food and Drug Administration.
www.fda.gov

This is a more technical medical site that contains "Ask the Mayo Physician."
www.mayohealth.org

This site includes a wide variety of material that is designed for consumers and medical practitioners.
www.webmd.com

This is a site for alternative medicine information.
www.alternativemedicine.com

This site helps you identify the better sites.
www.healthscout.com

Find out more information about food safety.
www.foodsafety.gov

This is the web site for the U.S. department of Agriculture (USDA).
www.fsis.usda.gov

Additional Medical Sources

American Journal of Gastroenterology
American Journal of Medicine
American Journal of Natural Medicine
Annals of Internal Medicine

Clinical Infectious Diseases
Emerging Infectious Diseases
Infectious Medicine
International Journal of Health Services
JAMA
Journal Immunology Methods
Journal of Infectious Diseases
Nature Biotechnology
Pediatrics
Science
Townsend Letter for Doctors & Patients
The New England Journal of Medicine
The Nutritional Supplement Advisor

Index

About the Author

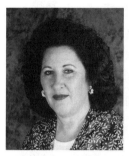

Skye Weintraub, N.D., has been in medical practice as a naturopathic physician for the last thirteen years and has researched and written books for the last seven years. She possesses a strong background in holistic health therapies, specializing in the treatment of chronic health concerns, especially allergies and digestive disorders.

Dr. Weintraub is the author of numerous books, including *Natural Healing with Cell Salts*, *Allergies and Holistic Healing*, *Natural Treatments for ADD and Hyperactivity*, and *The Parasite Menace*. She has also authored two booklets—*Selenium: The Health Connection* and *Natural Defenses for Bioterrorism*, and has contributed to other books, including *The Encyclopedia of Natural Healing*, by Alive Books, and *Alternative Cures*, by Rodale Press.

Dr. Weintraub is a frequent guest on radio programs exploring natural health topics, and travels nationwide, presenting and speaking on these topics. Additionally, she is a consultant for complementary health companies regarding the development of products, especially those concerning allergies, ADHD, and the overgrowth of disease-causing organisms in the digestive system. She may be reached at www.drskyeweintraub.com.

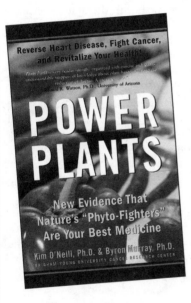
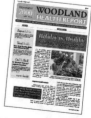